Case Studies in Obstetrics and Gynecology

Case Studies in Obstetrics and Gynecology

Editor: Romina Bailey

AMERICAN
MEDICAL PUBLISHERS
www.americanmedicalpublishers.com

AMERICAN
MEDICAL PUBLISHERS
www.americanmedicalpublishers.com

Cataloging-in-Publication Data

Case studies in obstetrics and gynecology / edited by Romina Bailey.
p. cm.
Includes bibliographical references and index.
ISBN 979-8-88740-609-1
1. Obstetrics. 2. Gynecology. 3. Obstetrics--Case studies.
4. Gynecology--Case studies. I. Bailey, Romina.
RG524 .O27 2023
618.2--dc23

American Medical Publishers,
41 Flatbush Avenue,
1st Floor, New York,
NY 11217, USA

ISBN 979-8-88740-609-1 (Hardback)

Contents

Preface

Obstetrics and gynecology is a medical specialty that focuses on the care of women's reproductive health. It deals with pregnancy, childbirth and postpartum care, while gynecology focuses on the health of the female reproductive system, including the uterus, ovaries, cervix, and vagina. Obstetrics is involved in providing comprehensive prenatal care to expectant mothers, monitor fetal development, and ensure the well-being of both the mother and the baby throughout the pregnancy. Gynecology focuses on the non-pregnancy-related aspects of women's health, encompassing issues such as reproductive health, menstrual disorders, contraception, menopause, sexually transmitted infections (STIs) and gynecological cancers. Obstetrics and gynecology aim to promote women's health and addresses the unique medical and emotional needs of women throughout their reproductive years. This book contains some path-breaking studies in the field of obstetrics and gynecology. Those in search of information to further their knowledge will be greatly assisted by it.

Significant researches are present in this book. Intensive efforts have been employed by authors to make this book an outstanding discourse. This book contains the enlightening chapters which have been written on the basis of significant researches done by the experts.

Finally, I would also like to thank all the members involved in this book for being a team and meeting all the deadlines for the submission of their respective works. I would also like to thank my friends and family for being supportive in my efforts.

Editor

1

A Successful Pregnancy with Amyotrophic Lateral Sclerosis

P. D. M. Pathiraja[1] and **S. K. Ranaraja**[2]

[1]*Obstetrics and Gynaecology, Ministry of Health, Sri Lanka*
[2]*Teaching Hospital Peradeniya, Sri Lanka*

Correspondence should be addressed to P. D. M. Pathiraja; madushan_pathi@yahoo.com

Academic Editor: Mehmet A. Osmanağaoğlu

Amyotrophic lateral sclerosis (ALS) is a degenerative motor neurone disease that is rarely seen in the obstetric population. We present a 32-year-old patient who presented in her fourth pregnancy with a background history of ALS. There was complete involvement of the upper and lower motor neurone system and bulbar system without involvement of the sensory system. At 34 weeks of gestation, she had a full course of steroids and an elective caesarian section under general anaesthesia due to extreme restricted mobility and difficulty of breathing. A multidisciplinary team managed the pregnancy, and both maternal and fetal outcomes were good.

1. Introduction

Amyotrophic lateral sclerosis is the most common and progressive motor neurone disease, and the prevalence is 2-4/100,000 in general population [1, 2]. The main problem during pregnancy is respiratory compromise. The mode of delivery and timing of delivery would be affected by the severity of the disease and other comorbid factors.

2. Case Report

A thirty-two-year-old lady in her fourth pregnancy came for her booking visit at ten weeks of gestation with a known history ALS for the last two years. Her obstetrics history included one previous vaginal delivery fifteen years prior, an emergency lower uterine segment caesarian section (LSCS) nine years prior for fetal distress, and two first trimester miscarriages in between these pregnancies. Four years following her emergency LSCS, she developed bilateral lower limb weakness and slurring of speech. Neurological examination showed generalized weakness with quadraparesis.

Routine investigations at presentation revealed a normal full blood count, serum biochemistry, serum vitamin B12, serum folate level, ferritin levels, and coagulation profile. Inflammatory markers such as ESR and CRP were normal. She had a negative rheumatoid factor, ANA, and ANCA. She had undergone an electromyelogram (EMG), which confirmed the presence of widespread anterior horn cell dysfunction consistent with ALS. Magnetic resonance imaging (MRI) of the spine revealed degenerative changes at C5/C6 and C6/C7 levels.

The current pregnancy was unplanned and her main problems during pregnancy were restricted mobility and shortness of breath. At booking, she was bed bound and reported generalized body weakness. On general examination, she had slurred speech, drooling of saliva, and no evidence of pallor or cyanosis. Her cardiovascular examination showed a heart rate of 76 beats per minute, blood pressure was 120/70 mmHg, and there were no audible murmurs. Her respiratory system examination revealed that respiratory rate of 26 breaths per minute with the use of accessory muscles. There was obvious intercostal and subcostal muscle recession during breathing with reduced air entry on both sides. On neurological assessment, both upper and lower limbs were wasted and fasciculation were noted. Assessment of power in all four limbs revealed 3/5, increased tone, with significant spasticity, and hyperreflexia. Her sensory function was unimpaired. Cranial nerve examination showed wasting of tongue muscles.

During the antenatal period, she was referred to a cardiologist and echocardiography was normal. She underwent serial lung function tests, which showed a severe restrictive type lung disease. With the help of a dietician and nutritionist, she continued with a semisolid diet. She had stockings and limb physiotherapy for prevention of deep vein thrombosis. The trained nursing staff regularly assessed her bowel and urinary habits while she is at home. She had muscle relaxant medication to relieve of her spasticity. Fetal anomaly ultrasound scan was normal and fetal growth was satisfactory. She was admitted to the ward at thirty weeks of gestation for close monitoring and further care.

At thirty-four weeks of gestation, the patient complained of progressive worsening of her shortness of breath. A multidisciplinary team (MDT) was gathered including a consultant obstetrician, neonatologist, anaesthetist, and neurologist to discuss the timing and mode of delivery. After the MDT meeting, a decision was made for an elective LSCS followed by monitoring at intensive care unit. Steroids were given for fetal lung maturity. The LSCS was performed without any complications, and the baby's birth weight was 2.4 kg and the Apgar score, neurological, and other system examination of the neonate was normal. The patient made quite an uneventful recovery with improvement in her lung functions and motor weakness remained stable. Both mother and baby were discharged home seven days post LSCS.

3. Discussion

The published literature of patients with ALS complicating pregnancy is very rare. This is partly because the incidence of the condition is highest among the elderly population particularly after the fifth decade. In addition, it is seen more commonly in men than women [1, 2]. The management of motor neurone disease in pregnancy especially ALS is challenging for both the obstetrician and patient. Pregnancy does not impact on with degenerative nature of the disease, however, both upper and lower motor neurone deficits can be seen [3].

Respiration is the main component, which get affected during pregnancy. In pregnancy, there is a 40% increase in minute ventilation, which is achieved exclusively by increased tidal volume. In ALS, diaphragmatic and costal muscles may be involved; thus, patient is unable to increase tidal volume. In the latter part of pregnancy, the diaphragmatic elevation caused by the enlarging uterus leads to a decrease in functional residual capacity. As a result, serial review of respiratory function by pulmonary function tests is recommended especially towards the end of pregnancy [4].

Riluzole is the only proven drug, which is effective in ALS and can be used during pregnancy. Food and Drug Administration (FDA) categorize it as a class C drug. It delays the requirement of ventilator dependency and may increase the duration of survival. The low birth weight has been reported when used during pregnancy [5]. Furthermore, liver functions need to be assessed every three months due to hepatotoxicity.

The mode of delivery in ALS is controversial. In normal pregnancy, the largest increase of cardiovascular and respiratory work occurs after birth and should be similar for either routes of delivery. Since motor neurone diseases do not affect the motor and sensory nerves of the uterus, a vaginal delivery is possible. However, if the patients have respiratory failure, she will need a cesarean section as spontaneous labour increases respiratory demand. Chio et al. report a case series of four patients of whom three had uncomplicated vaginal deliveries [6]. Sarfov et al. report a case of a single women with ALS, who delivered vaginally in her first pregnancy; however, she required a caesarian section in early third trimester due to worsening of the disease condition [7].

Choice of anaesthesia for patients with ALS is complicated. Regional anaesthesia offers the advantage of sustained pain relief and this together with general anaesthesia is associated with similar reductions in lung volume. However, the effects of regional anesthesia on intercostal muscles may impede expiratory flow that is of concern in patients with respiratory impairment. Xiao et al. report successful use of total intravenous short acting anesthesia without muscle relaxant. This would help to avoid any prolonged ventilation, therefore, prevent maternal respiratory compromise [8]. Corderio et al. present a case of noninvasive ventilation and spinal anaesthesia was used in a patient with rapid deterioration of ALS in pregnancy by avoiding intubation and total anaesthesia [9].

Since motor neurone disease does not affect fetal development, neonatal outcomes are generally good. Some case reports suggest an association of fetal growth restriction with Riluzole. There are other case series that have shown an association with congenital anomalies, such as anencephaly, cleft lip, and cleft palate, but this association is unclear [10].

The relationship between the hormonal change in pregnancy and increased susceptibility to ALS has been studied. A study done using patients who attend a neuromuscular clinic found mutation of the superoxide dismutase gene (SOD1) and vascular endothelial growth factor premotor gene (VEGF) could be a causative factor [11]. Both hormonal and inflammatory modification during pregnancy would result in oxidative stress, which leads to mutation of SOD 1 and VEGF molecules, which has toxic mediation and neuroprotective ability. There are some case reports that discuss the onset of ALS in the immediate postpartum period. Martinez et al. report a case of stem cell therapy in a patient who developed ALS during pregnancy. Bilateral autologous stem cell transplantation into the frontal motor cortex has been performed after delivery and disease progression was stabilized with improved quality of life [12]. By considering the long-term impact of the disease and complications could arise during pregnancy, it is advisable that proper counseling of the patient occur preconception.

4. Conclusion

ALS in pregnancy is very rare. Pregnancy in women with motor neurone diseases specifically ALS is a potentially dangerous event with respiratory compromise being the main problem encountered. Riluzole can be safely used during the pregnancy. MDT involvement is essential in optimizing care of patients with ALS in pregnancy with expected good maternal and fetal outcome.

References

[1] B. J. Traynor, M. B. Codd, B. Corr, C. Forde, E. Frost, and O. Hardiman, "Incidence and prevalence of ALS in Ireland, 1995-1997: a population-based study," *Neurology*, vol. 52, no. 3, pp. 504–509, 1999.

[2] C. Luneeta, V. Sansone, and M. Corbo, "Amyotrophic lateral sclerosis presenting during pregnancy: report of clinical and gentic features of three cases," *Journal of Neurology*, vol. 256, 2009.

[3] A. C. Guidon and E. W. Massey, "Neuromuscular disorders in pregnancy," *Neurologic Clinics*, vol. 30, no. 3, pp. 889–911, 2012.

[4] J. Faria, S. Pereira, and P. Castro, "Anesthetic management for caesarian section in a patient with amytrophic lateral sclerosis," *Regional Anaethesia and Pain Medicine*, vol. 37, 2012.

[5] R. S. Scalco, M. C. Vieira, E. V. da Cunha Filho, E. G. Lago, I. G. da Silva, and J. Becker, "Amyotrophic lateral sclerosis and Riluzole use during pregnancy: A case report," *Amyotrophic Lateral Sclerosis*, vol. 13, no. 5, pp. 471-472, 2012.

[6] A. Chiò, A. Calvo, N. di Vito et al., "Amyotrophic lateral sclerosis associated with pregnancy: report of four new cases and review of the literature," *Amyotrophic Lateral Sclerosis and Other Motor Neuron Disorders*, vol. 4, no. 1, pp. 45–48, 2003.

[7] S. Sarafov, M. Doitchinova, Z. Karagiozova et al., "Two consecutive pregnancies in early and late stage of amyotrophic lateral sclerosis," *Amyotrophic Lateral Sclerosis*, vol. 10, no. 5-6, pp. 483–486, 2009.

[8] W. Xiao, L. Zhao, F. Wang, H. Sun, T. Wang, and G. Zhao, "Total intravenous anesthesia without muscle relaxant in a parturient with amyotrophic lateral sclerosis undergoing cesarean section: a case report," *Journal of Clinical Anesthesia*, vol. 36, pp. 107–109, 2017.

[9] D. B. M. Kock-Cordeiro and A. J. Eggink, "Acute non invasive ventilation during pregnancy in a patient with amyotrophic lateral sclerosis," *European Respiratory Journal*, vol. 44, 2014.

[10] V. R. Lupo, J. H. Rusterholz, J. A. Reichert, and S. A. Hanson, "Amyotrophic lateral sclerosis in pregnancy," *The Obstetrician and Gynaecologist*, vol. 82, no. 4, pp. 682–685, 1993.

[11] C. Lunetta, V. A. Sansone, S. Penco et al., "Amyotrophic lateral sclerosis in pregnancy is associated with a vascular endothelial growth factor promoter genotype," *European Journal of Neurology*, vol. 21, no. 4, pp. 594–598, 2014.

[12] H. R. Martínez, S. S. Marioni, C. E. Escamilla Ocañas, M. T. Gonzalez Garza, and J. E. Moreno-Cuevas, "Amyotrophic lateral sclerosis in pregnancy: clinical outcome during the post-partum period after stem cell transplantation into the frontal motor cortex," *Cytotherapy*, vol. 16, no. 3, pp. 402–405, 2014.

2

A Case of Torsion in an Otherwise-Normal Ovary with a Giant Hematosalpinx Larger than Enlarged Ovary: Utilization of Diagnostic Laparoscopy for the Accurate Diagnosis

Sae Yu, Koji Yamanoi, Masumi Sunada, Sachiko Kitamura, Naoki Horikawa, Yoshitsugu Chigusa, Ken Yamaguchi, Akihito Horie, Junzo Hamanishi, Eiji Kondoh, and Masaki Mandai

Department of Gynecology and Obstetrics, Graduate School of Medicine, Kyoto University, 54 Shogoinkawahara-cho, Sakyo-ku, Kyoto City, Kyoto, Japan 606-8507

Correspondence should be addressed to Koji Yamanoi; kojiymni@kuhp.kyoto-u.ac.jp

Academic Editor: Kyousuke Takeuchi

We report a case of torsion in an otherwise-normal ovary with a giant hematosalpinx. A 23-year-old woman presented with complaints of abdominal pain and nausea. At initial visit, there was few abnormal findings of imaging tests, and we made a diagnosis of ovarian hemorrhage. Three days later, she came back with increased symptoms, and we detected the mass of a complex solid cystic structure with a unilocular cyst much larger than solid component. A diagnostic laparoscopy was performed immediately, and we could make a diagnosis of torsion in an otherwise-normal ovary with a giant hematosalpinx. We performed a salpingectomy and could preserve her ovary. This is the first case of torsion in an otherwise-normal ovary with a giant hematosalpinx which enlarged to a greater extent than the ovary.

1. Introduction

The adnexal torsion is one of the most common gynecological emergencies. The ovary without an apparent tumor can even undergo torsion, known as a torsion in otherwise-normal ovary [1]. Because of the low frequency and similarity of symptoms to more common disease including ovarian hemorrhage, it is often difficult to accurately diagnose, and the diagnosis is reported to be often delayed [2, 3].

It is common in clinical practice to perform imaging tests to help to make an accurate diagnosis preoperatively. Since the adnexa receives blood flow from both the uterus and the gonadal arteries, the adnexal torsion would not completely block the blood flow into ovaries, and partial blockage of blood flow causes the blood stagnation, frequently resulting in the enlargement of the ovaries [4]. Namely, when there is an enlarged ovary on imaging examination, torsion of the ovary is considered as a differential diagnosis [4, 5]. In fact, it is reported that there are some abnormal findings in imaging tests including enlargement of the ovaries even in the otherwise-normal ovary torsion, along with decreased blood flow and changes in the position [6]. However, the imaging findings of fallopian tubes that are involved in the otherwise-normal ovary torsion are still unclear. In some cases, the fallopian tubes have been reported to become swollen and edematous due to involvement of torsion [7, 8], but to date, there have been no reports showing that the fallopian tube got larger than the ovary itself in case of torsion of otherwise-normal ovary.

Herein, we report a case of torsion in an otherwise-normal ovary, occurring in a nonpregnant woman of reproductive age. Left adnexal enlargement to approximately 10 cm, with an enlarged ovary and an even larger, cystic fallopian tube was documented. We performed the literature search on PubMed, using the keywords "adnexal torsion," "hematosalpinx," and "reproductive age." However, we could not find any report of a markedly enlarged fallopian tube due to torsion in an otherwise-normal ovary. Because of these atypical imaging findings, we could not assume what the marked enlarged cystic tumor was derived from, and we could not understand the pathogenesis of her symptoms from imaging findings. A direct visual assessment with laparoscopy was performed, which enabled accurate diagnosis and prompt surgical treatment.

2. Case Report

A 23-year-old woman (gravida 0, para 0) presented to our emergency department with complaints of acute lower abdominal pain after sexual intercourse followed by nausea. She did not use any medication of contraception.

Physical examination revealed a soft and flat abdomen with no tenderness in the pouch of Douglas. Blood examination showed slightly elevated white blood cell (WBC) count 9550/μl, C-reactive protein (CRP) 2.3 mg/dl, and a negative human chorionic gonadotropin. On ultrasound, left adnexa was not enlarged, and a corpus luteum-like cyst, 3 cm in size, was detected inside the ovary. Small amount of ascites was also observed (Figures 1(a) and 1(b)).

Based on the above findings, provisional diagnosis of ovarian hemorrhage was made, and conservative treatment with oral painkillers was administered.

Three days later, the patient returned to the emergency department with increased intensity of lower abdominal pain along with strong nausea and diarrhea. Her vitals showed an increased pulse rate of 103 bpm and body temperature of 37.7°C. Her abdomen was generally soft, but there was moderate tenderness in the pouch of Douglas. Blood examination showed elevated inflammation-related factors (WBC 11,510/μl, CRP 12.0 mg/dl). Her platelet counts were kept in normal range ($21.6 \times 104/\mu l$ at her 1st visit and $25.6 \times 104/\mu l$ at her 2nd visit). Ultrasonography revealed a markedly enlarged adnexal mass (>10 cm × 15 cm) in the left lower abdomen. The mass had a complex solid cystic structure with a unilocular cyst much larger than solid component (Figure 1(c)). Contrast-enhanced computed tomography (CT) was then performed. The mass, located on the ventral side of the uterus, showed a weak contrast effect and a separate cystic compartment connected to the solid area with a band-like structure (Figures 1(d) and 1(e)).

Based on the above findings, adnexal torsion was suspected; however, the composition of enlarging cystic mass and the reason of rapid enlargement over a few days were unclear although we discussed it fully with radiologists. Nonetheless, to rule out ovarian torsion, a laparoscopic surgery was performed immediately.

On laparoscopic surgery, the whole left adnexa was found to be markedly swollen and twisted to at least 540 degrees (Figure 2(a)). Detorsion of the adnexa was performed, and separate cystic and solid masses were visualized. On aspirating fluid from the cystic mass, fimbria-like structure was observed on the surface of cystic mass (Figure 2(b)) suggesting that the cystic mass was a hematosalpinx and the solid mass, an enlarged ovary. A band-like tissue was connected the solid ovary to the fimbria (Figure 2(c)). A left salpingectomy was performed because of ischemic, irreversible changes in the enlarged left fallopian tube. Considering the young age of the patient and the weak contrast effect seen in CT, the ovary was preserved (Figure 2(d)). Total duration of the procedure was 1 h and 49 min, and total blood loss was 300 ml (including bloody ascites during laparoscopy).

After surgery, her symptoms (abdominal pain and nausea) disappeared quickly. Laboratory tests showed a rapid decrease in inflammatory markers. On the fifth postoperative day, the left ovary measured 62 × 36 mm (Figure 3(a)), and the patient was discharged on the same day. On 28th postoperative day, physical examination was unremarkable, and the left ovary had shrunk to 35 × 29 mm in size (Figure 3(b)).

Grossly, the cyst was unilocular, filled with blood, and had no obvious mass lesion (Figure 3(c)). Microscopically, extensive necrosis and congestion of the cyst wall with some preserved fallopian tube epithelium were observed (Figure 3d). Hence, a definitive diagnosis of fallopian tube hematoma due to adnexal torsion was made.

3. Discussion

We encountered a case of torsion in an otherwise-normal ovary in a nonpregnant woman of reproductive age with a marked enlarged hematosalpinx.

Especially in a nonpregnant woman of reproductive age, it is difficult to distinguish adnexal torsion from other common conditions with similar symptoms [9]. In this case, we first suspected ovarian hemorrhage because the patient was on cycle date 12 at the time of first visit and stated that she had sexual intercourse before development of symptoms. However, large ascites (intraperitoneal hemorrhage), which is often seen in ovarian hemorrhage [10], was not observed at this time. When a sudden abdominal pain occurs in a young woman and there remains some unclear findings, otherwise-normal ovarian torsion should be included in the differential diagnosis, and careful follow-up is recommended.

Because her left adnexa was not swollen at her first visit, her left fallopian tube as well as the ovary is thought to get very enlarged due to torsion. In a case report by Kamio et al., enlarged fallopian tube was seen as a separate structure from the ovary, but the size of the fallopian tube was smaller than that of the ovary [11]. In our case, on the contrary, the cystic fallopian tube formed an adnexal mass along with the ovary and was found to be enlarged to a greater extent than the ovary. Since the adnexa receive dual blood supply from the uterine and gonadal arteries, adnexal torsion can lead to partial block resulting in blood stagnation and enlargement of the ovaries [5, 12]. We propose that tube enlargement was the result of blood flow obstruction caused by adnexal torsion. Although the reason behind this marked fallopian tube hematoma formation due to congestion of blood flow still needs to be elucidated, it should be noted that the fallopian tubes can preferentially get enlarged when they are involved in the torsion of otherwise-normal ovary.

At first, the large cystic mass did not look like a fallopian tube, and it confused us a lot. In case of a torsion of otherwise-normal ovary, the imaging findings about fallopian tube can vary like our case. Clinically, it is very

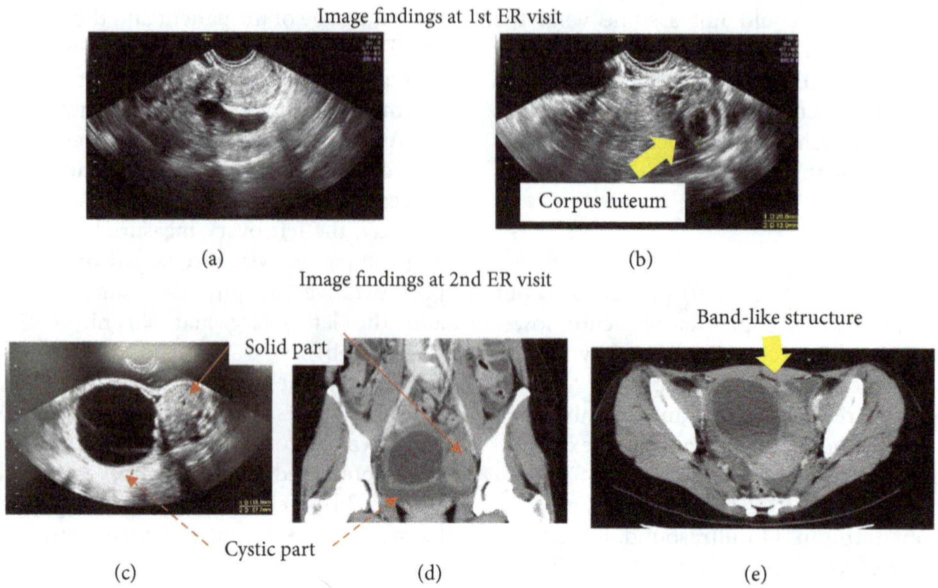

FIGURE 1: Image finding at 1st ER visit and 2nd ER visit. (a, b) Image findings at 1st ER visit. (a) Small amount of ascites on the left side. (b) A left adnexa 3 cm in size, and a small cyst inside that was suspected to be a corpus luteum. (c–e) Image findings at 2nd ER visit. (c, d) There are two-follicular enlargement. (e) A band-like structure between the solid and cystic parts. Arrows are indicated.

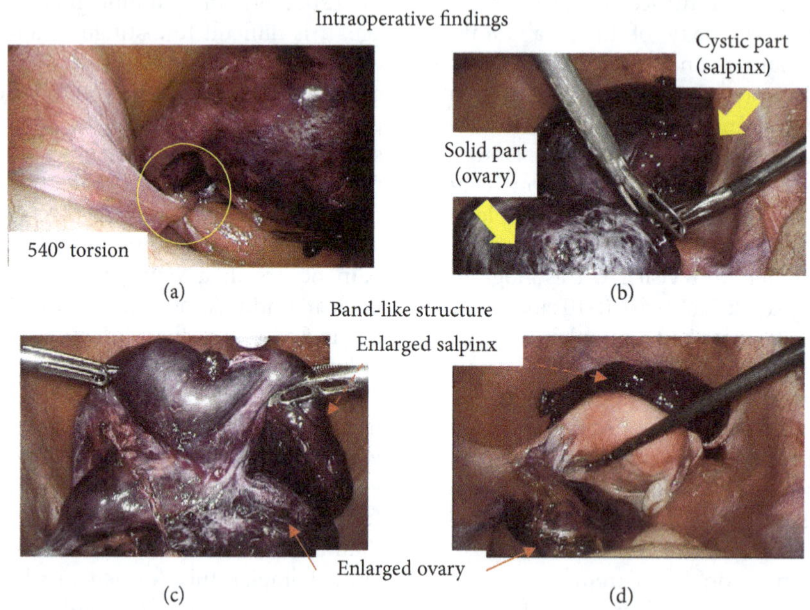

FIGURE 2: Intraoperative findings. (a) Adnexal torsion was observed. (b) Two-follicular enlargement was observed. (c) A band-like structure was observed. (d) Left salpingectomy was performed. Arrows are as indicated.

important to suspect a torsion of otherwise-normal ovary if we find the enlargement of ovary, decreased adnexal blood flow, and atypical position of the ovary [5, 13], regardless of other findings.

Whenever adnexal torsion is suspected, appropriate investigations are needed to rule out the condition. Delay in diagnosis and therapeutic intervention may lead to abolition of ovarian function. In case of adnexal torsion, we usually avoid oophorectomy to preserve ovarian function [14]. Especially in case of a relatively young age, we should try to preserve ovarian function to prevent loss of fertility [15].

Laparoscopy is a useful tool for the accurate evaluation of several intra-abdominal pathologies because it enables observation of the entire abdominal cavity with a relatively small wound [16, 17]. Also, emergency laparoscopy has the advantage of minimizing invasiveness and cost, as well as maximizing patient comfort in terms of pain control and postoperative recovery [18, 19]. However, as the field of view

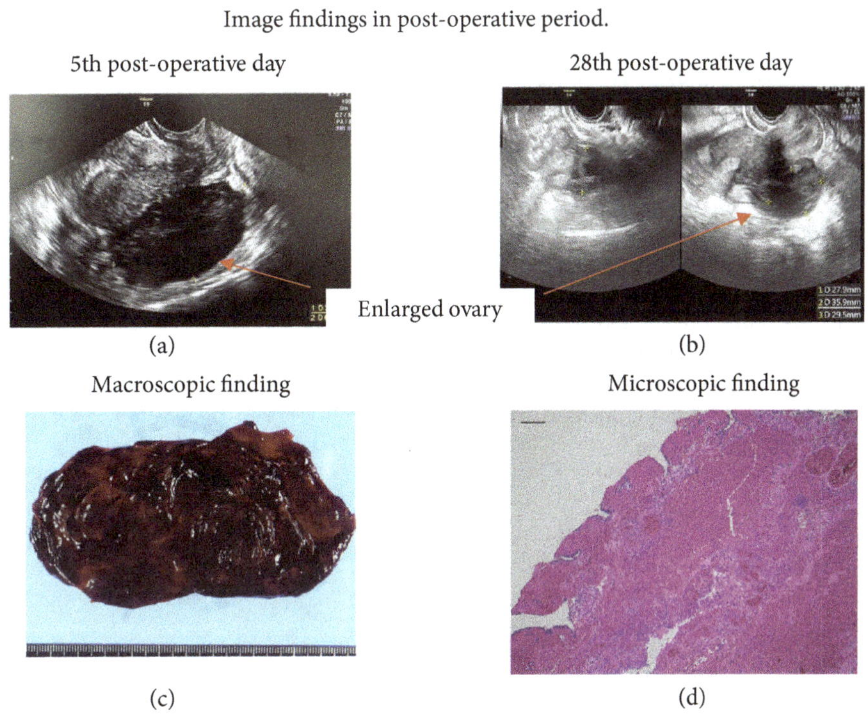

FIGURE 3: Image findings in postoperative period. (a, b) Ultrasonography findings. (a) An ultrasonography finding on 5th postoperative day. (b) An ultrasonography finding on 28th postoperative day. Arrows: left ovary. (c, d) Pathological findings. (c) Macroscopically, cyst was filled with blood. (d) Microscopically (40x), extensive necrosis and congestion of the cyst wall with some preserved fallopian tube epithelium were observed. Scale bar: 100 μm.

is limited, it can be difficult to observe the large structures fully, as in our case. In addition, if the tissue is highly fragile due to torsion, as in our case, rough handling may result in inadequate observation of the lesion due to contusion or bleeding from the tissue. Hence, it is important to carefully handle the tissues to maintain a clear field of vision. Additionally, in case of cystic structures, aspirating the cyst fluid may enhance visualization of the target tissue and associated unique structures, hence providing a diagnostic clue.

4. Conclusion

We encountered a case of torsion in an otherwise-normal ovary with a giant hematosalpinx. A marked cystically enlarged fallopian tube made it difficult to fully understand the actual pathophysiology. Because diagnosis of otherwise-normal ovary torsion is often difficult, we should not rule out its possibility. If we suspect it from any reason, we should consider treating it without delay to preserve their fertility. For treatment, laparoscopic surgery is useful because the lesion can be observed in detail with a small wound, and treatment can be performed sequentially.

Consent

Written informed consent was obtained from the patient for the publication of this case report and its accompanying images. Patient anonymity is preserved.

References

[1] Z. Tsafrir, J. Hasson, I. Levin, E. Solomon, J. B. Lessing, and F. Azem, "Adnexal torsion: cystectomy and ovarian fixation are equally important in preventing recurrence," *European Journal of Obstetrics, Gynecology, and Reproductive Biology*, vol. 162, no. 2, pp. 203–205, 2012.

[2] J. J. Robertson, B. Long, and A. Koyfman, "Myths in the evaluation and management of ovarian torsion," *The Journal of Emergency Medicine*, vol. 52, no. 4, pp. 449–456, 2017.

[3] E. Karaman, B. Beger, O. Çetin, M. Melek, and Y. Karaman, "Ovarian torsion in the normal ovary: a diagnostic challenge in postmenarchal adolescent girls in the emergency department," *Medical Science Monitor*, vol. 23, pp. 1312–1316, 2017.

[4] M. Graif, "Sonographic evaluation of ovarian torsion in childhood and adolescence," *AJR. American Journal of Roentgenology*, vol. 150, no. 3, pp. 647–649, 1988.

[5] G. Ssi-Yan-Kai, A. L. Rivain, C. Trichot et al., "What every radiologist should know about adnexal torsion," *Emergency Radiology*, vol. 25, no. 1, pp. 51–59, 2018.

[6] S. Servaes, D. Zurakowski, M. R. Laufer, N. Feins, and J. S. Chow, "Sonographic findings of ovarian torsion in children," *Pediatric Radiology*, vol. 37, no. 5, pp. 446–451, 2007.

[7] M. Toyoshima, H. Mori, K. Kudo et al., "Isolated torsion of the fallopian tube in a menopausal woman and a pre-pubertal girl: two case reports," *Journal of Medical Case Reports*, vol. 9, no. 1, 2015.

[8] H. M. Richard, R. B. Parsons, K. F. Broadman, R. S. Shapiro, and H. C. Yeh, "Torsion of the fallopian tube: progression of

sonographic features," *Journal of Clinical Ultrasound*, vol. 26, no. 7, pp. 374–376, 1998.

[9] D. Houry and J. Abbott, "Ovarian torsion: a fifteen-year review," *Annals of Emergency Medicine*, vol. 38, no. 2, pp. 156–159, 2001.

[10] M. V. Medvediev, A. Malvasi, S. Gustapane, and A. Tinelli, "Hemorrhagic corpus luteum: clinical management update," *Journal of Turkish Society of Obstetric and Gynecology*, vol. 17, no. 4, pp. 300–309, 2020.

[11] M. Kamio, T. Oki, Y. Inomoto, T. Tsuji, M. Yoshinaga, and T. Douchi, "Torsion of the normal ovary and oviduct in a pre-pubertal girl," *The Journal of Obstetrics and Gynaecology Research*, vol. 33, no. 1, pp. 87–90, 2007.

[12] C. Moore, A. B. Meyers, J. Capotasto, and J. Bokhari, "Prevalence of abnormal CT findings in patients with proven ovarian torsion and a proposed triage schema," *Emergency Radiology*, vol. 16, no. 2, pp. 115–120, 2009.

[13] A. Sintim-Damoa, A. S. Majmudar, H. L. Cohen, and L. S. Parvey, "Pediatric ovarian torsion: spectrum of imaging findings," *Radiographics*, vol. 37, no. 6, pp. 1892–1908, 2017.

[14] B. H. Al Wattar and Y. Afifi, "Untwist and keep: appraising evidence for conservative management of ovarian torsion," *BJOG : An International Journal of Obstetrics and Gynaecology*, vol. 127, no. 8, p. 966, 2020.

[15] A. Shevach Alon, R. Kerner, S. Ginath, G. Barda, J. Bar, and R. Sagiv, "Clinical characteristics of women with isolated fallopian tube torsion compared with adnexal torsion," *The Israel Medical Association Journal*, vol. 21, no. 9, pp. 575–579, 2019.

[16] S. Shitanaka, K. Yamanoi, J. Ogura et al., "A case of synchronous primary corpus and ovarian cancer with Pseudo-Meigs syndrome: utilization of a diagnostic laparoscopy for the accurate diagnosis," *Gynecol Minim Invasive Ther.*, vol. 8, no. 4, pp. 188–191, 2019.

[17] K. J. Sasaki and C. E. Miller, "Adnexal torsion: review of the literature," *Journal of Minimally Invasive Gynecology*, vol. 21, no. 2, pp. 196–202, 2014.

[18] M. Mandrioli, K. Inaba, A. Piccinini et al., "Advances in laparoscopy for acute care surgery and trauma," *World Journal of Gastroenterology*, vol. 22, no. 2, pp. 668–680, 2016.

[19] S. Di Saverio, "Emergency laparoscopy," *Journal of Trauma and Acute Care Surgery*, vol. 77, no. 2, pp. 338–350, 2014.

3

A Rare Disease Presenting Postpartum: Acute Fatty Liver of Pregnancy

Sofía Córdoba-Vives,[1,2] Patricia Pérez-Rodríguez,[2,3] Astrid Marín-Delgado,[2,4] Miguel Matus-Vargas,[2] and Adriana Arias-González[2,4]

[1]*Department of Maternal Fetal Medicine, Rafael Angel Calderón Guardia Hospital, San José, Costa Rica*
[2]*University of Costa Rica, San José, Costa Rica*
[3]*Department of Obstetrics and Gynecology, Rafael Angel Calderón Guardia Hospital, San José, Costa Rica*
[4]*Department of Pathology, Rafael Angel Calderón Guardia Hospital, San José, Costa Rica*

Correspondence should be addressed to Sofía Córdoba-Vives; soficv@gmail.com

Academic Editor: A. O. Awonuga

Acute fatty liver of pregnancy is a rare but highly fatal disease affecting women most frequently during the third trimester of pregnancy or in the postpartum period. It is considered a diagnosis of exclusion and requires a timely diagnosis to avoid maternal mortality. We present the case of a 33-year-old primigravida who required an emergency cesarean section due to fetal bradycardia. On postoperative day one, the patient was noted jaundiced, oliguric, and hypoglycemic. Laboratory tests revealed important hepatic dysfunction, coagulopathy, and renal failure. She was admitted to the Intensive Care Unit with the suspicion of acute fatty liver of pregnancy. Plasma exchange was started on postoperative day 5 with major clinical and laboratory improvement. A transjugular hepatic biopsy confirmed the diagnosis. The patient had satisfactory evolution and was discharged 15 days after delivery. Acute fatty liver of pregnancy is a highly morbid disease that needs a high index of suspicion to be diagnosed. Admission to an Intensive Care Unit to ensure maximum supportive care is mandatory in this disease.

1. Introduction

Acute fatty liver of pregnancy (AFLP) is a rare but highly morbid disease. The majority of AFLP cases are diagnosed in the third trimester of pregnancy or during the early postpartum period with some isolated reports occurring in the second trimester of pregnancy [1]. The disease is characterized by jaundice, coagulopathy, and signs and symptoms of hepatic and renal failure [2]. Diagnostic criteria for AFLP, known as the Swansea criteria, have been proposed to distinguish AFLP from other causes of liver dysfunction, including HELLP syndrome [3]. Accurate and timely diagnosis is fundamental to ensure good maternal and fetal outcomes.

In the last years, maternal mortality has been reduced due to the implementation of new therapies such as artificial liver support therapy (ALST). We present the case of a patient presenting with AFLP in the immediate postpartum who was admitted to the Intensive Care Unit (ICU) and received plasma exchange (PE) with excellent results.

2. Case Report

A 33-year-old primigravida consulted the emergency department with a 40-week pregnancy and history of spontaneous rupture of membranes (SROM). The diagnosis of SROM was confirmed, and she was admitted to labor and delivery. Augmentation of labor was initiated, and approximately 2 hours after admission, fetal bradycardia was observed, and she was taken to an emergency cesarean delivery. During surgery, about 50% of placental abruption was diagnosed. No important bleeding was reported afterwards, and no surgical complications were reported. A healthy female newborn was obtained, who weighed 3.3 kgs, Apgar score was 8-9, and no neonatal complications were reported.

Table 1: Swansea criteria for AFLP.

Clinical symptoms
(i) Nausea and vomiting
(ii) Abdominal pain
(iii) Encephalopathy
(iv) Polydipsia or polyuria
Laboratory findings
(i) Bilirubin greater than 0.8 mg/dL
(ii) Glucose less than 72 mg/dL
(iii) WBC greater than 11 000/microliter
(iv) AST or ALT greater than 42 units/L
(v) AKI or creatinine greater than 1.7 mg/dL
(vi) Ammonia greater than 47 micromoles/L
(vii) Coagulopathy or PT greater than 14 s
(viii) Urea greater than 340 micromoles/L
Ultrasonographic features
(i) Ascites
(ii) Echogenic liver
Histologic features
(i) Microvesicular steatosis

Source: Nelson et al. [14].

Fourteen hours after the surgery, the patient was noted jaundiced, oliguric, and hypoglycemic (glycemia: 40 mg/dL). She was conscious and alert, and no important obstetric bleeding was evidenced at the time. Her vital signs at that moment were the following: heart rate: 120 beats per minute (BPM), peripheral capillary oxygen saturation (SpO_2): 95%, respiratory rate: 16 respirations per minute (RPM), temperature 36.3 degree Celsius, and blood pressure: 74/48 mmHg.

Laboratory tests evidenced important hepatic dysfunction (Total Bilirubin (TB) 7.9 mg/dL, Indirect Bilirubin (IB) 2.7 mg/dL, direct bilirubin (DB) 5.149 mg/dL, Aspartate Aminotransferase (ASAT) 170 U/L, and Alanine Aminotransferase (ALAT) 149 U/L), coagulopathy (prothrombin time (PT) 27 seconds, International Normalized Ratio (INR) 2.56, and fibrinogen 71 mg/dL), acute kidney injury (creatine 2.7 mg/dL) as well as hyperammonemia (126 μmol/L), low platelets (95 000), and leukocytosis (33 030/microliter). At this point, her hemoglobin level was 9.9 mg/dL, hematocrit 27.8%, and lactate dehydrogenase (LDH) 432 IU/L. Due to the laboratory anomalies, an abdominal ultrasound was ordered. The ultrasound revealed an echogenic liver with fatty infiltrates and mild hepatic steatosis.

It is important to note that on the days prior to her hospital admission, the patient had not presented with any symptoms suggesting hepatic failure, and she had no known exposure to virus or medications that could explain the clinical alterations. At this moment, the patient was considered to have 7 Swansea criteria and was admitted to the ICU with suspicion of AFLP.

In the ICU, resolution of the coagulopathy was initiated with blood products. The transfusion was guided by rotational tromboelastography (ROTEM). She required platelets (1 pool), fresh frozen plasma (1 unit), and cryoprecipitates (1 unit). The patient remained stable for the next 3 days.

On postoperative day 5, the patient deteriorated importantly. She turned disoriented and encephalopathic; she was coagulopathic (prolonged PT and INR > 5) once more and persistently hypoglycemic despite an adequate diet. Other causes of hepatic failure in pregnancy and postpartum were discarded, such as viral hepatitis. At this point, the decision to start plasma exchange therapy was made, she received a total of three sessions (one daily) of PE, and recovery of her neurological status and laboratory tests was reached on postoperative day 9.

Once the coagulation disorder was reversed, she was taken to a transjugular hepatic biopsy. The biopsy reported microvesicular steatosis, ballooning degeneration of hepatocytes, canalicular cholestasis, and cholangiolitis, findings suggesting AFLP considering the clinical context. On postoperative day 15, the patient was discharged home, with complete resolution of symptoms and normalization of hepatic and renal functions.

3. Discussion

AFLP is a rare and serious liver pregnancy-related disease with an incidence of 1 per 6500 to 20 000 pregnancies [4]. Publications in the 1980s suggested mortality rates as high as 70%; more recent studies, suggest lower mortality rates: approximately 20% in some centers in low-income countries or even less than 10% in high-income countries. This reduction in mortality is due to the better understanding of the disease, recognition of milder presentations, early intervention and delivery, as well as aggressive management of complications, and the implementation of new treatment modalities, like artificial liver support therapy (ALST), which includes plasma exchange (PE) [5].

Perinatal mortality for infants born to affected mothers is highly variable. Data show a perinatal mortality rate of 10 to 20%, with the majority of reported cases caused by a stillbirth. Perinatal morbidity has been related to fetal acidosis and prematurity [5].

Pathogenesis of AFLP is not completely elucidated, but it is related to an abnormal beta-oxidation of fatty acids in fetal mitochondria that is probably caused by a genetic mutation in long-chain 3-hydroxyl coenzyme A dehydrogenase; this mutation contributes to microvesicular fatty infiltration of the liver of the mother [2].

Patients with AFLP typically present with a story of 1–2 weeks of nausea and vomiting; this prodromal symptom has an incidence that varies from 60 to 100% [6]. The clinical diagnosis is made by the application of the Swansea criteria (Table 1), which have a high negative predictive value. Six of the fourteen criteria are required to confirm the diagnosis of AFLP, once other causes of liver disease are excluded [3]. Although her clinical presentation was atypical, our patient had 7 Swansea criteria when the initial suspicion of AFLP was raised.

The definitive and confirmatory diagnosis of this clinical entity remains to be made histologically [7]. However, liver biopsy is not always performed routinely to establish the diagnosis of AFLP, due to coagulation disorders that usually manifest and the consequent bleeding complications that a patient undergoing the procedure could present [8]. To avoid these complications, in some hospitals, hepatic

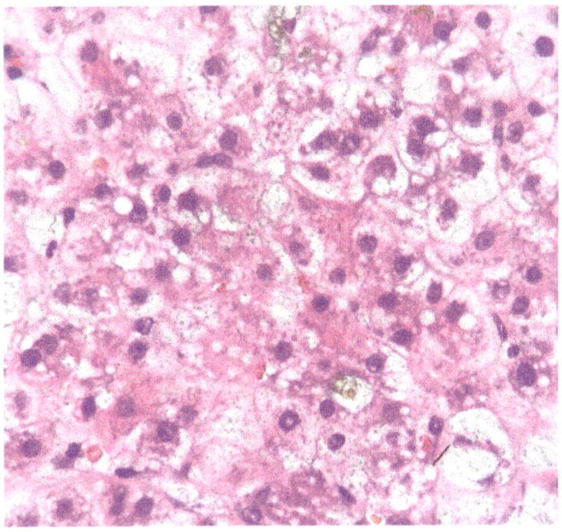

FIGURE 1: Microvesicular steatosis. Note the small white intracytoplasmic vesicles in the hepatocytes (400x, H&E staining). *Source: own.*

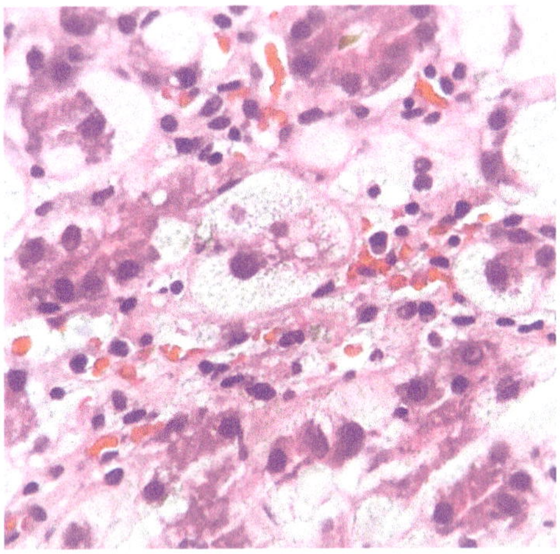

FIGURE 2: Ballooning degeneration. Note swollen hepatocytes with abundant and clear cytoplasm (400x, H&E staining). *Source: own.*

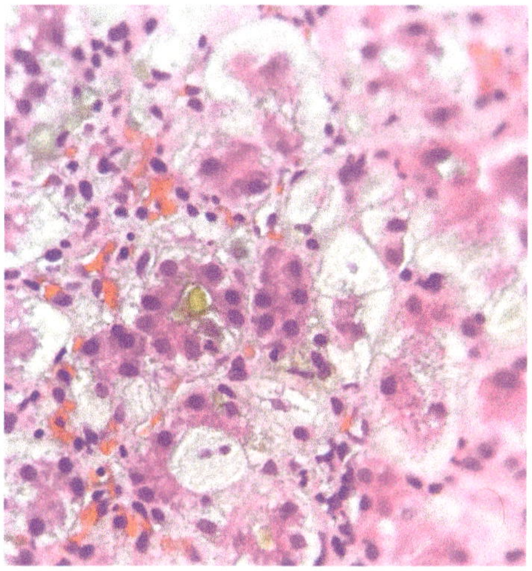

FIGURE 3: Canalicular cholestasis. Note the green-orange pigment located inside the canaliculus. On the right, ballooned hepatocytes (400x, H&E staining). *Source: own.*

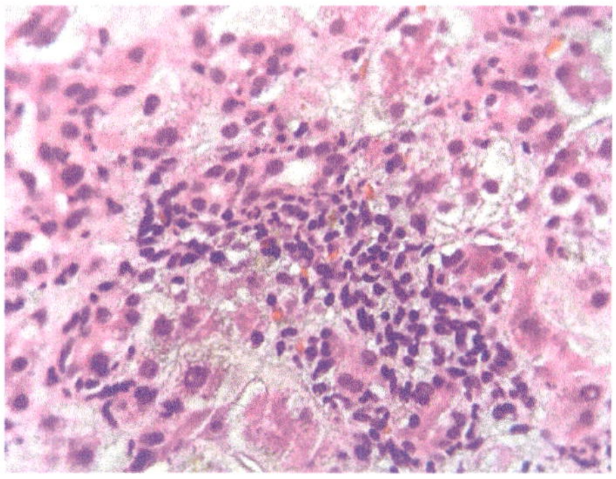

FIGURE 4: Cholangiolitis. Presence of polymorphonuclear intraepithelial leukocytes in the bile duct (400x, H&E staining). *Source: own.*

biopsies are done percutaneously, such is the case of our patient who underwent a transjugular hepatic biopsy.

Histologically, AFLP is mainly characterized by a diffuse microvesicular steatosis pattern (Figure 1), predominantly in the pericentral area and unusually in the periportal area [9]. Hepatocytes may look normal or pale and swollen (ballooning degeneration) (Figure 2), the cytoplasm is foamy and granular, and the nuclei are centrally located [10]. Other histological findings could be seen, such as bile canalicular plugs (Figure 3) and cholangiolitis (Figure 4), both signs of intrahepatic cholestasis. The accompanying inflammatory infiltrate is usually minimal, and hepatocyte necrosis occurs only in severe cases [10].

The main histopathological differential diagnosis includes pregnancy-induced hypertensive disorders, where the clinical manifestations are similar to AFLP; however, in hypertensive disorders, it is expected to find sinusoidal fibrin deposits or hemorrhage in the periportal areas [11] and in hepatic steatosis due to alcohol, where perivenular and periportal fibrosis, sclerosing hyaline necrosis, venulo-occlusive lesions, and canalicular cholestasis are present [12]; it is important to note that the biopsy findings must be interpreted based on the clinical context of the pregnant patient.

In patients diagnosed with AFLP, morbidity and mortality are secondary to hepatic dysfunction that can affect multiple organs and systems. The time to recovery after delivery depends on the severity of the disease and if there are other complications. The majority of patients will have clinical recovery within 3 to 4 days after delivery, but normalization of laboratory parameters lags frequently [5]. In our case, recovery was reached 9 days after delivery, and the patient required three plasma exchange sessions.

Treatment of AFLP is largely supportive and best carried in a critical care environment with a multidisciplinary team [5]. Artificial liver support therapy (ALST) has been widely used in the management of acute or chronic liver failure caused by various etiologies. This therapy improves liver injury and provides a homeostatic environment for hepatocyte regeneration. Available ALST includes hemoperfusion, plasma exchange (PE), continuous renal replacement therapy, Molecular Adsorbent Recycling System, and Plasma Perfusion (PP). Combining PE and PP in patients with liver disease allows to remove a large number of toxic substances and improve clotting factors and albumin [13]. Some patients will have persistent hepatic failure and acidosis and may be candidates for liver transplantation [14]. Fortunately, our patient recovered normal liver and renal function after PE.

4. Conclusion

AFLP is a highly morbid disease that needs a high index of suspicion to be diagnosed. An adequate and timely diagnosis to allow early admission to an ICU to ensure maximum supportive care is essential to reduce maternal mortality. The definitive diagnosis of this disease remains to be made histologically. ALST and PE have been widely recognized as effective therapies in patients complicated by this entity.

Abbreviations

AFLP: Acute fatty liver of pregnancy
ALST: Artificial liver support therapy
ICU: Intensive Care Unit
PE: Plasma exchange
PROM: Premature rupture of membranes
PP: Plasma Perfusion.

Consent

Informed consent was obtained from the subject in this case report.

References

[1] J. J. Byrne, A. Seasley, D. B. Nelson, D. D. Mcintire, and F. Gary, "Comparing acute fatty liver of pregnancy from hemolysis, elevated liver enzymes, and low platelets syndrome," *The Journal of Maternal-Fetal & Neonatal Medicine*, vol. 12, pp. 1–11, 2020.

[2] Z. Wu, P. Huang, Y. Gong, J. Wan, and W. Zou, "Treating acute fatty liver of pregnancy with artificial liver support therapy," *Medicine*, vol. 97, no. 38, p. e12473, 2018.

[3] L. C. Casey, R. J. Fontana, A. Aday et al., "Acute liver failure (ALF) in pregnancy: how much is pregnancy related?," *Hepatology*, vol. 72, no. 4, pp. 1366–1377, 2020.

[4] L. Chang, M. Wang, H. Liu et al., "Pregnancy outcomes of patients with acute fatty liver of pregnancy: a case control study," *BMC pregnancy and childbirth*, vol. 20, no. 1, pp. 1–8, 2020.

[5] E. E. Naoum, L. R. Leffert, H. V. Chitilian, K. J. Gray, and B. T. Bateman, "Acute fatty liver of pregnancy," *Anesthesiology*, vol. 130, no. 3, pp. 446–461, 2019.

[6] P. V. Gracia and C. Montufar-Rueda, "Acute fatty liver of pregnancy: diagnosis, treatment, and outcome based on 35 consecutive cases," *J Matern Fetal Neonatal Med*, vol. 24, no. 9, pp. 1143–1146, 2011.

[7] C. R.-B. V. Gómez-Hernández, "Hígado graso agudo en el embarazo," *Crónicas Científicas*, no. 15, pp. 39–49, 2020.

[8] R. H. Westbrook, G. Dusheiko, and C. Williamson, "Pregnancy and liver disease," *Journal of Hepatology.*, vol. 64, no. 4, pp. 933–945, 2016.

[9] B. Gasmi and D. E. Kleiner, "Liver histology diagnostic and prognostic features," *Clinics in liver disease*, vol. 19, 2021.

[10] B. K. WJ, *Odze and Goldblum Surgical Pathology of the GI Tract, Liver, Biliary Tract and Pancreas*, Elsevier, Philadelphia, 3d ed edition, 2015.

[11] K. J. T. Rodríguez, "¿Qué hay en común entre el hígado graso agudo del embarazo y la preeclampsia? Subdiagnóstico clínico de alta mortalidad," *Revista Med*, vol. 27, no. 1, pp. 61–72, 2020.

[12] E. N. Eduardo-Pino, J. A. Viruez-Soto, M. A. Aliaga-Aguilar et al., "Hígado Graso Agudo Del Embarazo," *Cuadernos Hospital de Clínicas*, vol. 57, p. 6, 2016.

[13] J. Ding, L. P. Han, X. P. Lou et al., "Effectiveness of combining plasma exchange with plasma perfusion in acute fatty liver of pregnancy: a retrospective analysis," *Gynecol Obstet Invest*, vol. 4.

[14] D. B. Nelson, J. J. Byrne, and F. G. Cunningham, "Acute fatty liver of pregnancy," *New England Journal of Medicine*, vol. 137, no. 3, p. 12, 2021.

4

Challenging Obstetrical Management in Generalized Peritonitis during Pregnancy

Susana Patrícia Lima Oliveira, Ana Isabel Sousa, and Nuno Nogueira Martins

Department of Obstetrics and Gynecology, Centro Hospitalar Tondela-Viseu, Viseu, Portugal

Correspondence should be addressed to Susana Patrícia Lima Oliveira; susana.limaoliveira91@gmail.com

Academic Editor: Kyousuke Takeuchi

Acute abdomen in pregnancy represents a diagnostic and therapeutic challenge, despite the current advances in modern medicine, since the typical symptoms and altered laboratory parameters mimic normal pregnancy. Acute appendicitis is the most common nonobstetric surgical emergency during pregnancy, with an incidence of 1 per 500-2000 pregnancies. Delayed diagnosis and reluctance to operate on a pregnant woman predispose to adverse maternal and fetal outcomes. The elective termination of pregnancy or interventions to prolong it in the presence of appendicitis is controversial. We present a case of a 38-year-old Caucasian woman, G2P0, admitted to the Obstetric Emergency Department at 13 4/7 weeks of gestation with a primary complaint of severe nausea and vomiting associated with progressive diffuse abdominal pain which had started 7 days before. After the difficulty of inherent differential diagnosis, she was diagnosed with generalized peritonitis due to acute perforated appendicitis. Prompt exploratory laparotomy with appendectomy and drainage of multiple abscesses were performed. Conservative obstetrical management was assumed, with subsequent periodic monitoring of the fetal focus. Due to abdominal compartment syndrome, the abdomen was left open for 4 days. After 7 days in the intensive care unit, recovery was favorable, pregnancy remained uneventful, and a healthy full-term baby was born 27 weeks later. This case represents a successful example of how the cooperation of the obstetrics and general surgery teams and the decision of conservative obstetrical management in the surgical environment contributed to optimizing maternal health, achieving the best obstetrical outcome.

1. Introduction

Acute abdomen in pregnancy represents one of the most confronting diagnostic and therapeutic contemporaneous dilemmas, challenging modern medicine [1, 2] . Appendicitis occurs in approximately 1 out of every 500 to 2000 gestations, most commonly seen in the second trimester [3, 4]. It is the main cause of nonobstetrical emergency requiring surgery in pregnancy, representing 25% of all causes [2, 5]. Overall, the prevalence of appendicitis is the same in pregnant and nonpregnant patients [3, 6].

Reaching the correct diagnosis could be laborious due to physiologically anatomical and biochemical adjustments occurring during pregnancy [7]. The classic symptoms—anorexia, nausea, and vomiting—may easily be mistaken for hyperemesis *gravidarum*; pain in the right lower quadrant could be assumed as round ligament pain; and mild leukocytosis is a common laboratory finding in normal gestation [8, 9]. Even though the appendix ascends in the abdominal cavity as the uterus enlarges modifying the location of symptoms, pain in the right lower quadrant of the abdomen is the most common presenting complaint regardless of gestational age [3, 10, 11].

Delays in diagnosis and reluctance to perform surgery on pregnant women confer a greater risk of developing appendicular perforation and subsequent peritonitis, which may lead to other complications including sepsis, abortion, premature labor, and maternal mortality [1, 2, 12].

Unruptured appendicitis is associated with a fetal loss rate of 2% compared to more than 30% in pregnant women with a perforated appendix [13]. Sepsis in pregnancy represents one of the leading causes of death in the intensive care setting, with maternal mortality ranging from 1.8 to 11% and fetal mortality from 10 to 40% depending on gestational age [14].

A high index of suspicion and a low threshold to decide for surgery remains paramount in the management of this potentially life-threatening condition [11, 15]. Evidence does not support that surgery during pregnancy results in an increased incidence of congenital abnormalities [16].

Multidisciplinary cooperation between surgical and obstetrics teams is the cornerstone in ensuring optimal care for the pregnant and the fetus [7]. Clinical decision-making regarding termination or proceeding pregnancy in a critical illness is a controversial issue with arguments on both sides [17, 18].

A case of septic shock in the context of the acute abdomen during pregnancy with successful step-by-step coordination of obstetrics and general surgery teams achieving the best obstetrical outcome despite the difficulty in diagnosis, management, and decision is presented below.

2. Case Presentation

A 38-year-old Caucasian woman, G2P0, presented to the Obstetric Emergency Department at 13 4/7 weeks of gestation with a primary complaint of severe nausea and vomiting associated with progressive diffuse abdominal pain which had started 7 days before. She had a history of medicated and clinically controlled bipolar disorder and hypothyroidism and had no relevant family history. She had been to the Obstetric Emergency Department twice before with similar but milder complaints and was discharged with the diagnosis of hyperemesis *gravidarum* and clinical improvement under antiemetic drugs. At readmission, the patient referred progression of emesis to complete oral intolerance and worsening pain in the right lower quadrant in the absence of diarrhea, constipation, dysuria, or anomalous vaginal discharge or bleeding.

She was admitted to the obstetrical observation room, and her vital signs upon arrival were a tympanic temperature of 37.5°C, a blood pressure of 133/81 mmHg, a heart rate of 124 bpm, a respiratory rate of 19 breaths/min, and a 0_2 saturation of 98% on room air. Generalized muscle guarding was observed on abdominal examination along with a positive *Blumberg* sign.

Obstetrical ultrasound revealed an intrauterine gestational sac containing a fetus with a crown-rump length compatible with 13 4/7 weeks and fetal heart rate (FHR) was 159 bpm. Laboratory findings reported a white blood count of 9.9×10^9/L, and increased values of C-reactive protein (30.94 mg/dL), procalcitonin (144.30 ng/mL), and creatinine (1.6 mg/dL). Arterial blood sample results revealed hyperlactatemia (5.8 mmol/L), hypocalcemia (2 mEq/L), and hyperglycemia (320 mg/dL). The renal ultrasound was normal. Abdominal ultrasound described a moderate amount of peritoneal fluid dispersed into the abdominal cavity, including perihepatic and perisplenic recesses, not referring to the appendix.

Prompt collaboration of the General Surgery Department was requested, and the diagnosis of septic shock in relation to an acute abdomen was confirmed. At that time, blood pressure became immeasurable, and the patient was immediately taken to the operating room for exploratory laparotomy. Under general anesthesia, through a midline incision along the full length of the abdomen, intraoperative findings included a multiperforated and gangrenous appendix and abundant purulent ascites. Multiple abscesses were drained, and after the main surgical procedure, the abdomen was irrigated with copious isotonic fluid.

At that moment, the obstetrics team was confronted with the challenging decision of termination or continuation of the pregnancy. Conservative obstetrical management was assumed, with subsequent periodic monitoring of the fetal focus. Due to severe peritonitis with massive bowel distension and presumed abdominal compartment syndrome, the abdomen was left open and a temporary closure with transparent adherent film and gauze was made (Figure 1).

In the immediate postoperative period, the patient was transferred to the intensive care unit (ICU). Intravenous fluid resuscitation, vasopressors, combined antibiotics, and sedatives were administered. Mechanical ventilation and hemodialysis were required. An intravenous piperacillin/tazobactam antibiotic regimen was used, started on postoperative day 0, and replaced by amoxicillin/clavulanate on postoperative day 6 after microbiological results of the peritoneal fluid collected during surgery that identified *Escherichia coli, Streptococcus mitis, Streptococcus oralis*, and *Streptococcus constellatus ssp constellatus*, all multisensitive. Antibiotic therapy was continued until postoperative day 14.

A first laparostomy revision was performed on postoperative day 2, with mild infection signs and significant bowel edema again preventing abdominal closure. Laparostomy was reconstructed with a polypropylene mesh and delayed primary fascial closure was achieved on postoperative day 4.

During the stay in the ICU, daily FHR was obtained at the bedside by the obstetrics team, assuring fetal vitality. The patient became progressively less dependent on supportive therapy, with no fever records since postoperative day 5 and extubated on day 7. Complete recovery occurred, and she was discharged home on postoperative day 15. No more adverse or unanticipated events occurred.

Pregnancy was then uneventfully carried to full term, with referral to periodic prenatal visits at the hospital. The labor was induced with prostaglandin E2 at 41 0/7 weeks. Due to a nonreassuring fetal status (prolonged deceleration), an emergent cesarean section with midline vertical suprapubic incision and hysterotomy with low-transverse incision was performed. A male weighing 3150 g with an Apgar score of 5/8/10 was born. He was admitted to the Special Newborn Care Unit with a diagnosis of sepsis, but evolution under antibiotic therapy, double intravenous antibiotic therapy with ampicillin and gentamicin from day 1 to day 11 of life, revealed favorable. Vaginal or placental swabs were not collected after the cesarean section because there was no evidence before delivery or during delivery of an infectious condition. The placenta was submitted for histopathological analysis revealing mild vasculitis and funiculitis phenomena. The blood culture of the newborn's first day of life did not identify microorganisms.

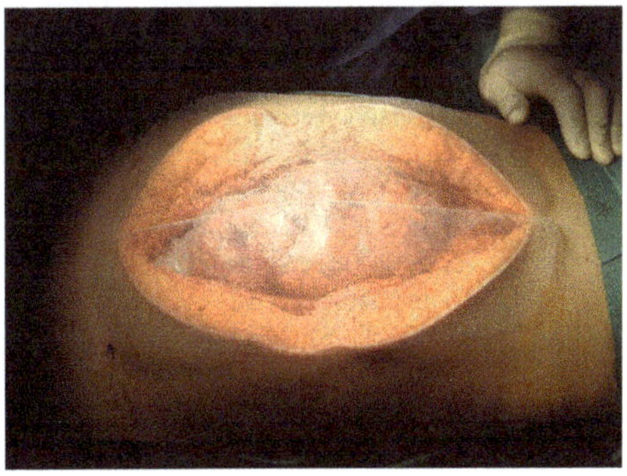

FIGURE 1: Confection of temporary abdominal closure due to abdominal compartment syndrome.

In a developmental appointment in Pediatrics, the mother revealed that she was very satisfied with the conduct of the team that provided her with life without serious sequelae and a healthy child. In the first year of life, the boy achieved all developmental milestones.

Nine months after the intervention, surgery records of the mother documented an incisional hernia, lacking plastic repair indication due to its large dimensions.

3. Discussion

More than a century has passed since *Edmund A. Babler* (1874-1930) declared *"the mortality of appendicitis complicating pregnancy and the puerperium is the mortality of delay"*. Even so, this statement remains valid nowadays, proven by several cases of a perforated appendix with increased maternal and fetal mortality [19].

In the extreme critical scenario, maternal sepsis is an uncommon complication of pregnancy demanding expeditious diagnosis, prompt identification of the source of infection, and targeted management [20].

The presence of a second dependent patient—the fetus in a life-threatening maternal condition may generate a conflicting obstetrical issue concerning induction of abortion in early pregnancy and timing of delivery in late pregnancy [17, 21].

For previable pregnancies, there is no clear evidence in favor of interrupting an early pregnancy to improve the mother's health [22]. Radical termination of pregnancy to execute an appendicectomy is not evidence-based, and optimizing maternal status is paramount [14, 17, 18]. Likewise, in advanced pregnancy, a concomitant cesarean is not recognized as a part of treatment for the surgical condition and should only be performed for obstetrical reasons. The use of tocolytics is controversial, as studies have failed to prove benefits with an increased risk of pulmonary lesion [23]. For a pregnant woman dealing with serious cardiovascular compromise due to sepsis, a delivery/induction of abortion could lead to higher maternal and fetal mortality, unless chorioamnionitis or septic abortion has occurred [24]. Except after 38 weeks, a c-section represents a transference of the maternal problems to the newborn, exposing it to the unnecessary risks of premature birth, like respiratory distress syndrome [17].

However, there are advocates of elective termination of pregnancy complicated by appendicitis, but this controversial subject is notably scarce in the literature. *Horntrich* et al. stated that *"caesarean section should be precedent to appendectomy, at least in cases of advanced appendicitis and when the foetus is viable"* [25]. *Ford* et al., in a recent review, affirmed that in pregnancy before viability when the mother becomes ill termination of pregnancy is mandatory, preventing the septic status [26].

A few cases of induction of abortion following diagnosis of an acute abdomen in pregnancy can be found. *Cohen-Kerem* et al., in a systematic review, concluded that the rate of elective termination of pregnancy in a sequence of nonobstetrical surgery was 1.3% [27]. A paper included in this review conducted by *Tamir* et al. studied 84 pregnant women who underwent laparotomy after the diagnosis of acute appendicitis and determined 7 therapeutic abortions in that population [15]. Another paper integrated into the review that followed 44 pregnant patients with a diagnosis of biliary colic or cholecystitis stated that 3 patients interrupted their pregnancy during the first trimester because of persistent symptoms and the priority of an earlier cholecystectomy [28]. *Ueberrueck* et al. retrospectively analyzed 94 appendicectomies for suspected acute appendicitis during pregnancy and reported that the rate of therapeutic or requested abortion was 21.7% in the first trimester [29]. *Qihui* et al. investigated retrospectively 26 pregnant women with acute pancreatitis and declared that 9 cases requested termination of pregnancy and 5 cases were submitted to induction of abortion [30].

The rationale for the termination of pregnancy was not established in most papers. Some reasons mentioned are related to the concern with pregnancy gradually complicating the critical condition and to the fear of teratology as a result of medications administered, allegedly harmful to the fetus [30].

Our case report shows that conservative obstetrical behaviour carried out since the beginning, facing the threatening diagnosis of maternal shock septic, allowed the achievement of well-being for the mother and the fetus. Another feature highlighted in our case is the successful management of gestational abdominal compartment syndrome, whose evidence is practically absent in the literature. Few cases reported treatment of abdominal compartment syndrome in pregnancy. *Turnock* et al. described a case of acute perforated second-trimester appendicitis associated with intraabdominal sepsis and abdominal compartment syndrome. They applied a temporary abdominal closure with negative pressure wound therapy for nearly 1 week with excellent surgical and obstetrical results [31]. In our report, the abdomen was left open for 4 days despite the gravid uterus, and the cooperation between surgical and obstetrics teams, with intensive care support, made the complete restoration of maternal health possible, reaching the best obstetrical outcome.

A comparative table of previous studies on appendicitis in pregnancy is presented below (Table 1).

We also question whether the two sepsis clinical pictures (maternal and newborn) are related or whether they are

Table 1: Comparative table of previous studies reporting appendicitis in pregnancy..

Reference	Type of study	Pain location/other symtoms	Trimester	Management	Maternal outcomes	Fetal or neonatal outcomes
Babler 1908 [19]	Case report	Sudden, progressive, severe right lower abdominal pain becoming excruciating associated with vomiting	Third (30 weeks)	Open surgery	Perforated appendix; large appendiceal abscess (discharged on postoperative D35); phlebitis in the left thigh (1 week after discharge)	Preterm labor (D2)
Tamir et al. 1990 [15]	Case series (84 patients; 54 patients with appendicitis pathologically confirmed)	Diffuse or periumbilical pain migrating to the right lower abdominal quadrant (48%); right lower quadrant pain only (28%); nausea/ vomiting (91/81%); anorexia (70%); diarrhea (31%); constipation (4%)	First (32%); second (44%); third (16%)	Open surgery: right transverse muscle-spitting incision over the point of maximum tenderness (79%); low midline vertical incisions (13%); laparoscopic surgery: completed (1%), initially underwent diagnostic laparoscopy (4%) in the first trimester	Confirmed appendicitis: perforation rate: 43% (all with symptoms >24 h); periappendiceal or pelvic abscess: 22%; wound infection: 13% (11% perforated); no long-term maternal morbidity or mortality	Spontaneous abortion (2%); preterm labor (27%); failure of tocolysis (5%); Apgar score at 5 min <7 (5%); negative laparotomies: perinatal death (17%); extreme perinatal morbidity (3%)
Turnock et al. 2016 [31]	Case report	Progressive right/left lower and right upper quadrant abdominal pain associated with dysuria, nausea, and vomiting with oral intolerance in the previous 5 days	Second (15 weeks)	Laparoscopic approach with conversion to laparotomy (due to massive bowel distention and purulent ascites); temporary abdominal closure due to acute compartment syndrome with saline-dampened surgical towel placed over cassette cover; peritoneal toilet with inspection of the ileocolic anastomosis (D4); fascial closure (D6); delayed primary closure of the laparotomy incision (D12)	Ileocecum abscess; perforation of the appendiceal base with extension into the cecum; cecal necrosis (discharged on postoperative D15); no surgical complications at 5 years postdelivery	Term spontaneous vaginal delivery; child obtained all developmental milestones
Tase et al. 2017 [4]	Systematic review (43 articles)	Right lower quadrant pain (60-100%); nausea, vomiting, and anorexia common and indistinguishable from pregnancy related symptoms	First (30%); second (45%); third (25%)	Both open and laparoscopic surgery safe without statistically significant difference in perioperative obstetric or neonatal outcomes; no advisable medical management due little evidence on safety	Perforation rate: 20.3-43% (66% if delay in surgery >24 h; 8.7% first trimester, 12.5% second trimester, 26.1% third trimester)	Fetal loss: 1.5% delayed diagnosis, nonperforated; 35-55% delayed diagnosis, perforated appendix; delivery rate: 15-45% (preterm labor highest in the first week following surgery)
Hata et al. 2020 [32]	Case report	Acute epigastralgia, followed by right	Third (27 weeks)	Laparoscopic surgery with reduced-port approach	None (discharged on postoperative D8)	Vaginal delivery at term

Table 1: Continued.

Reference	Type of study	Pain location/other symtoms	Trimester	Management	Maternal outcomes	Fetal or neonatal outcomes
		lower abdominal pain and vomiting				
Tavakoli et al. 2020 [33]	Case report	Acute onset of sharp right abdominal pain associated with nausea and a single episode of vomiting	Third (37 weeks)	Conservative: intravenous antibiotics with complete resolution of abdominal pain; induction of labor (D3)	None (patient's pain and clinical status stable on D3 and discharged on postoperative D6 with a 10-day course of oral antibiotic; patient denied elective appendectomy at 20-months)	Uncomplicated vaginal delivery (D4)
Matsui et al. 2020 [34]	Case report	Diffuse abdominal pain migrating to the right lower abdominal quadrant started the day before admission	Second (20 weeks; dichorionic diamniotic twin pregnancy)	Laparoscopic surgery (3 trocars; insufflation pressure 10 mm Hg; left lateral tilt; ultrasonic energy)	None (discharged on postoperative D9)	Uncomplicated elective cesarean section (38 weeks)
Saleh et al. 2020 [35]	Case report	Persistent, severe, exacerbated by movement lower abdominal pain associated with loss of appetite in the previous 2 days	Second (17 weeks)	Laparoscopic surgery	Acute, nonperforated appendix; pelvic abscess; peritoneovaginal fistula (discharged on postoperative D5; endometriosis and decidualization on pathological examination of the appendix)	Uncomplicated spontaneous vaginal delivery (40 1/7 weeks)
Ghannouchi et al. 2021 [36]	Case report	Right iliac fossa pain in the previous 2 days	Third (32 weeks)	Planned appendectomy	None (discharged on postoperative D2; appendicular deciduosis on microscopical examination)	Uncomplicated delivery (39 weeks)
Sanders-Davis et al. 2021 [37]	Case report	Generalized abdominal pain migrating to right lumbar region associated with loss of appetite and vomiting; no respiratory symptoms (PCR SARS-CoV-2 infection positive)	Third (33 1/7 weeks)	Open surgery: right-sided transverse incision guided by the available imaging to allow access to the cranially displaced appendix	Perforated appendix with local peritonitis (worsening respiratory function after appendectomy with a diagnosis of bilateral pneumonia; discharged on postoperative D7)	Emergent cesarean section (33 6/7 weeks); neonatal respiratory distress syndrome with oxygen requirement at high pressures on mechanical ventilation, extubated at 24 hours of age (PCR SARS-CoV-2 negative at D3 and D5)

D: day.

independent. Considering that the maternal infectious condition resolved at the transition to second trimester, that the pregnancy continued uneventfully to term, and that 27 weeks separate the resolution of maternal and newborn sepsis, with no prebirth signs indicating intra-amniotic infection before the diagnosis of neonatal sepsis (no leukocytosis, maintenance of apyrexia during labor, absence of purulent vaginal discharge or pain on uterine palpation, absence of fetal/maternal tachycardia, intact membranes at the beginning of cesarean section, and artificial rupture of membranes intraoperatively with liquid clear amniotic), the hypothesis that they are two independent infectious situations seems to be the most likely.

As strengths of the study, the authors mention the fact that there was successful management in terms of several successive and rapidly deteriorating complex pathologies of the maternal clinical condition, such as acute appendicitis, generalized peritonitis, and abdominal compartment syndrome as a complication of laparotomy, aggravated and with mutual potential for atrocity by a fetus that was developing in this environment in the final stage of the first trimester. In addition, there was also an efficacious approach to emergent delivery and treatment of neonatal sepsis. All this effective management with the best maternal and perinatal outcome was based on the step-by-step coordination and communication of an in-hospital multidisciplinary team, consisting of obstetricians, general surgeons, intensivists, neonatologists, specialists in maternal-fetal medicine, and anaesthesiologists who joined knowledge and efforts in a common objective, the achievement of maternal stability with preservation of gestational and neonatal integrity. This article also emphasizes the importance of the low threshold of suspicion of appendicitis, even when the symptoms are confused with the normal ones of the pregnancy state or others that do not fit the usual clinical picture of acute appendicitis. In addition, it is a warning to raise awareness of the scarce literature on appendicitis in pregnancy, reinforcing the need for an active and critical discussion of these rare cases among the teams to promote further theoretical-practical knowledge, namely, about the management of the infectious pathology of appendicitis, peritonitis, sepsis, and abdominal compartment syndrome and how to manage the pregnancy itself in the limbo of these potentially fatal diagnoses.

As a limitation of this study, the authors cite the difficulty in diagnosing an acute abdominal process in pregnant women, either because of the anatomical changes that modify the appendicular location or because of the typical symptoms of pregnancy that camouflage a true pathology in aggravation. This obstacle explains the high rate of peritonitis in this population. Theoretically, emergent surgery should not be delayed in pregnant women as in nonpregnant women. However, the uncertainty of the diagnosis and the concern with fetal integrity during and after the surgical procedure generates a postponement in the decision of urgent intervention in the pregnant woman. Another potential limitation is related to the scarce literature regarding the characteristics, pathophysiology, epidemiology, risk factors, and management of appendicitis, peritonitis, and abdominal compartment syndrome in pregnancy, due to the very small number of inherent studies published, while those that exist have high variability in the diagnostic methods and surgical techniques used, potentially reflecting local practical experience and individual surgeon preference. And the emergency scenario itself dictates that not much time is wasted on audio-visual documentation that could help both "predict the unpredictable" and expedite practical approaches to similar cases in the future. A meta-analysis of all existing studies could serve to create a uniform protocol that facilitates clinical decisions in emergency medicine for pregnant women.

In conclusion, acute appendicitis is the main nonobstetrical cause for surgical intervention in pregnancy. A high index of suspicion, a low threshold to perform a life-saving operation, and the conservative obstetrical patterns carried out by surgical and obstetrics teams were the cornerstones for the improvement of mother's health, allowing her to proceed with the pregnancy and ultimately have a full-term newborn.

References

[1] G. Augustin and M. Majerovic, "Non-obstetrical acute abdomen during pregnancy," *European Journal of Obstetrics, Gynecology, and Reproductive Biology*, vol. 131, no. 1, pp. 4–12, 2007.

[2] S. K. Zachariah, M. Fenn, K. Jacob, S. A. Arthungal, and S. A. Zachariah, "Management of acute abdomen in pregnancy: current perspectives," *International Journal of Women's Health*, vol. 11, pp. 119–134, 2019.

[3] D. J. Selzer and D. Stefanidis, "Surgical emergencies in the pregnant patient," *Advances in Surgery*, vol. 53, pp. 161–177, 2019.

[4] A. Tase, M. F. Kamarizan, and K. Swarnkar, "Appendicitis in pregnancy: difficulties in diagnosis and management. Guidance for the emergency general surgeon: a systematic review," *International Journal of Surgery Open*, vol. 6, pp. 5–11, 2017.

[5] A. P. Carrillo and A. Chandraharan, "Abdominal pain in pregnancy: a rational approach to management," *Obstetrics, Gynaecology and Reproductive Medicine*, vol. 27, no. 4, pp. 112–119, 2017.

[6] N. B. Gilo, D. Amini, and H. J. Landy, "Appendicitis and cholecystitis in pregnancy," *Clinical Obstetrics and Gynecology*, vol. 52, no. 4, pp. 586–596, 2009.

[7] S. M. Flexer, N. Tabib, and M. B. Peter, "Suspected appendicitis in pregnancy," *The Surgeon*, vol. 12, no. 2, pp. 82–86, 2014.

[8] H. W. Jones, "Gynecologic Surgery," in *Sabiston Textbook of Surgery: The Biological Basis of Modern Surgical Practice [Internet]*, C. M. Townsend, R. D. Beauchamp, M. B. Evers, and K. L. Mattox, Eds., pp. 2027–2052, Elsevier, Philadelphia, PA, 2016.

[9] B. Richmond, "The Appendix," in *Sabiston Textbook of Surgery: The Biological Basis of Modern Surgical Practice [Internet]*, C. M. Townsend, R. D. Beauchamp, M. B. Evers, and K. L. Mattox, Eds., pp. 1296–1311, Elsevier, Philadelphia, PA, 2016.

[10] R. J. Vissers and W. B. Lennarz, "Pitfalls in appendicitis," *Emergency Medicine Clinics*, vol. 28, no. 1, pp. 103–118, 2010.

[11] T. F. Kelly and T. J. Savides, "Gastrointestinal Disease in Pregnancy," in *Creasy and Resnik's Maternal-Fetal Medicine: Principles and Practice [Internet]*, R. Resnik, C. J. Lockwood, T. R. Moore, M. F. Greene, J. A. Copel, and R. M. Silver, Eds., pp. 1164-1165, Elsevier, Philadelphia, PA, 2018.

[12] K. Mahomed, "Abdominal pain," in *High-risk pregnancy: management options [Internet]*, D. James, P. Steer, C. Weiner, and B. Gonik, Eds., pp. 1019–1021, Elsevier, St. Louis, MO, 2010.

[13] D. R. Wenzke, J. E. Jacobs, E. J. Balthazar, and N. Wehrli, "Diseases of the Appendix," in *Textbook of Gastrointestinal Radiology [Internet]*, R. M. Gore and M. S. Levine, Eds., pp. 955–971, Elsevier, Philadelphia, PA, 2014.

[14] A. M. Kendle and J. Louis, "Recognition and treatment of sepsis in pregnancy," *Journal of Midwifery & Women's Health*, vol. 63, no. 3, pp. 347–351, 2018.

[15] I. L. Tamir, F. S. Bongard, and S. R. Klein, "Acute appendicitis in the pregnant patient," *American Journal of Surgery*, vol. 160, no. 6, pp. 571–576, 1990.

[16] J. R. Bauchat and M. Van de Velde, "Nonobstetric Surgery during Pregnancy," in *Chestnut's Obstetric Anesthesia: Principles and Practice [Internet]*, D. H. Chestnut, C. A. Wong, A. Cynthia, L. C. Tsen, W. D. Ngan Kee, Y. Beilin, J. Mhyre, B. T. Bateman, and N. Nathan, Eds., pp. 358–379, Elsevier, Philadelphia, PA, 2019.

[17] R. B. Sanda and S. E. Garba, "Acute appendicitis in pregnancy," *Archives of International Surgery*, vol. 3, no. 1, pp. 6–10, 2013.

[18] D. A. Guinn, D. E. Abel, and M. W. Tomlinson, "Early goal directed therapy for sepsis during pregnancy," *Obstetrics and Gynecology Clinics of North America*, vol. 34, no. 3, pp. 459–479, 2007.

[19] E. A. Babler, "Perforative appendicitis complicating pregnancy," *Journal of the American Medical Association*, vol. LI, no. 16, pp. 1310–1314, 1908.

[20] J. van Dillen, J. Zwart, J. Schutte, and J. van Roosmalen, "Maternal sepsis: epidemiology, etiology and outcome," *Current Opinion in Infectious Diseases*, vol. 23, no. 3, pp. 249–254, 2010.

[21] P. J. Neligan and J. G. Laffey, "Clinical review: special populations- critical illness and pregnancy," *Critical Care*, vol. 15, no. 4, p. 227, 2011.

[22] U. Nair, "Acute abdomen and abdominal pain in pregnancy," *Obstetrics, Gynaecology and Reproductive Medicine*, vol. 15, no. 6, pp. 359–367, 2005.

[23] U. Retzke, H. Graf, and M. Schmidt, "Appendicitis in pregnancy," *Zentralblatt für Chirurgie*, vol. 123, Supplement 4, pp. 61–65, 1998.

[24] C. E. Burlinson, D. Sirounis, K. R. Walley, and A. Chau, "Sepsis in pregnancy and the puerperium," *International Journal of Obstetric Anesthesia*, vol. 36, pp. 96–107, 2018.

[25] J. Horntrich, M. Hinkel, G. Haring, and H. Radzuweit, "Acute appendicitis in pregnancy," *Zentralblatt für Chirurgie*, vol. 111, no. 13, pp. 788–793, 1986.

[26] J. M. Ford and H. Scholefield, "Sepsis in obstetrics: cause, prevention, and treatment," *Current Opinion in Anesthesiology*, vol. 27, no. 3, pp. 253–258, 2014.

[27] R. Cohen-Kerem, C. Railton, D. Oren, M. Lishner, and G. Koren, "Pregnancy outcome following non-obstetric surgical intervention," *American Journal of Surgery*, vol. 190, no. 3, pp. 467–473, 2005.

[28] N. P. Dixon, D. M. Faddis, and H. Silberman, "Aggressive management of cholecystitis during pregnancy," *American Journal of Surgery*, vol. 154, no. 3, pp. 292–294, 1987.

[29] T. Ueberrueck, A. Koch, L. Meyer, M. Hinkel, and I. Gatinger, "Ninety-four appendectomies for suspected acute appendicitis during pregnancy," *World Journal of Surgery*, vol. 28, no. 5, pp. 508–511, 2004.

[30] C. Qihui, Z. Xiping, and D. Xianfeng, "Clinical study on acute pancreatitis in pregnancy in 26 cases," *Gastroenterology Research and Practice*, vol. 2012, Article ID 271925, 5 pages, 2012.

[31] A. R. Turnock, B. P. Fleischer, M. J. Carney, and W. B. Vanderlan, "Perforated second trimester appendicitis with abdominal compartment syndrome managed with negative pressure wound therapy and open abdomen," *Journal of Surgical Case Reports*, vol. 2016, no. 6, article rjw101, 2016.

[32] T. Hata, N. Hayashi, S. Urabe et al., "Reduced-port laparoscopic appendectomy for acute appendicitis in pregnancy," *Journal of Surgical Case Reports*, vol. 2020, no. 6, article rjaa097, 2020.

[33] A. Tavakoli, P. Wadensweiler, E. Blumenthal, E. Kuncir, R. Houshyar, and T. Brueseke, "Medical management of appendicitis in early-term pregnancy," *BML Case Reports*, vol. 13, no. 8, article e234252, 2020.

[34] S. Matsui, T. Tanioka, Y. Kamata et al., "Laparoscopic appendectomy during the second trimester of a twin pregnancy," *Asian Journal of Endoscopic Surgery*, vol. 14, no. 3, pp. 594–597, 2021.

[35] M. Saleh, A. F. Kim, A. Gardner, K. Sun, and S. Brubaker, "Peritoneovaginal fistula and appendicitis-related pelvic abscess in pregnancy," *American Journal of Perinatology Reports*, vol. 10, no. 2, pp. e129–e132, 2020.

[36] M. Ghannouchi, K. Nacef, M. B. KHlifa et al., "Acute abdomen during pregnancy: appendicular deciduosis-a case report," *Journal of Surgical Case Reports*, vol. 2021, no. 10, article rjab477, 2021.

[37] L. J. Sanders-Davis and J. Ritchie, "Appendicitis with concurrent COVID-19 infection in a patient during the third trimester of pregnancy," *BML Case Reports*, vol. 14, no. 6, article e242651, 2021.

5

Laparoscopic Adnexal Detorsion in a 20-Week Pregnant Patient: A Case Report and Literature Review

Rawad Halimeh [1], Serge Tomassian [2], Maria El Hage [2], Nicole Metri [2], Marianne Bersaoui [1], Rafi Daou [3], and Elie Anastasiadis [1]

[1] *Obstetrics and Gynecology Department, Saint George Hospital University Medical Center, Beirut, Lebanon*
[2] *Faculty of Medicine and Medical Sciences, University of Balamand, El-Koura, Lebanon*
[3] *Faculty of Medicine, University of London, St. Georges, Nicosia, Cyprus*

Correspondence should be addressed to Rawad Halimeh; rawad.halimeh@gmail.com

Academic Editor: Erich Cosmi

Adnexal torsion is a cause of severe pelvic pain in reproductive aged women and during pregnancy. Adnexal torsion occurs when there is a complete turn of the ovary, tube, or both resulting in impaired blood flow to the ovary. The diagnosis of adnexal torsion is sometimes challenging due to the enlarged effect of the uterus, the displacement of abdominal and pelvic structures and the nonspecific symptoms in pregnancy. Therefore, prompt diagnosis is essential for better maternal and neonatal outcomes. The gold standard for confirmation and treatment of ovarian torsion is surgery. Laparoscopy and Laparotomy are surgical options with defined risks and benefits. Therefore, choosing the best surgical technique and surgical procedure are of utmost importance to decrease the chances of adverse events intra and postoperatively. Little literature exists regarding the laparoscopic approach of an ovarian torsion during the second trimester. Our case is a 20-week pregnant patient who had a 1080 degree rotation of the left adnexa. She required laparoscopy for adnexal detorsion and had good intraoperative, postoperative, maternal, and neonatal outcomes following management.

1. Introduction

The diagnosis of acute pelvic pain in pregnancy is often challenging [1]. Difficulties in diagnosing pelvic pain during pregnancy is mostly due to several pregnancy related factors [1]. These factors include the displacement of abdominal and pelvic structures by the enlarging gravid uterus, the nonspecific gastric symptoms, and the difficult abdominal examination in pregnancy [2]. Acute pelvic pain can present with nonspecific signs and symptoms that are associated with numerous conditions which can be grouped into different categories [1]. These categories include: (1) Non obstetrical-non gynecological causes such as urolithiasis, appendicitis, cholecystitis, and intestinal obstruction. (2) Obstetrical causes such as placental abruption, abnormally invasive placentas, and uterine rupture. (3) Gynecologic causes such as ovarian torsion, pain resulting from adnexal masses, and degeneration or necrosis of uterine fibroids [1]. Adnexal torsion occurs when the adnexa, ovary, or fallopian tube completes at least a full turn around a centre-line axis formed by the infundibulopelvic ligament and tubo-ovarian ligament [3]. This leads to an impaired venous flow, possibly followed by impaired arterial flow to the ovary. The lack of blood flow results in stromal edema, hemorrhagic infarction and necrosis respectively [4]. It accounts for approximately 3% of all gynecologic surgical emergencies in women and 80% of these instances happen in the reproductive age group [5]. Ovarian torsion is rare during gestation, developing in only 1 in 5000 pregnancies [6].

2. Case Presentation

A 32-year-old Lebanese female patient G2P0010 (spontaneous pregnancy), who was at 20 weeks and 2 days of gestation as per last menstrual period, presented to the emergency room for the evaluation of same day pelvic pain. The pain began 3 hours prior to presentation and was described as severe, stabbing in nature, nonradiating, and intermittent. The patient

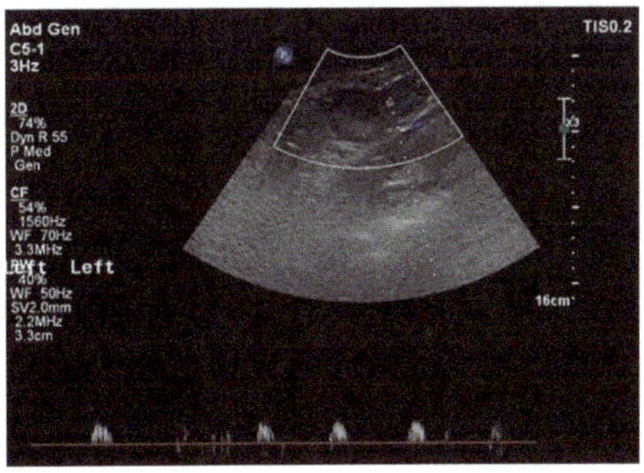

Figure 1: Absent Doppler flow to the enlarged left ovary.

reported normal fetal movements and denied feeling contractions; she did not have any other associated symptoms.

Past medical and surgical histories were unremarkable. Patient denied cigarette smoking, alcohol intake, or any exposure to illicit drugs. She did not have any known food or drug allergies. Patient had a routine transabdominal obstetrical ultrasound at 12 weeks of gestation; No adnexal abnormalities were noted. The patient was only taking vitamins. Review of systems was negative as she denied any recent illness, fever, chills, night sweats, nausea or vomiting, suspicious food intake, or recent sick contact.

The patient had stable vitals in the emergency room with a blood pressure of 120/80 mmHg, heart rate of 80 beats per minute and a temperature of 37.3 degrees Celsius. Physical examination revealed positive active bowel sounds, no epigastric, left or right upper quadrant tenderness. Costovertebral angle signs were negative bilaterally, Mc Burney's point tenderness was negative, and Murphy sign was also negative. Cervical exam was done showing a cervix which was closed, posterior, and long. The patient had severe left lower quadrant tenderness with guarding that was not radiating on physical exam. No vaginal discharge was noted. Her pain was not relieved by intravenous pain medications.

Laboratory workup showed a complete blood count which was within normal ranges: WBC 10,400/mm^3 (Neutrophils 86.2%, Lymphocytes 9.3%), Hemoglobin 11.3 g/dL, Platelets 180,000/mm^3, SGPT 45 U/L, GGT 7 U/L, PT-INR 1.1, PTT 29.86 seconds, C-Reactive Protein 0.9 mg/L; creatinine 0.51 mg/dL, Urine analysis: RBC 1/mm^3, WBC 14/mm^3, Urine culture: no growth after 48 hours of incubation.

After a primary assessment, the patient had an abdomino-pelvic ultrasound performed. Abdominal ultrasound was normal; however, the pelvic ultrasound showed an enlarged left ovary (59 × 51 × 54 mm) with diffuse hyperechogenic-stroma, peripheral displacement of the follicles, and a hypoechoic rim and minimal fluid in the pelvis (Figure 1). Doppler was done and showed a nearly absent flow to the left ovary (Figure 1). This clinical scenario combined with the ultrasound result was compatible with the diagnosis of left sided adnexal torsion. Of note, fetal heart rate was normal at 157 beats per minute.

The decision for urgent laparoscopic detorsion was made to try to preserve ovarian function and prevent any adverse maternal or neonatal effects.

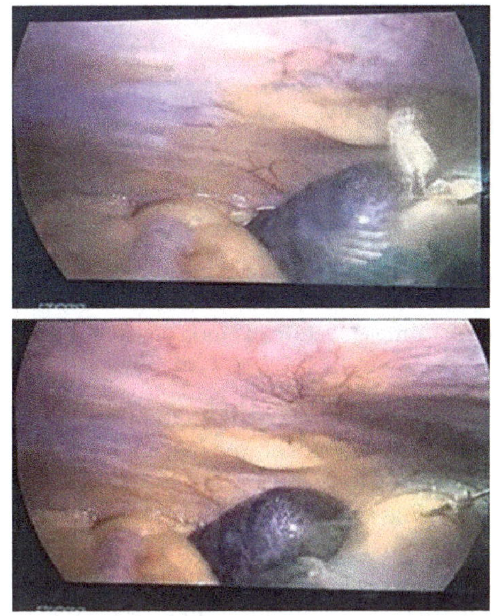

Figure 2: Dark purple discoloration of left ovary.

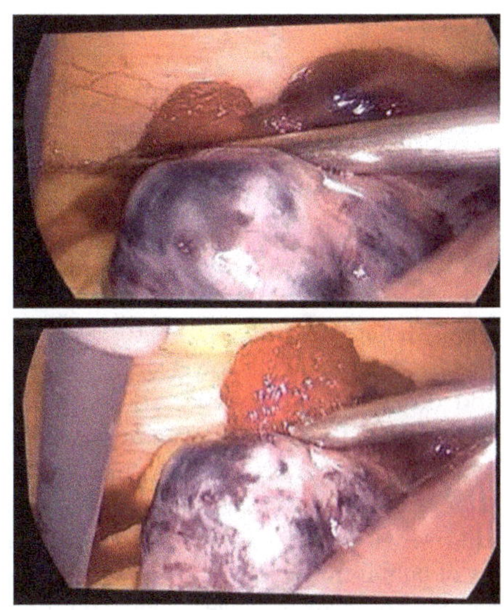

Figure 3: Gradual return of blood flow to the left ovary.

Entry to the pelvis was challenging due to the enlarged uterus at 20 weeks of gestation; therefore, a Veres needle was introduced at Palmer's point. The abdomen was insufflated using CO_2 with a pressure of 12 mmHg followed by insertion of trocars number ten at the supraumbilicus, and two number fives at the left lower quadrant and suprapubic area, respectively. A 20-week-sized uterus and the left adnexal torsion (ovary and tube) were visualized with dark purple discoloration of the ovary (Figure 2). Adnexal detorsion was completed with removal of the necrotic ovarian tissue and any blood clots. This was done with meticulous conservation of the ovarian parenchyma. A gradual return to normal coloration of the ovary was noted 6 minutes after detorsion (Figure 3). This was followed by a complete return to normal coloration after 10 minutes (Figure 4) with sufficient hemostasis assured. No intraoperative complications were encountered with a

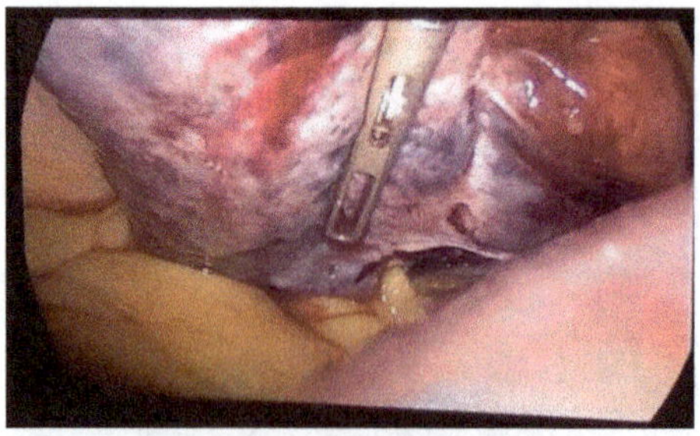

FIGURE 4: Complete return of blood flow to the left ovary.

procedure time of 45 minutes. Postoperative Doppler ultrasound of the left adnexa showed normal flow. The patient presented for induction of labor at 39 weeks and 6 days of gestation following an uncomplicated pregnancy after surgery. She had an operative vaginal delivery (Forceps delivery) of a healthy baby boy (Weight 3810 g, Height 52 cm) with an Apgar of 9/10 and 10/10 at 1 and 5 minutes, respectively, and was discharged home on day 2 post-delivery.

3. Discussion

Most cases of ovarian torsion in pregnancy occur during the first trimester [5], but can also happen to a lesser degree in the second or third trimester [7]. According to Yen et al. 60% of ovarian torsion occurred between the 10th and 17th weeks of gestation, whereas only 5.9% took place after 20 weeks [8]. The risk factors for adnexal torsion include an enlarged ovary, ovarian tumors, ovarian hyperstimulation syndrome, and pregnancy [9–12]. Patients with ovarian torsion usually present with a sudden onset acute lower abdominal pain with guarding and other various nonspecific symptoms such as nausea and vomiting [13]. The pain can be constant or intermittent. There may be a history of transient episodes of pain, which indicate previous partial torsions since the ovary may torse and untorse with sudden change in position or activity. The intensity of pain is not severe in most of these intermittent episodes, which can occur for several days to months before admission. Occlusion of the vascular pedicle leads to hypoxia which causes this pain [14]. Since it is a surgical emergency, prompt diagnosis should be made to preserve residual function of the ovary [7]. The first step in diagnosing torsion is with imaging by an abdominal ultrasound [7]. In the case of ovarian torsion, almost all patients have an enlarged ovary on ultrasound; [7] "Whirlpool sign" is usually observed which is the main hallmark seen on imaging [15]. Doppler flow of the ovary may be normal or abnormal [16] and, therefore, does not improve accuracy of diagnosis due to the high false negative rates [6]. However, clinicians can predict the nonviability of the ovary with the presence or absence of arterial and venous blood flow on Doppler [17] making it a viable prognostic tool. Unfortunately, in some cases, the ultrasound result is equivocal and may not be sufficient for diagnosis of the torsion [18]. In such cases an MRI is helpful for diagnosis and can demonstrate the components of the mass in a clearer fashion than the ultrasound. An MRI can show the twisting of the pedicle [19] more so during the second and third trimesters due to the enlarged uterus [17]. Diagnosis of ovarian torsion with ultrasonography had overall accuracy of 96.0% with the sensitivity of 72.1% and the specificity of 99.6%, respectively [20]. Abnormal ovarian blood flow using Doppler was the most diagnostically accurate isolated sonographic sign with PPV 80.0% [21]. On the other hand, MRI has a sensitivity of 77.2% and a specificity of 86.1% for the diagnosis of adnexal torsion. The probability of adnexal torsion was increased six times in case of visualization of the whirpool sign and eight times higher in cases of visualization of tubal thickening [22].

The gold standard for confirmation and treatment of ovarian torsion is surgery whether laparoscopy or laparotomy [11]. The viability of the ovary is usually assessed by direct visualization of the ovary [11]. Dark (black or blue) and enlarged ovaries are usually associated with nonviability of the ovary; however, most of the times, they may retain function following detorsion [24]. Conservative surgical treatment is usually considered regardless of the color of the ovary since the clinical appearance does not correlate well with the residual function [23–25]. This logic counters the traditional method of managing ovarian torsion with removal of the adnexa [26], which was done due to the false belief that detorsion would pose a higher risk of thromboembolic events [27]. However, detorsion will carry a higher risk of recurrence [28].

3.1. Laparoscopy vs. Laparotomy for Management of Ovarian Torsion in Pregnancy. There are limited data available regarding the best surgical method for treating ovarian torsion in pregnancy. There are many maternal and fetal advantages of laparoscopy. The main maternal advantages are less operative blood loss, less postoperative pain, shorter hospital stay, and a decreased risk of preterm labor [29, 30]. However, fetal loss has always been a major concern when choosing the surgical approach. The main risk with laparoscopy is that it poses a risk on the fetus since it utilizes carbon dioxide for pneumoperitoneum, which can decrease the blood flow in the uterine arteries and maternal circulation causing intrauterine hypoxia [31, 32]. It can also increase the carbon dioxide absorption by the fetus leading to fetal acidosis [33]. Thus, having an intraperitoneal pressure of less than 12 mmHg and performing laparoscopy with an estimated time of less than thirty minutes is considered safe in pregnancy [34].

Nevertheless, the laparoscopic technique during pregnancy is challenging and risky [35]. Visualization of the surgical field may be compromised by the increasing size of the gravid uterus, which could lead to Trocar injury to the uterus [35, 36]. Therefore, either Veres needle insertion or Hasson technique (open technique) could be used depending on the surgeons' skills and preference. Trocar sites should be limited to subxiphoid, left upper quadrant, or right upper quadrant access points which will aid in avoiding uterine injury [35]. In addition, a sufficient distance between the uterus and the tip of the laparoscope can be obtained by placing a supraumbilical primary trocar allowing for an ideal visual field [35] especially during the second and third trimesters. In our case, it was difficult to place the trocar in the infrumbilical site due to the enlarged uterus reaching past the umbilicus, so we opted for the supraumbilical site. It is worthy to note that the uterus should never be manipulated by a transcervical device [35].

Moreover, the positioning of the patient is an important factor to consider in laparoscopic ovarian detorsion. As previously mentioned, carbon dioxide in the pneumoperitoneum affects the maternal venous blood flow causing a decrease in the preload and an increase in the afterload and systemic vascular resistance. Thus, placing the patient on her left lateral side with a 30-degree angle in Trendelenburg position would relieve the compression on the inferior vena cava, increase the venous return to the maternal heart, normalize the pulmonary pressure, and increase the cardiac output during surgery [37]. It would also help us get a better visual field through displacing the abdominal structures cephalad.

3.2. Role of Gaseless Laparoscopy for Management of Ovarian Torsion in Pregnancy. The gasless laparoscopy, a surgery done with a vertical midline umbilical skin incision is made with the abdominal wall lifted anteriorly to achieve exposure [38]. A laparoscope is then introduced into the abdominal cavity for inspection [38].

Gasless laparoscopy was shown to be a safer approach than CO2 laparoscopy, especially in patients with a history of previous abdominal surgery, and resulted in excellent cosmetic results since the single surgical wound was limited to the umbilicus [38]. Problems that could arise in CO2 laparoscopy such as bradyarrhythmias, venousstasis, gasembolism, subcutaneous emphysema and hypercarbia were not observed in gasless laparoscopy [38]. The CO2 laparoscopy resulted in an increase in elevation in the central venous pressure, respiratory function, and stress response in contrast with gasless laparoscopy [39]. Postoperative recovery time of borborygmus and the incidence of postoperative nausea, vomiting, and shoulder pain were much lower in gasless than CO2 laparoscopy [39].

Moving on to the postoperative and obstetric care, it is recommended that fetal heart rate is to be measured and documented postoperatively alongside monitoring of uterine contractions. They will be used to assess for early signs of preterm labor [37]. However, the systematic use of tocolysis is to be avoided [37], unless signs of preterm labor are evident. Intraoperative pneumatic compression devices are to be used to prevent any thromboembolic event during surgery especially since the patient is already at a high risk of hypercoagulable diseases during her pregnancy. Early ambulation is to be advised as well to decrease the risk of deep vein thrombosis [37].

4. Conclusion

It is becoming evident that laparoscopic surgery for ovarian torsion during pregnancy is safe and feasible, does not increase maternal or fetal complications [40], and shows no significant difference regarding gestational age at delivery or mode of delivery [40]. Therefore, laparoscopy can be done throughout all trimesters with no differences in outcomes from laparotomy. However, the complexity of the laparoscopy increases with the increasing gestational age so it should only be done by experienced surgeons who take into careful consideration the operative time, the intraperitoneal pressure, the positioning of the patient, and the placement of the trocars to decrease risks and complications [37]. In our case, gasless laparoscopy was not done mainly because of the safety of CO2 laparoscopy when done with a short surgical time, appropriate pressure, and expertise.

References

[1] G. Masselli, M. Derme, F. Laghi, M. Framarino-dei-Malatesta, and G. Gualdi, "Evaluating the acute abdomen in the pregnant patient," *Radiologic Clinics of North America*, vol. 53, no. 6, pp. 1309–1325, 2015.

[2] L. Spalluto, C. Woodfield, C. DeBenedectis, and E. Lazarus, "MR imaging evaluation of abdominal pain during pregnancy: appendicitis and other nonobstetric causes," *RadioGraphics*, vol. 32, no. 2, pp. 317–334, 2012.

[3] C. Huchon and A. Fauconnier, "Adnexal torsion: a literature review," *European Journal of Obstetrics & Gynecology and Reproductive Biology*, vol. 150, no. 1, pp. 8–12, 2010.

[4] G. Ssi-Yan-Kai, A. Rivain, C. Trichot et al., "What every radiologist should know about adnexal torsion," *Emergency Radiology*, vol. 25, no. 1, pp. 51–59, 2018.

[5] L. Hibbard, "Adnexal torsion," *American Journal of Obstetrics and Gynecology*, vol. 152, no. 4, pp. 456–461, 1985.

[6] J. Hasson, Z. Tsafrir, F. Azem et al., "Comparison of adnexal torsion between pregnant and nonpregnant women," *American Journal of Obstetrics and Gynecology*, vol. 202, no. 6, pp. 536.e1–536.e6, 2010.

[7] S. Chang, C. Yen, L. Lo, C. Lee, and C. Liang, "Surgical intervention for maternal ovarian torsion in pregnancy," *Taiwanese Journal of Obstetrics and Gynecology*, vol. 50, no. 4, pp. 458–462, 2011.

[8] C. Yen, S. Lin, W. Murk et al., "Risk analysis of torsion and malignancy for adnexal masses during pregnancy," *Fertility and Sterility*, vol. 91, no. 5, pp. 1895–1902, 2009.

[9] E. Damigos, J. Johns, and J. Ross, "An update on the diagnosis and management of ovarian torsion," *The Obstetrician & Gynaecologist*, vol. 14, no. 4, pp. 229–236, 2012.

[10] T. Johnson and J. Woodruff, "Surgical emergencies of the uterine adnexae during pregnancy," *International Journal of Gynecology & Obstetrics*, vol. 24, no. 5, pp. 331–335, 1986.

[11] D. Ding, C. Huang, and M. Hong, "A review of ovary torsion," *Tzu Chi Medical Journal*, vol. 29, no. 3, p. 143, 2017.

[12] N. Gil Navarro, E. Garcia Grau, S. Pina Pérez, and L. Ribot Luna, "Ovarian torsion and spontaneous ovarian hyperstimulation syndrome in a twin pregnancy: a case report," *International Journal of Surgery Case Reports*, vol. 34, pp. 66–68, 2017.

[13] Z. Sidiropoulou, "Acute abdomen in pregnancy due to isolated fallopian tube torsion: the laparoscopic treatment of a rare case," *World Journal of Clinical Cases*, vol. 2, no. 11, p. 724, 2014.

[14] D. Nichols and P. Julian, "Torsion of the adnexa," *Clinical Obstetrics and Gynecology*, vol. 28, no. 2, pp. 375–380, 1985.

[15] S. Vijayaraghavan, "Sonographic whirlpool sign in ovarian torsion," *Journal of Ultrasound in Medicine*, vol. 23, no. 12, pp. 1643–1649, 2004.

[16] M. Mathew, S. Jesrani, and S. Mubarak, "Conservative management of twisted ischemic adnexa in early pregnancy," *Annals of Medical and Health Sciences Research*, vol. 5, no. 2, p. 142, 2015.

[17] J. Bouquet de Joliniere, J. Dubuisson, F. Khomsi et al., "Laparoscopic adnexectomy for ovarian torsion during late pregnancy: case report of a nonconservative treatment and literature analysis," *Frontiers in Surgery*, vol. 4, 2017.

[18] S. Rha, J. Byun, S. Jung et al., "CT and MR imaging features of adnexal torsion," *RadioGraphics*, vol. 22, no. 2, pp. 283–294, 2002.

[19] C. Li, S. Wang, X. Tao, Y. Hu, X. Li, and X. Xiao, "Torsion of normal-sized ovary during late pregnancy: a case report and review of the literature," *Journal of Obstetrics and Gynaecology Research*, vol. 44, no. 11, pp. 2110–2114, 2018.

[20] A. Rostamzadeh, S. Mirfendereski, M. J. Rezaie, and S. Rezaei, "Diagnostic efficacy of sonography for diagnosis of ovarian torsion," *Pakistan Journal of Medical Sciences*, vol. 30, no. 2, 1969.

[21] R. Mashiach, N. Melamed, N. Gilad, G. Ben-Shitrit, and I. Meizner, "Sonographic diagnosis of ovarian torsion," *Journal of Ultrasound in Medicine*, vol. 30, no. 9, pp. 1205–1210, 2011.

[22] S. Béranger-Gibert, H. Sakly, M. Ballester et al., "Diagnostic value of MR imaging in the diagnosis of adnexal torsion," *Radiology*, vol. 279, no. 2, pp. 461–470, 2016.

[23] J. Shalev, M. Goldenberg, G. Oelsner et al., "Treatment of twisted ischemic adnexa by simple detorsion," *New England Journal of Medicine*, vol. 321, no. 8, pp. 546–546, 1989.

[24] G. Oelsner, "Minimal surgery for the twisted ischaemic adnexa can preserve ovarian function," *Human Reproduction*, vol. 18, no. 12, pp. 2599–2602, 2003.

[25] M. Mathew, "Untwisting and fixation of ovarian torsion in early pregnancy," *JABHS*, vol. 9, pp. 65–67, 2008.

[26] J. Anders and E. Powell, "Urgency of evaluation and outcome of acute ovarian torsion in pediatric patients," *Archives of Pediatrics & Adolescent Medicine*, vol. 159, no. 6, p. 532, 2005.

[27] P. McGovern, R. Noah, R. Koenigsberg, and A. Little, "Adnexal torsion and pulmonary embolism," *Obstetrical & Gynecological Survey*, vol. 54, no. 9, pp. 601–608, 1999.

[28] M. Pansky, N. Smorgick, A. Herman, D. Schneider, and R. Halperin, "Torsion of normal adnexa in postmenarchal women and risk of recurrence," *Obstetrics & Gynecology*, vol. 109, no. 2, Part 1, pp. 355–359, 2007.

[29] H. Al-Fozan and T. Tulandi, "Safety and risks of laparoscopy in pregnancy," *Current Opinion in Obstetrics and Gynecology*, vol. 14, no. 4, pp. 375–379, 2002.

[30] P. Ye, N. Zhao, J. Shu et al., "Laparoscopy versus open surgery for adnexal masses in pregnancy: a meta-analytic review," *Archives of Gynecology and Obstetrics*, vol. 299, no. 3, pp. 625–634, 2019.

[31] A. Westerband, J. M. Van de water, M. Amzallag et al., "Cardiovascular changes during laparoscopic cholecystectomy," *Survey of Anesthesiology*, vol. 39, no. 6, pp. 328–329, 1993.

[32] W. Kammerer, "Nonobstetric surgery during pregnancy," *Medical Clinics of North America*, vol. 63, no. 6, pp. 1157–1164, 1979.

[33] N. Soper, J. Hunter, and R. Petrie, "Laparoscopic cholecystectomy during pregnancy," *Surgical Endoscopy*, vol. 6, no. 3, pp. 115–117, 1992.

[34] M. Curet, D. Vogt, O. Schob, C. Qualls, L. Izquierdo, and K. Zucker, "Effects of CO_2 Pneumoperitoneum in Pregnant Ewes," *Journal of Surgical Research*, vol. 63, no. 1, pp. 339–344, 1996.

[35] A. Dizon and E. Carey, "Minimally invasive gynecologic surgery in the pregnant patient," *Current Opinion in Obstetrics and Gynecology*, vol. 30, no. 4, pp. 267–271, 2018.

[36] M. Fatum and N. Rojansky, "Laparoscopic surgery during pregnancy," *Obstetric and Gynecologic Survey*, vol. 56, no. 1, pp. 50–59, 2001.

[37] J. Estadella, P. Español, B. Grandal, M. Gine, and J. Parra, "Laparoscopy during pregnancy: case report and key points to improve laparoscopic management," *European Journal of Obstetrics & Gynecology and Reproductive Biology*, vol. 217, pp. 83–88, 2017.

[38] A. Takeda, S. Imoto, M. Mori, T. Nakano, and H. Nakamura, "Early experience with isobaric laparoendoscopic single-site surgery using a wound retractor for the management of ectopic pregnancy," *European Journal of Obstetrics & Gynecology and Reproductive Biology*, vol. 154, no. 2, pp. 209–214, 2010.

[39] S. Li, J. Deng, F. Huang, X. Gan, and Y. Cao, "Impact of gasless laparoscopy on circulation, respiration, stress response, and other complications in gynecological geriatrics," *International Journal of Clinical and Experimental Medicine*, vol. 7, no. 9, pp. 2877–2882, 2014.

[40] Y. Daykan, R. Bogin, M. Sharvit et al., "Adnexal torsion during pregnancy: outcomes after surgical intervention—a retrospective case-control study," *Journal of Minimally Invasive Gynecology*, vol. 26, no. 1, pp. 117–121, 2019.

Conservative Management of Cervical Pregnancy with the Administration of Methotrexate and Potassium Chloride: A Case Report

Mojgan Javedani Masroor,[1] Anna Zarei,[1] and Hossein Sheibani[2]

[1]*Shahid Akbar Abadi Clinical Research Development Unit, School of Medicine, Iran University of Medical Sciences, Tehran, Iran*
[2]*Clinical Research Development Unit, Imam Hossein Hospital, Shahroud University of Medical Sciences, Shahroud, Iran*

Correspondence should be addressed to Mojgan Javedani Masroor; mojgan.javedani.masroor@gmail.com

Academic Editor: Maria Grazia Porpora

Background. Cervical pregnancy is a rare form of ectopic pregnancy in which the fetus implants and grows inside the endocervical canal. This report aims at introducing a case of successful conservative management of cervical ectopic pregnancy. *Case presentation.* The patient was a 35-year-old woman, who had received treatment for primary infertility for 5 years. She complained of painless bleeding on day 37 of gestational age with a start point from 10 days before. The patient had stable vital signs and was referred to Shahid Akbar Abadi Hospital in Tehran affiliated with the Iran University of Medical Sciences. In the ultrasonography, the pregnancy sac and the yolk sac with the embryonic pole with a positive fetal heart rate were presented and located near the internal os, so the cervical pregnancy was diagnosed, and after treatment with intramuscular methotrexate and intra-amniotic administration of potassium chloride, a gradual decrease in β-HCG levels was observed without the need for additional interventional treatment. *Conclusion.* The primary takeaway of our report is that the conservative treatment, including intramuscular methotrexate and intrauterine potassium chloride administration, may be effective in treating cervical pregnancy that can be detected early without the use of curettage.

1. Background

Cervical pregnancy (CP) is a rare form of ectopic pregnancy (EP) in which the fetus implants and grows inside the endocervical canal. Nontubular EPs make up less than 1% of all EPs, although their occurrence has increased in recent years [1, 2]. The incidence of CP varies between one in 1000 and one in 18000 pregnancies and 1% of all EPs [2].

Although the cause of CP is unknown, it has increased in recent years due to the increasing use of assisted reproductive techniques (in vitro fertilization). Other predisposing factors include previous cesarean section delivery, cervical surgery, previous dilatation and curettage, smoking, and the use of intrauterine devices [3].

Patients present with painless vaginal bleeding, but there have been reports of pain and cramps. Clinical diagnostic criteria for the diagnosis of cervical pregnancy are shown in Table 1 [4–6].

Ultrasound has been described as helpful in differentiating a true cervical pregnancy from developing spontaneous abortion. In such cases, magnetic resonance imaging (MRI) of the pelvis can be used as a compliment when the diagnosis is unclear. Ultrasound criteria for diagnosing cervical pregnancy are presented in Table 2 [5, 7].

Clinical diagnosis of CP is difficult. Other items that could be included in the list of differential diagnoses of cervical pregnancy include cervical carcinoma, cervical leiomyoma or protruding leiomyoma, trophoblastic tumor, and placenta previa [7].

If the diagnosis is delayed, severe vaginal bleeding and acute abdominal/pelvic pain may occur. Diagnosis often occurs late and due to massive blood loss in 50% of cases, an emergency

Table 1: Clinical diagnostic criteria for the diagnosis of the cervical pregnancy.

1	Painless bleeding from the uterus after a period of amenorrhea
2	The uterus is smaller than the enlarged cervix, which dilates and surrounds it.
3	The internal os may not be dilated. The closed internal os with partially open external os.
4	Bulky cervical speculum with bluish mucosa. The ovular tissue is completely placed in the endocervix
5	Severe bleeding due to cervical manipulation.

Table 2: Ultrasound criteria for diagnosing cervical pregnancy.

1	Observation of pregnancy sac in the cervix
2	Heart movement should be detected below the surface of the internal opening.
3	Absence of intrauterine pregnancy
4	Observing the uterus in the form of an hourglass with an enlarged cervix
5	No movement of the pregnancy sac due to the pressure of the vaginal probe (i.e., no sliding sign, which is usually seen in incomplete abortions.

hysterectomy is required [6]. Recently, the recommended protocol for the treatment of cervical ectopic pregnancy is fertility preservation rather than invasive surgery and hysterectomy [7].

Treatment for cervical ectopic pregnancies includes medical treatment with methotrexate and surgical treatment. The best treatment regimen for medical treatment has not yet been determined, but evidence suggests that single-dose or multidose regimens of methotrexate have been successful. In the cases of advanced pregnancies, especially if associated with fetal heart activity, the combined use of multiple doses of methotrexate (MTX) and potassium chloride (KCl) injections into the fetus or the amniotic fluid might be used. However, these injections must be done by a well-specialized person to avoid rupturing the membranes during the procedure [8]. Methotrexate is a folic acid analog that has been used successfully for the treatment of ectopic pregnancy ad blocks trophoblast cell division and prevents trophoblast proliferation [9].

In the current study, we described a case of cervical pregnancy that was managed with the intramuscular (IM) administration of methotrexate and intra-amniotic injection of KCl without the need for additional interventional treatment. This report aims at introducing a case of successful conservative management of cervical ectopic pregnancy.

2. Case Presentation

The patient was a 35-year-old woman, who had received treatment for primary infertility for 5 years. She had menarche at the age of 17, and her menstrual cycles were regular. The patient had a follicle-stimulating hormone (FSH) level of 1.613 (IU/L) and a luteinizing hormone (LH) level of 0.6 (IU/L) and was treated with letrozole over five days from the third to the seventh day of the menstrual cycle and then became pregnant.

She complained of painless bleeding on day 37 of gestational age with a start point from 10 days before. The patient had stable vital signs and was referred to Shahid Akbar Abadi Hospital in Tehran affiliated with the Iran University of Medical Sciences. Beta human chorionic gonadotropin (BHCG) was checked and was 6000 IU/l.

In physical examination, the abdomen was soft without distension and tenderness. Speculum examination was done slowly. Bleeding was less than that of the menstruation, and the cervix was completely closed. Hegar's sign and Chadwick's sign were both positive.

In the transvaginal ultrasonography, the pregnancy sac and the yolk sac with the embryonic pole with a positive fetal heart rate (FHR) were presented and located near the internal os, at the beginning of the cervical canal. The crown-rump length (CRL) was 4 mm, and the patient had normal endometrial thickness. Most of the pregnancy sac was seen in the proximal cervix, and there was a small part in the lower segment. The pregnancy bag had more blood than the other areas. There was a mild decidual reaction around the amniotic sac. Therefore, a cervical pregnancy was diagnosed, and the patient was hospitalized for further treatment (Figure 1).

Due to the stable vital signs, clinical condition of the patient, and the presence of embryonic echo, treatment with intramuscular MTX was selected. Potential risks and alternative therapies were explained to the patient, and informed written consent was obtained. Treatment consisted of intramuscular injection of MTX 5 mg/kg and folic acid 0.1 mg/kg alternately every other day for 4 days.

Serial ultrasonography was done, and there was a fetal echo (with FHR +) in the pregnancy bag on days 7 and 14 (Figures 2 and 3), so one cc KCL was injected into the pregnancy bag under the guidance of ultrasound.

After treatment with 4 doses of MTX, a gradual decrease in β-HCG levels was observed (Figure 4). The patient reported minimal vaginal discharge, with no pain or other symptoms, so she was discharged after 14 days with the recommendation of weekly follow up until the β-HCG levels decreased under the 10 IU/L.

Serial ultrasonography was done. As in the 3rd ultrasonography, there was a fetal echo (with FHR +) in the pregnancy bag (Figure 3).

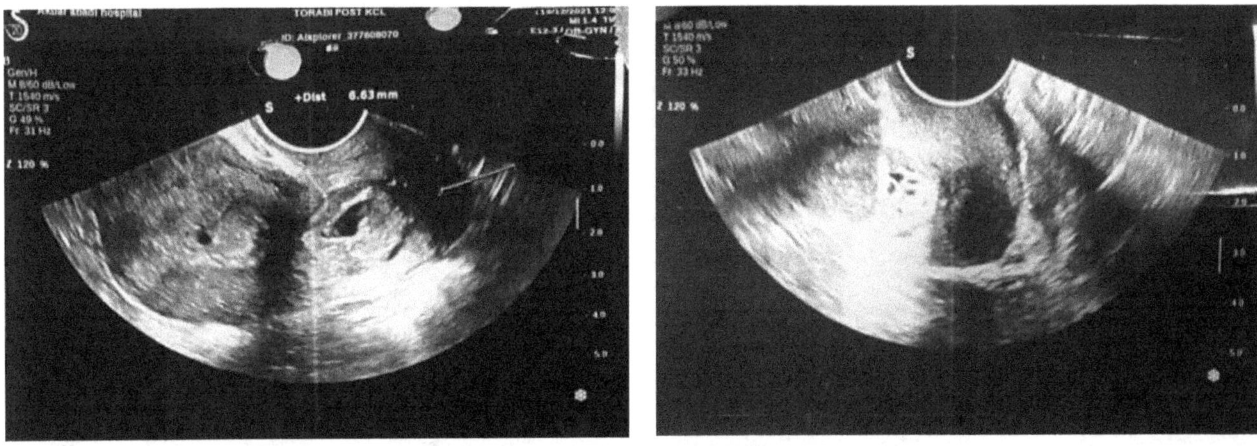

(a) (b)

FIGURE 1: The obstetric ultrasonography shows the pregnancy sac and the yolk sac with the embryonic pole located near the internal os.

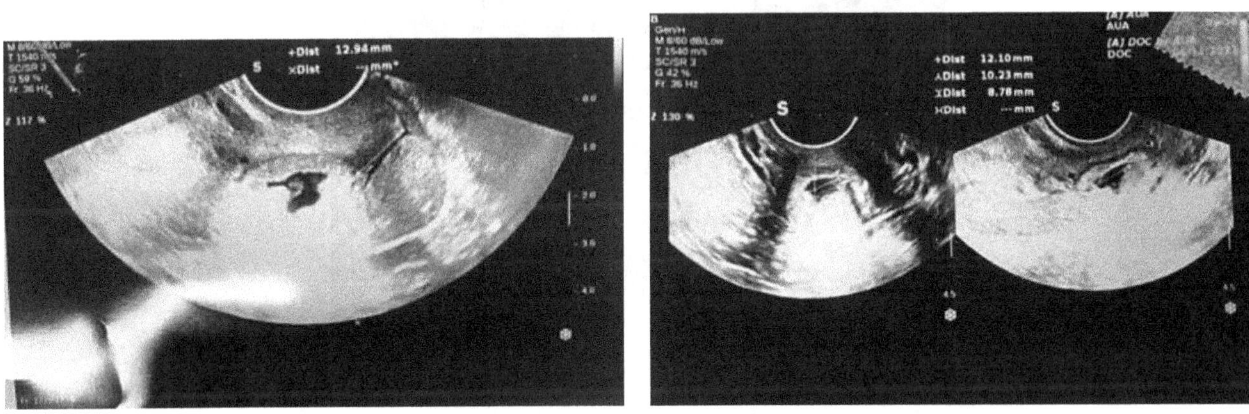

(a) (b)

FIGURE 2: The 2nd ultrasonography, a fetal echo (with FHR +) in the pregnancy bag.

3. Discussion

Cervical pregnancies are rare in naturally conceived pregnancies and even after assisted reproductive technology. One of the differential diagnoses of cervical pregnancies is Cesarean scar pregnancies (CSPs). Cesarean scar pregnancies are more commonly seen today, both in the East and the West, as a result of a significant increase in the proportion of Cesarean deliveries over the last three decades [10].

The exact mechanism of ectopic pregnancy is unknown. The rapid migration of fertilized eggs through the uterus and changes in the ability of the endometrial lining to accept implantation and damage to the endometrial canal may all be the causative factors [11]. In the current study, in the past medical history, the patient was only treated with an ovulation-stimulating drug and did not receive intrauterine insemination (IUI) or in vitro fertilization (IVF).

The cause of pregnancy after IVF is not well understood. It is believed that it is related to the increase in contractions of the uterine gap junction in the luteal phase. This increase in contractions is due to an increase in progesterone [12, 13]. Authors such as Bennett et al. have accepted this hypothesis but continued to point out that women undergoing assisted reproductive techniques often have other risk factors for cervical pregnancy [14]. In the current study, there were no other risk factors for cervical pregnancy. However, the prevalence of cervical ectopic pregnancy has increased with assisted reproductive technologies [3]. It should be noted that cervical pregnancy is very dangerous if not considered correctly. If left untreated, it can eventually lead to a hysterectomy. However, in most women, the risk factor is unknown [15].

The ultrasonographic diagnosis of cervical pregnancy is to find the trophoblastic invasion of the cervix below the internal os [12]. In the current study, cervical ectopic pregnancy was diagnosed early based on the transvaginal and ultrasound examination of the patient.

In a study done by Vela et al., twelve cases of cervical pregnancy with the early diagnosis were evaluated, of whom none resulted in a hysterectomy, so the earlier diagnosis the less likely complications are [16].

We successfully treated one case of cervical pregnancy with an intramuscular injection of MTX combined with an

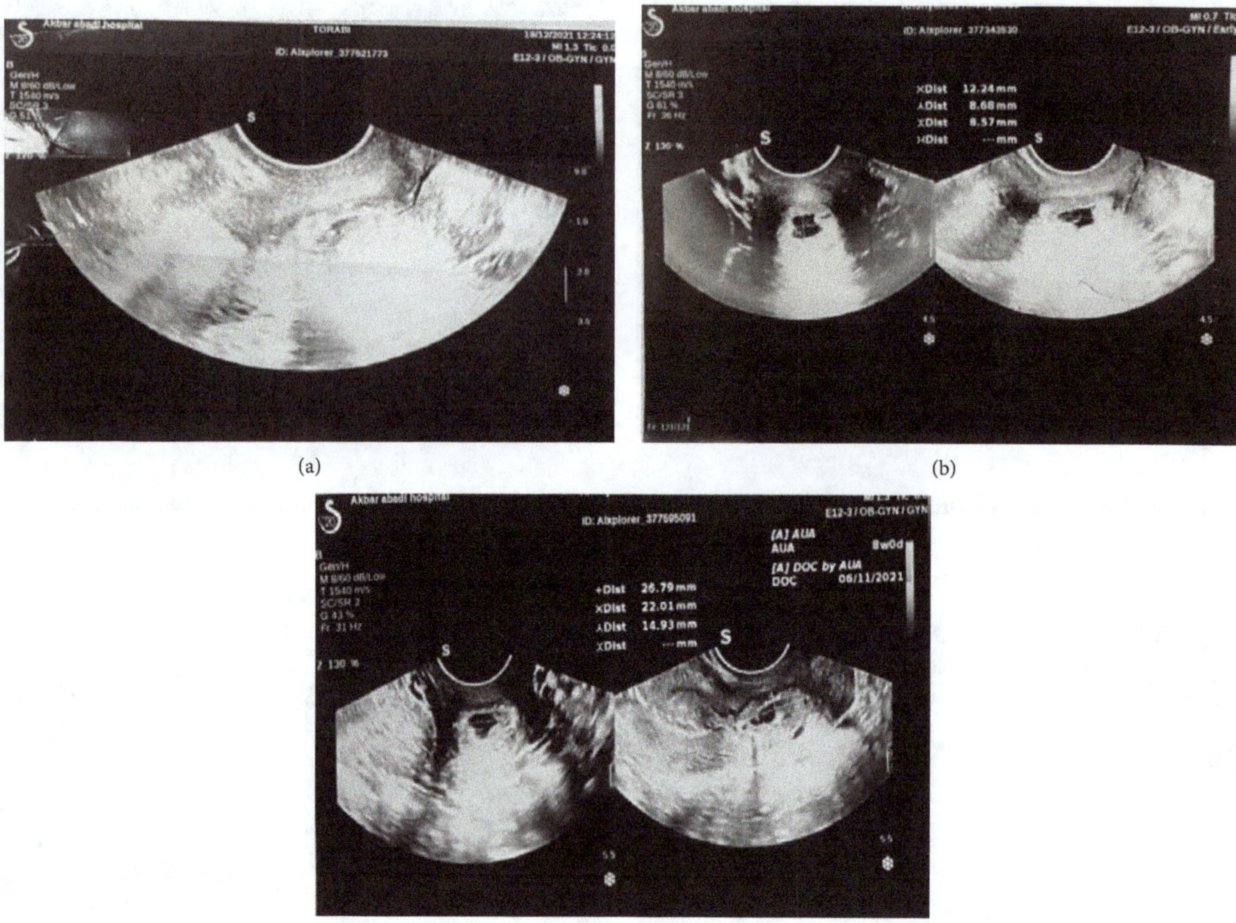

(a) (b) (c)

FIGURE 3: The 3rd ultrasonography, a fetal echo (with FHR +) in the pregnancy bag.

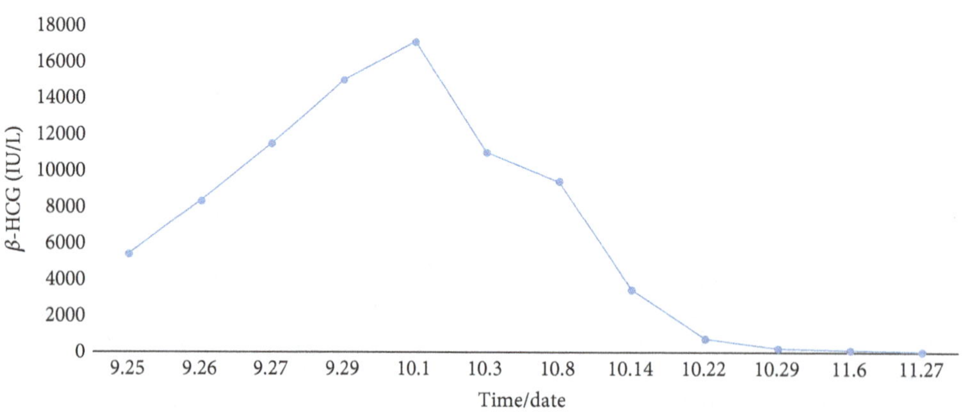

FIGURE 4: Changes in β-HCG levels during treatment.

intra-amniotic injection of potassium chloride without the need for further treatment with curettage and additional interventions.

The presence of a large number of management options highlights the fact that there is no standardized protocol, or we could say that no agreement has yet been reached on the optimal treatment for cervical pregnancy and CSP management. Several options have been used over the last three decades for the conservative nonoperative management of cervical pregnancy [10].

However, there are scientific limitations due to the rarity of cases; the trend of modern clinical practice is more towards conservative nonoperative management [12, 17]. Management of ectopic pregnancy depends on several factors including gestational age, fetal heart activity, patient stability, interest in maintaining fertility, and availability of medical and specialized facilities. Conservative nonoperative treatment includes administration of methotrexate in case of advanced gestational age and presence of FHR. Failure in conservative management, severe bleeding, and unstable hemodynamics requires surgical intervention including curettage with a Foley catheter for uterine tamponade, topical injection of prostaglandins, uterine artery embolization, bilateral ligation of the uterine or iliac artery, and hysterectomy for patients who are no longer interested in pregnancy [18, 19]. According to operative management, laparoscopic surgery and suturing is the single most effective treatment of CSP. Optimal repair of the uterine defect is essential for the prevention of another CSP [10].

In a study done by Samal et al. in 2015, a successful case of conservative treatment in a 29-year-old woman with GA = 7 who was treated with a combination of methotrexate and intra-amniotic injection KCL and curettage suction was presented [20]. A study done by Kadija et al. in 2016 showed efficient fertility-sparing conservative treatment, dilatation, and curettage, of a 13-week cervical pregnancy followed by systemic methotrexate [21].

Hamouda et al. discussed the relative effectiveness and positive efficacy of intramuscular and single-dose MTX administration without the need for curettage in cervical pregnancy [22]. In a study done by Petousis et al. in 2015, a cervical pregnancy was successfully treated with the intramuscular injection of methotrexate (MTX) and intraamniotic administration of potassium chloride in a 41-year-old woman with a gestational age of 54 days.

According to the administration of an intra-amniotic feticide using potassium chloride (KCL), it may be effective in the treatment of cervical pregnancy without the need for performing curettage. Indeed, the effectiveness of exclusive administration of MTX has been reported to be as high as 81.3%, while the percentage is increased to 90% when MTX is combined with additional conservative methods [16].

Our patient was ideal for conservative management. However, the most important point in treating cervical pregnancy with MTX is patient selection and identification. These patients should be hemodynamically stable; the ectopic pregnancy should not be ruptured; there should be no complaints of severe bleeding and severe pelvic pain; the CRL size should not exceed 3.5_3 cm; the BHCG level should be less than 5000 IU/L, and the patient should be willing to participate in the next follow-up visits [23–25]. In our patient, the length of CRL was 4 mm; the maximum BHCG level was 160000 IU/L, and vital signs were stable. After intraamniotic administration of the KCL, a decrease in BHCG level was seen.

The effectiveness of the administration of MTX for cervical pregnancy has been reported to be as high as 81.3%. without the need for curettage, while a combination of systemic MTX along with additional conservative methods has a better prognosis and was found to be effective in 91% of cases [26].

4. Conclusion

The primary takeaway of our report is that the conservative treatment, including IM MTX and intrauterine KCL administration, may be effective in treating cervical pregnancy that can be detected early without the use of curettage.

5. Recommendation

Further multicenter observational or even randomized studies should be done to evaluate the relative effectiveness of various therapeutic protocols and also assess the issue of cost-effectiveness of invasive vs. conservative management.

Abbreviations

(BHCG): Beta human chorionic gonadotropin
(CP): Cervical pregnancy
(EP): Ectopic pregnancy
(FHR): Fetal heart rate
(FSH): Follicle-stimulating hormone
(IM): Intramuscular
(IUI): Intrauterine insemination
(IVF): In vitro fertilization
(LH): Luteinizing hormone
(MRI): Magnetic resonance imaging
(MTX): Methotrexate.

Consent

Written informed consent was obtained from the patient for participation. Written informed consent was obtained from the patient for publication of this case report and any accompanying images. A copy of the written consent is available for review by the Editor-in-Chief of this journal.

Authors' Contributions

MJM evaluated the patient clinically and prepared the first and draft revision of the paper. AZ prepared the first and draft revision of the paper. HS revised the paper. All authors read and approved the final manuscript.

Acknowledgments

We all express our gratitude to the patient who kindly gave consent for this case to be presented in this paper.

References

[1] H.-C. Chang, T.-H. Chiu, and L.-M. Lo, "Early cervical ectopic pregnancy: a case report and review of the literature," *Journal of Medical Ultrasound*, vol. 22, no. 2, pp. 117–119, 2014.

[2] M. Yitzhak, R. Orvieto, S. Nitke, M. Neuman-Levin, Z. Ben-Rafael, and A. Schoenfeld, "Case report: cervical pregnancy a conservative stepwise approach," *Human Reproduction (Oxford, England)*, vol. 14, no. 3, pp. 847–849, 1999.

[3] P. Bianchi, M. M. Salvatori, F. Torcia, G. Cozza, and B. Mossa,

"Cervical pregnancy," *Fertility and Sterility*, vol. 95, no. 6, pp. 2123.e3–2123.e4, 2011.

[4] A. Dobrosavljevic, B. Nikolic, A. Jurisisc, N. Zečević, R. Aničić, and M. Jeftović, "Diagnosis and treatment of cervical ectopic pregnancy - case report," *Clinical and Experimental Obstetrics & Gynecology*, vol. 46, no. 1, pp. 139-140, 2019.

[5] S. K. Samal and S. Rathod, "Cervical ectopic pregnancy," *Journal of Natural Science, Biology, and Medicine*, vol. 6, no. 1, p. 257, 2015.

[6] R. J. Paalman and T. W. McElin, "Cervical pregnancy: review of the literature and presentation of cases," *American Journal of Obstetrics and Gynecology*, vol. 77, no. 6, pp. 1261–1270, 1959.

[7] D. Chrestiana, A. B. Cheng, N. L. Panebianco, and A. J. Dean, "Pitfalls in cervical ectopic pregnancy diagnosis by emergency physicians using bedside ultrasonography," *The American Journal of Emergency Medicine*, vol. 32, no. 4, pp. 397.e1–397.e3, 2014.

[8] S. Petousis, C. Margioula-Siarkou, I. Kalogiannidis et al., "Conservative management of cervical pregnancy with intramuscular administration of methotrexate and KCl injection: case report and review of the literature," *World Journal of Clinical Cases*, vol. 3, no. 1, pp. 81–84, 2015.

[9] J. A. DeLoia, A. M. Stewart-Akers, and M. D. Creinin, "Effects of methotrexate on trophoblast proliferation and local immune responses," *Human Reproduction*, vol. 13, no. 4, pp. 1063–1069, 1998.

[10] K. Jameel, G. E. Abdul Mannan, R. Niaz, and D. E. Hayat, "Cesarean scar ectopic pregnancy: a diagnostic and management challenge," *Cureus*, vol. 13, no. 4, article e14463, 2021.

[11] Y. Khatib, A. Khashikar, R. Wani, and R. D. Patel, "Cervical ectopic pregnancy: a case report of missed diagnosis," *DY Patil University*, vol. 9, no. 6, p. 741, 2016.

[12] D. K. Pandher and A. Shehgal, "Diagnosis and management of cervical ectopic pregnancy-report of three cases," *Nepal Medical College Journal*, vol. 11, pp. 64-65, 2009.

[13] P. Lesny, S. R. Killick, J. Robinson, and S. D. Maguiness, "Transcervical embryo transfer as a risk factor for ectopic pregnancy," *Fertility and Sterility*, vol. 72, no. 2, pp. 305–309, 1999.

[14] S. Bennett, J. Waterstone, J. Parsons, and S. Creighton, "Two cases of cervical pregnancy following in vitro fertilization and embryo transfer to the lower uterine cavity," *Journal of Assisted Reproduction and Genetics*, vol. 10, no. 1, pp. 100–103, 1993.

[15] K. Surampudi, "A case of cervical ectopic pregnancy: successful therapy with methotrexate," *The Journal of Obstetrics and Gynecology of India*, vol. 62, no. S1, pp. 1–3, 2012.

[16] G. Vela and T. Tulandi, "Cervical pregnancy: the importance of early diagnosis and treatment," *Journal of Minimally Invasive Gynecology*, vol. 14, no. 4, pp. 481–484, 2007.

[17] T. Yamagami, R. Yoshimatsu, T. Matsumoto et al., "Fertility after uterine artery embolization: investigation using a sheep model," *Reproductive Sciences*, vol. 17, no. 4, pp. 350–357, 2010.

[18] B. Rizk, C. P. Holliday, S. Owens, and M. Abuzeid, "Cervical and cesarean scar ectopic pregnancies: diagnosis and management," *Middle East Fertility Society Journal*, vol. 18, no. 2, pp. 67–73, 2013.

[19] M. Yitzhak, R. Orvieto, S. Nitke, M. Neuman-Levin, Z. Ben-Rafael, and A. Schoenfeld, "Case report: cervical pregnancy—a conservative stepwise approach," *Human Reproduction*, vol. 14, no. 3, p. 847-849.20, 1999.

[20] S. Samal, S. Ghose, P. Pallavee, and P. Porkkodi, "Successful management of live cervical ectopic pregnancy: a case report," *Journal of Clinical and Diagnostic Research: JCDR*, vol. 9, p. QD03, 2015.

[21] S. Kadija, A. Stefanovic, K. Jeremic et al., "Successful conservative treatment of a cervical ectopic pregnancy at 13 weeks, clinical experimental," *Obstetrics & Gynecology*, vol. 43, pp. 291–293, 2016.

[22] B. Hamouda, N. Ouerdiane, W. Daaloul, A. Masmoudi, B. Bouguerra, and R. Sfar, "Conservative management of cervical pregnancy. a case-report," *La Tunisie Medicale*, vol. 86, no. 9, pp. 827–829, 2008.

[23] P. J. Hajenius, F. Mol, B. W. J. Mol, P. M. Bossuyt, W. M. Ankum, and F. Van der Veen, "Interventions for tubal ectopic pregnancy," *Cochrane Database of Systematic Reviews*, vol. 1, article CD000324, 2007.

[24] G. H. Lipscomb, "Medical management of ectopic pregnancy," *Clinical Obstetrics and Gynecology*, vol. 55, no. 2, pp. 424–432, 2012.

[25] H. Fernandez, P. Bourget, C. Lelaidier, S. Doumerc, and R. Frydman, "Methotrexate treatment of unilateral twin ectopic pregnancy: case report and pharmacokinetic considerations," *Ultrasound in Obstetrics and Gynecology*, vol. 3, no. 5, pp. 357–359, 1993.

[26] J. Yavanasuriya, A. Keepanasseril, N. S. Kubera, D. K. Maurya, and G. Dorairajan, "Management of cervical pregnancy with a combination of systemic methotrexate and ultrasound-guided local instillation of methotrexate and potassium chloride: a case report and review of the literature," *Journal of Gynecologic Surgery*, vol. 32, no. 5, pp. 290–292, 2016.

7

Laparoscopic Vessel Endometriosis Resection Surgery: A Case Report and Review of Literature

Shadi Rezai[1] **Richard A. Giovane**[2] **Tiffanie Mann,**[2] **Ninad M. Patil,**[3] **Elise Bardawil,**[1] **Cassandra E. Henderson**[4] **and Xiaoming Guan**[1]

[1]*Division of Minimally Invasive Gynecologic Surgery, Department of Obstetrics and Gynecology, Baylor College of Medicine, 6651 Main Street, 10th Floor, Houston, TX 77030, USA*
[2]*University of Alabama, Department of Family Medicine, 801 Campus Drive, Tuscaloosa, AL 35487, USA*
[3]*Department of Pathology & Immunology, Baylor College of Medicine, 6651 Main Street, Suite F0455.10, Houston, TX 77030, USA*
[4]*Maternal and Fetal Medicine, Department of Obstetrics and Gynecology, Lincoln Medical and Mental Health Center, 234 East 149th Street, Bronx, NY 10451, USA*

Correspondence should be addressed to Xiaoming Guan; xiaoming@bcm.edu

Academic Editor: Maria Grazia Porpora

Background. Endometriosis usually occurs in the pelvis and often involves the ovaries, the uterosacral and broad ligaments, and the pelvic peritoneum. In rare instances, it can occur in the vasculature of the pelvis. Patients with endometriosis present with abnormal pain, menstrual cycle disruption and infertility. Management of endometriosis is usually surgical with excision of the tissue via laparoscopic means. *Case.* A 42-year-old Gravida 5, Para 2-0-3-2 patient with a 22 year history of endometriosis, who had had multiple laparoscopic endometriosis resections, total abdominal hysterectomy, and an exploratory laparotomy with bilateral salpingo-oophorectomy, presented with left pelvic pain when standing, dyspareunia, and a 3.7 cm cyst on ultrasound. The patient underwent laparoscopic vessel endometriosis resection and excision of endometriotic nodules from external iliac vessels. Final pathology report showed evidence of old endometriosis in all locations. On interval follow-up, the patient reported sustained relief from pain. *Conclusion.* Complete resection of endometriosis from large vessels can be successfully achieved laparoscopically by a well-experienced surgeon with delicate, proper techniques.

1. Background

Endometriosis is defined as the presence of endometrial tissue, including glands and/or stroma, occurring anywhere outside of the uterine cavity [1]. The ectopic tissue embeds and infiltrates itself into nearby structures and responds cyclically to sex hormones, eliciting an inflammatory response. Over time, there may be fibrosis in the surrounding tissue. Occasionally, the endometriotic tissue may be replaced by collagen and scar tissue, referred to as "burnt-out endometriosis" [1, 2]. While the precise etiology of endometriosis is unclear, retrograde menstruation and/or metaplasia of the peritoneal lining are postulated mechanisms in most cases. It remains one of the most common gynecological disorders of the female reproductive tract [2]. In symptomatic women, it classically presents with chronic pelvic pain and infertility [2]. Endometriosis is graded in severity using surgical staging: from stage I correlated with minimal disease, to stage 4 signifying severe or complex disease [3].

While endometriotic lesions usually develop within the pelvic cavity, affecting the ovaries and the ligamentous structures between the uterus and the peritoneum, it is not uncommon to identify lesions beyond these structures [1]. Vessel endometriosis is a rare phenomenon of severe endometriosis whereby fibrotic endometriotic nodules appear in the vasculature of the pelvis [4]. Endometriosis has a preponderance for recurrence, as retreatment is evidenced in many cases as the primary reasoning for surgical procedures such as laparoscopy [5]. Additionally, rates of retreatment appear to be significantly reduced following excision and removal via laparoscopy [5]. Hence, a more definitive treatment must be used to decrease recurrence. Laparoscopy is a less invasive surgical

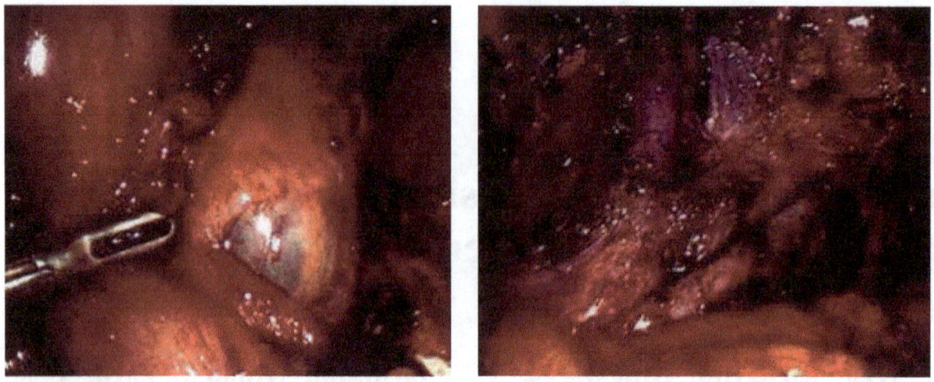

(a) (b)

FIGURE 1: Intraoperative images: (a) left pelvic cyst (a 4 cm ovarian remnant cyst) was identified and the entire ovary was removed; (b) endometriotic nodules and endometriosis on left external iliac artery and vein.

approach utilized to eradicate endometriotic lesions [5, 6]. It also drastically reduces the amount of time necessary for adequate postoperative healing and recovery [7, 8]. The objective of our review of the literature is to demonstrate the benefits of laparoscopic resection in a novel case of complex endometriosis affecting the external iliac vasculature, ureter, bowel and rectum.

2. Presentation of the Case

The patient, is a 42-year-old white female Gravida 5, Para 2-0-3-2, with a past medical history of endometriosis, diagnosed since age 19.

The patient presented to our clinic with severe pelvic pain, particularly on the left side, with associated dysmenorrhea, dyschezia and dyspareunia. The patient reported that this pain was constant and had been ongoing for a few months. Pelvic pain was exacerbated upon standing; there were no alleviating factors. Her physical exam revealed positive pelvic pain preponderant on the left side. No nodularity was palpable on rectal examination. The rest of the physical exam was unremarkable. Based on the patient's presentation and physical exam, it was decided to do a pelvic ultrasound. The ultrasound showed a 3.7 cm septated cystic mass in the left adnexa (ovarian remnant cyst) on ultrasound.

Upon further chart review, the patient had multiple previous surgeries. These include two cesarean deliveries, two laparoscopic endometriosis resections and fulguration of endometriotic implants. The patient also had a laparoscopic left ovarian cystectomy for a 10 cm endometrioma (which recurred as a 5 cm endometrioma within 6 months), two exploratory laparotomies, including a total abdominal hysterectomy (TAH) and an exploratory laparotomy with bilateral salpingo-oophorectomy (BSO).

The patient underwent laparoscopic resection of endometriotic implants and nodules from left external iliac artery and vein (Figure 1(b)), bowel resection, ureteral lysis, left pelvic cyst (ovarian remnant cyst) removal (Figure 1(a)), left pelvic nodule resection, lysis of adhesions (Figure 2(a)), cystoscopy and stent placement for management of endometriosis (Figure 2(b)) and pelvic pain.

2.1. Operative Technique (17). The Enseal device was used to lyse omental adhesions and cold scissors were used to lyse bowel adhesions. A 4 cm ovarian remnant was identified and the entire ovary was removed (Figure 1(a)). The left ureter was completely dissected out in order to completely remove the left ovarian remnant cyst. The endo-GIA stapler was used to transect the bowel. Bowel endometriosis was resected with the TA stapler though the 5 cm umbilical incision (Figure 2(c)). A rigid nodule was detected at the left external iliac vessels and was dissected out and removed using sharp and blunt dissection. The harmonic was used to transect the fibrotic tissues of the endometriosis nodule. The ureteral endometriosis was also transected. A left ureteral stent was placed and left in for 4 weeks.

The final pathology report (Figures 3(a) and 3(b)) confirmed evidence of burnt-out endometriosis in all locations including bowel and external iliac nodule. In the left external iliac vessel, residual endometrial-type stroma, vasculature, and hemosiderotic macrophages were seen on H&E stain (Figure 3(a)), and highlighted by CD10 immunohistochemical stain (Figure 3(b)).

On interval follow-up, the patient reported sustained relief from pain, last recorded at 9 months intraoperatively.

3. Discussion

Review of the literature shows that complete resection of endometriotic lesions from the affected vasculature can be utilized to successfully treat chronic pelvic pain secondary to severe endometriosis [9, 10]. Pelvic pain usually returns within one year of treatment in patients receiving medical therapy such as GnRH agonists; conversely, Sutton et al. showed that 90% of patients receiving laparoscopy for endometriosis were symptom-free at one year [5]. While endometriosis is a common finding in chronic pelvic pain and a known factor affecting fecundity, a small subset of women have deeply infiltrating endometriosis, affecting distant organs and structures [4]. Such patients with severe disease are often plagued with high rates of recurrence as it can be difficult to (1) identify all lesions during one laparoscopic procedure and/or (2) resect and completely remove endometriotic implants involving more delicate

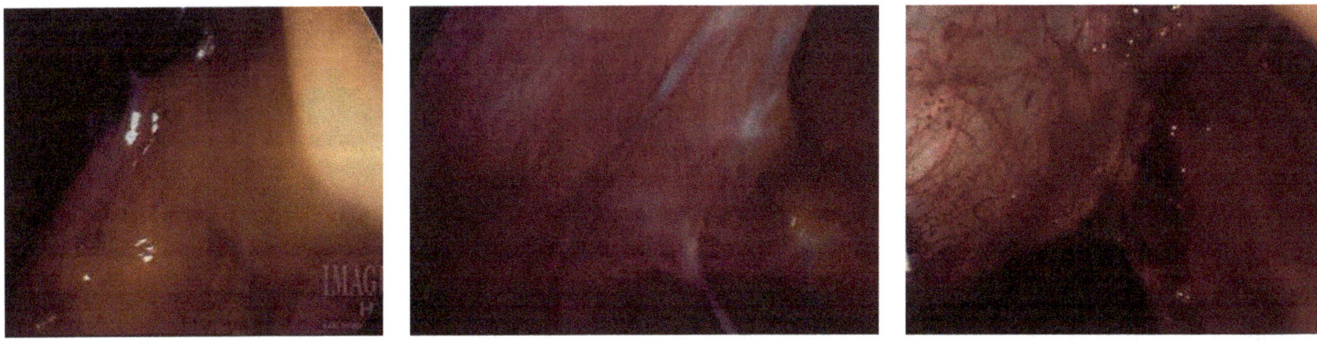

(a) (b) (c)

FIGURE 2: Intraoperative images: (a) adhesion of bowel and omentum to anterior abdominal wall; (b) white patches of endometriotic implants; (c) endometriotic implants on the large bowel (left), adhesions of omentum to large bowel (right).

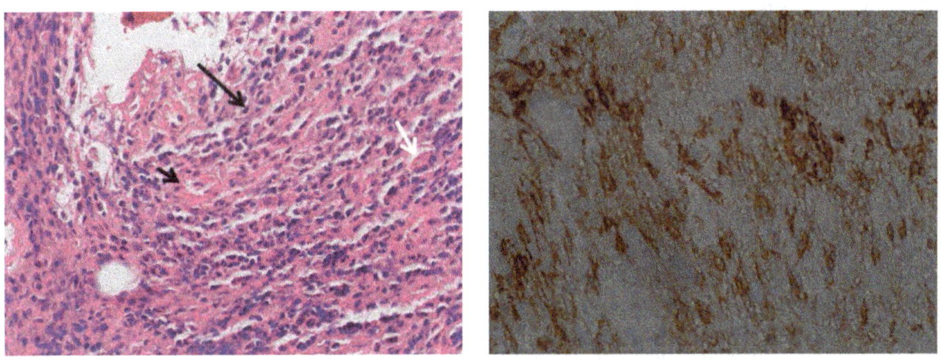

(a) (b)

FIGURE 3: Pathology slides: left external iliac nodule biopsy: (a) endometrial-type stroma (long black arrow) and capillary (short black arrow) with hemosiderin-laden macrophage (white arrow). (H&E stain); (b) endometrial-type stroma is positive for CD10 (CD10 immunohistochemical stain).

structures (i.e., bowel, ureter and vessels), requiring extreme skill and anatomical knowledge [11, 12]. In this case, the patient had a history of chronic, debilitating endometriosis despite numerous surgeries designed to substantially reduce or eliminate symptoms.

Overall, laparoscopic procedures are associated with a shorter hospital stay, faster healing time, and decreased morbidity. However, morbidity may be increased in patients who undergo repeat procedures when prior surgical treatment has been unsuccessful [10, 13–15]. In our case, the patient did not report complete pain resolution until after complete resection of the fibrotic nodules lining the external iliac artery and vein. In patients with known severe disease who report persistent pain despite multiple medical and surgical therapies, it may prove worthwhile to thoroughly investigate less commonly affected structures to identify fibrotic nodules and other pathologic changes associated with endometriosis.

4. Conclusion

Complete resection of endometriosis, including from large vessels may be the key to successful surgical treatment. With sufficient experience, knowledge of anatomy, and precise dissection technique, endometriomas can be safely removed from large vessels [15].

Disclosure

Presented, in part, as surgical video presentation format (16, 17) at the 45th AAGL Global Congress on Minimally Invasive Gynecology, the Rosen Hotel at Shingle Creek, Orlando, Florida, November 14–18, 2016.

References

[1] L. C. Giudice, "Clinical practice. Endometriosis," *The New England Journal of Medicine*, vol. 362, no. 25, pp. 2389–2398, 2010.

[2] P. Vercellini, P. Viganò, E. Somigliana, and L. Fedele, "Endometriosis: pathogenesis and treatment," *Nature Reviews Endocrinology*, vol. 10, no. 5, pp. 261–275, 2014.

[3] American Society for Reproductive Medicine, "Revised american society for reproductive medicine classification of endometriosis: 1996," *Fertility and Sterility*, vol. 67, no. 5, pp. 817–821, 1997.

[4] A. J. Dwivedi, S. N. Agrawal, and Y. J. Silva, "Abdominal wall endometriomas," *Digestive Diseases and Sciences*, vol. 47, no. 2, pp. 456–461, 2002.

[5] C. J. Sutton, A. S. Pooley, S. P. Ewen, and P. Haines, "Follow-up report on a randomized controlled trial of laser laparoscopy in the treatment of pelvic pain associated with minimal to moderate endometriosis," *Fertility and Sterility*, vol. 68, no. 6, pp. 1070–1074, 1997.

[6] C. J. Sutton, S. P. Ewen, N. Whitelaw, and P. Haines, "Prospective, randomized, double-blind, controlled trial of laser laparoscopy in the treatment of pelvic pain associated with minimal, mild, and moderate endometriosis," *Fertility and Sterility*, vol. 62, no. 4, pp. 696–700, 1994.

[7] A. N. Fader, K. L. Levinson, C. C. Gunderson, A. D. Winder, and P. F. Escobar, "Laparoendoscopic single-site surgery in gynecology: A new frontier in minimally invasive surgery," *Journal of Minimal Access Surgery*, vol. 7, no. 1, pp. 71–77, 2011.

[8] P. F. Escobar, D. Starks, A. N. Fader, M. Catenacci, and T. Falcone, "Laparoendoscopic single-site and natural orifice surgery in gynecology," *Fertility and Sterility*, vol. 94, no. 7, pp. 2497–2502, 2010.

[9] A. N. Fader, L. Rojas-Espaillat, O. Ibeanu, F. C. Grumbine, and P. F. Escobar, "Laparoendoscopic single-site surgery (LESS) in gynecology: a multi-institutional evaluation," *American Journal of Obstetrics & Gynecology*, vol. 203, no. 5, pp. 501.e1–e6, 2010.

[10] A. N. Fader, S. Cohen, P. F. Escobar, and C. Gunderson, "Laparoendoscopic single-site surgery in gynecology," *Current Opinion in Obstetrics and Gynecology*, vol. 22, no. 4, pp. 331–338, 2010.

[11] P. F. Escobar, A. N. Fader, M. F. Paraiso, J. H. Kaouk, and T. Falcone, "Robotic-assisted laparoendoscopic single-site surgery in gynecology: initial report and technique," *The Journal of Minimally Invasive Gynecology*, vol. 16, no. 5, pp. 589–591, 2009.

[12] S. A. Scheib and A. N. Fader, "Gynecologic robotic laparoendoscopic single-site surgery: prospective analysis of feasibility, safety, and technique," *American Journal of Obstetrics & Gynecology*, vol. 212, no. 2, pp. 179.e1–e8, 2015.

[13] M. A. Bedaiwy, T. Farghaly, W. Hurd et al., "Laparoendoscopic single-site surgery for management of ovarian endometriomas," *Journal of the Society of Laparoendscopic Surgeons*, vol. 18, no. 2, pp. 191–196, 2014.

[14] M. A. Bedaiwy, D. Sheyn, L. Eghdami et al., "Laparoendoscopic single-site surgery for benign ovarian cystectomies," *Gynecologic and Obstetric Investigation*, vol. 79, no. 3, pp. 179–183, 2015.

[15] P. F. Escobar, M. A. Bedaiwy, A. N. Fader, and T. Falcone, "Laparoendoscopic single-site (LESS) surgery in patients with benign adnexal disease," *Fertility and Sterility*, vol. 93, no. 6, pp. 2074.e7–e10, 2010.

8

Pregnancy Outcome after Exposure to Migalastat for Fabry Disease: A Clinical Report

Natalja Haninger-Vacariu [1] **Sarah El-Hadi,** [1] **Udo Pauler,** [2] **Marina Foretnik,** [1] **Renate Kain** [3] **Zoltán Prohászka,** [4] **Alice Schmidt,** [1] **Nina Skuban,** [5] **Jay A. Barth,** [5] **and Gere Sunder-Plassmann** [1]

[1] *Division of Nephrology and Dialysis, Department of Medicine III, Medical University of Vienna, Vienna, Austria*
[2] *Department of Medicine I, University Hospital St. Pölten, Lower Austria, Austria*
[3] *Department of Pathology, Medical University of Vienna, Vienna, Austria*
[4] *Semmelweis University, Research Laboratory, Third Department of Internal Medicine, Budapest, Hungary*
[5] *Amicus Therapeutics, Inc., Cranbury, NJ, USA*

Correspondence should be addressed to Natalja Haninger-Vacariu; natalja.haninger@meduniwien.ac.at

Academic Editor: Yossef Ezra

Our patient was a 37-year-old woman with Fabry disease (*GLA* p.R112H) with a medical history of recurrent headache, nausea, vomiting, vertigo, and tobacco use (20 cigarettes/day). Fabry disease was diagnosed in 2005 when she experienced proteinuria, preeclampsia, and hypertension (201/130 mm Hg) during pregnancy (delivered 50 cm, 3.4 kg healthy boy; *GLA* wild type [WT]). Enzyme replacement therapy was initiated in 2009. The patient enrolled in the phase 3 ATTRACT trial (ClinicalTrials.gov; NCT01218659) and started migalastat in May 2012 while taking hormonal contraceptives. Two years after initiating migalastat, the patient had proteinuria (2166 mg/24 h) without hypertension (131/68 mm Hg), which persisted (788 mg/24 h a month later). Kidney biopsy results were consistent with existing Fabry disease. A serum pregnancy test and ultrasound confirmed pregnancy (18 weeks' gestation). Migalastat and hormonal contraceptives were stopped; the patient continued to smoke. Fetal MRI was normal at ~29 weeks' gestation. In October 2014, at 37+ weeks' gestation, the patient delivered a 45-cm, 2.29-kg healthy girl (*GLA* WT). Excepting low birth weight, which may be related to the patient's smoking, pregnancy outcome was normal despite exposure to migalastat for 18 weeks. Migalastat therapy during pregnancy is not advised.

1. Introduction

Fabry disease is a rare, X-linked lysosomal storage disorder caused by deficiency of α-galactosidase A (α-Gal A), encoded by the *GLA* gene [1]. The resulting accumulation of globotriaosylceramide (GL-3) produces a wide variety of debilitating signs and symptoms, including cardiomyopathy, renal failure, cerebrovascular events, and gastrointestinal manifestations [2]. The first clinical symptoms of Fabry disease typically occur during childhood, and, if left untreated, the burden of the disease increases over time [3].

Until recently, enzyme replacement therapy (ERT), consisting of lifetime infusions of agalsidase alfa or agalsidase beta, was the only treatment approach for patients with Fabry disease [4–6]. ERT is associated with several limitations, including the burden of frequent infusions and disease progression despite adherence to therapy [7]. Migalastat is a small-molecule pharmacological chaperone designed to bind selectively and reversibly to the active sites of amenable variants of α-Gal A [7]. It is estimated that approximately 35%–50% of patients with Fabry disease worldwide have amenable *GLA* variants [8]. Migalastat binding stabilizes mutant forms of α-Gal A and facilitates trafficking to lysosomes, where dissociation of migalastat endogenous α-Gal A activity is restored, leading to the catabolism of GL-3 and other disease substrates [9].

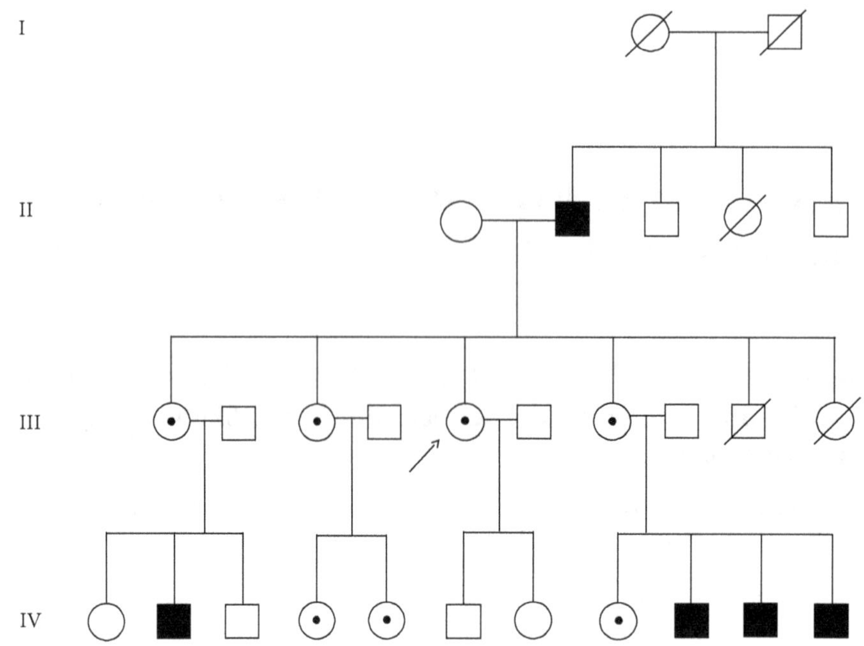

Figure 1: Pedigree analysis. The patient is indicated by the arrow. Black boxes represent males with Fabry disease; circles with black dots represent females with Fabry disease. Slash indicates deceased.

In two phase 3 trials (FACETS [NCT00925301] and ATTRACT [NCT01218659]), migalastat was shown to provide clinical benefits for patients with Fabry disease and amenable *GLA* variants and was generally well tolerated [8, 10]. Migalastat is now approved for the treatment of Fabry disease in patients ≥16 years old with amenable *GLA* variants in the European Union, Switzerland, Israel, Australia, Republic of Korea, and Japan, and in adult patients in the United States and Canada [7, 9]. Because developmental toxicity was observed in rabbits who received maternally toxic doses of migalastat in preclinical studies [9] it is recommended that migalastat not be given during pregnancy. Herein, we describe the medical history and outcome of a white woman with Fabry disease who became pregnant, despite hormonal contraception, while being treated with migalastat during the phase 3 ATTRACT trial [8].

2. Case Presentation

2.1. Study Background. ATTRACT was a phase 3, randomized, open-label, active-controlled study designed to evaluate the efficacy and safety of migalastat HCl (150 mg every other day [QOD]) and ERT in patients with Fabry disease who were receiving ERT and who had an amenable *GLA* variant [8]. Full methodology is described in Hughes et al. [8]. Briefly, eligible patients were randomly assigned to either continue ERT or switch to migalastat HCl (150 mg QOD) for 18 months [8]. After completing the randomized treatment period, patients could participate in a 12-month open-label extension of migalastat HCl (150 mg QOD) [8]. Patients of reproductive potential agreed to use medically accepted methods of contraception throughout the duration of the study and for up to 30 days after the last dose of migalastat.

Written informed consent was obtained from all study participants before initiating any study-related procedures. The appropriate ethics committee approved the clinical study protocol at each site and the trial was conducted in accordance with the Declaration of Helsinki.

All clinical chemistry analyses were performed in an International Standardization Organization (ISO) 15189 accredited clinical laboratory at the Department of Laboratory Medicine, Medical University of Vienna. Glomerular filtration rate was estimated (eGFR) using the Chronic Kidney Disease Epidemiology Collaboration (CKD-EPI) equation. Analyses of complement-related proteins was performed at the third Department of Internal Medicine, Semmelweis University, Budapest, Hungary. Genetic testing for rare variants in *GLA* and complement-related genes was performed as previously described [11].

2.2. Patient History. The patient is a white woman who was diagnosed with Fabry disease in 2005 at 28 years of age. Her father had Fabry disease (generation II), and all 3 surviving siblings (all females) also had Fabry disease (generation III) (Figure 1). The patient's medical history prior to migalastat treatment was significant for headache (beginning at 12 years of age), psoriasis (beginning at 17 years of age), and nausea, vomiting, and vertigo (beginning at 18 years of age). The patient had a history of smoking (since the age of 14) and smoked 20 cigarettes per day. Her first pregnancy, which occurred in 2002 at the age of 25, resulted in a miscarriage during the fifth month (18 weeks' gestation) after having a traffic accident (Table 1). At 26 years of age, the patient was hospitalized for strong headache and neck pain. At 27, the patient had a second pregnancy. An emergency cesarean delivery was performed at 38+ weeks of gestation due to preeclampsia (blood pressure ≥140/90 mm Hg), proteinuria (urine test for

TABLE 1: Overview of pregnancies.

Pregnancy	Year of delivery	Age of mother at delivery (years)	Outcome	Sex of child	Gestational age at birth (weeks)	Mode of delivery	Birth weight (kg)	Birth height (cm)	Head circumference at birth (cm)	Assessment[a]	*GLA*
1	2002	25	Miscarriage	N/A	±18	Vaginal	N/A	N/A	N/A	N/A	N/A
2	2005	27	Live birth	Male	38 + 6	Emergency C-section	3.40	50	33.3	AGA	WT
3	2014	37	Live birth	Female	37 + 1	C-section	2.29	45	32	SGA	WT

AGA, appropriate gestational age; N/A, not available; SGA, small for gestational age; WHO, World Health Organization; WT, wild type. [a]According to WHO child growth standards. SGA is defined as infants with a birth weight below the 10th percentile for gestational age [26].

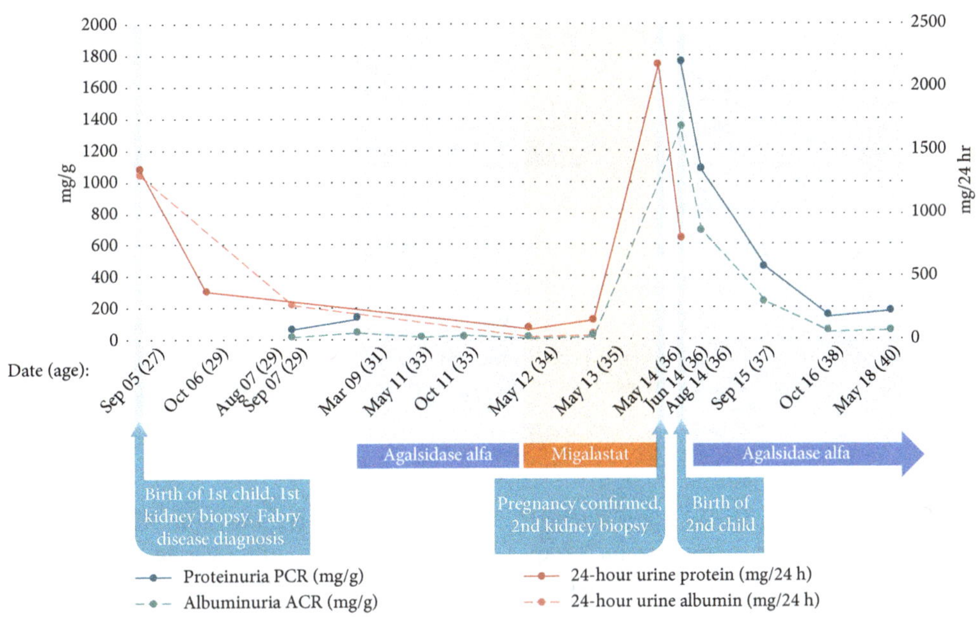

(a)

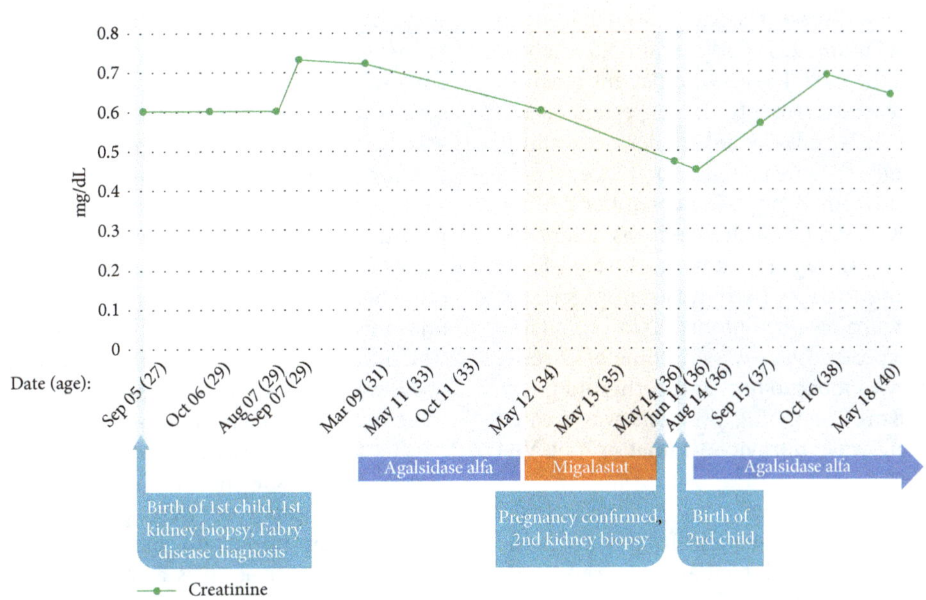

(b)

FIGURE 2: Continued.

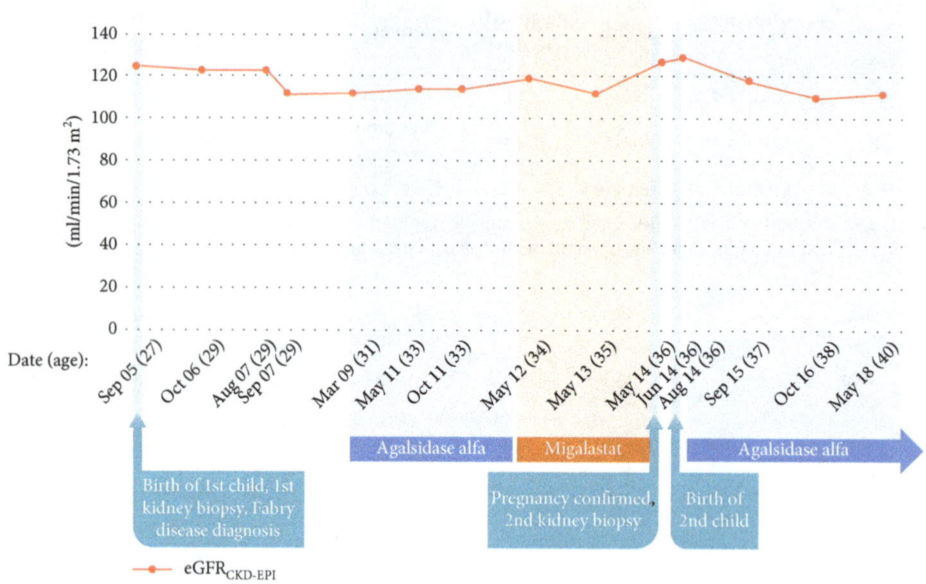

(c)

FIGURE 2: Time course of (a) proteinuria and albuminuria, (b) creatinine, and (c) $eGFR_{CKD\text{-}EPI}$. ACR, albumin-to-creatinine ratio; $eGFR_{CKD\text{-}EPI}$, estimated glomerular filtration rate chronic kidney disease epidemiology collaboration; PCR, protein-to-creatinine ratio.

proteinuria was positive), and pelvic abnormalities, which resulted in delivery of a healthy male infant (50 cm, 3.4 kg, *GLA* WT) (Table 1). Twenty days postpartum, an increase in 24-hour urine protein (935.9 mg/24 h) was recorded. Then, 1-month postpartum, an increase in 24-hour urine protein (1340 mg/24 h, Figure 2), hypertension (210/130 mm Hg), severe neck pain, headache, and edema resulted in a 7-day hospital stay and consultation with a nephrologist. During this time, Fabry disease was diagnosed based on kidney biopsy results (Figure 3(a)) and mutational analysis (*GLA* p.R1112H). For the next 4 years, the patient received no specific Fabry disease treatment, and experienced the occasional occurrence of leg edema and moderate swelling. In March 2009, at the age of 31, the patient experienced a mild increase of proteinuria (from 59 mg/g in September 2007 to 132 mg/g in March 2009) and headaches and was diagnosed with depression. The patient began treatment with agalsidase alfa via infusion; during therapy, there was no progression of renal, cardiac, or neurologic symptoms. Two years later, in 2011, the patient experienced new symptoms of chronic pharyngitis (secondary to tobacco use) and euthyroid goiter (thyroid volume, 31.8 mL). Ongoing psoriasis was treated with psoralen and long-wave ultraviolet radiation (PUVA) phototherapy.

2.3. Migalastat Treatment and Pregnancy. In May 2012, the patient enrolled in the ATTRACT trial and was randomly assigned to migalastat HCl (150 mg QOD) [8]. At enrollment, 24-h urine protein was 83 mg/24 h. In accordance with the study protocol, the patient agreed to use hormonal contraceptives (Diane mite; ovulation inhibitor) for the duration of the study. While enrolled in the study, renal, cardiac, and neurologic assessments conducted through February 2014 showed no evidence of disease progression. In May 2014, after 2 years of migalastat treatment, proteinuria increased sharply from 78 mg/24 h (in February 2014) to 2166 mg/24 h, without hypertension (131/68 mm Hg). A urine pregnancy test was negative. The following month, ongoing proteinuria (788 mg/24 h, Figure 2) prompted kidney biopsy, which showed cellular characteristics consistent with existing Fabry disease (Figure 3(b)). A serum pregnancy test result was positive, and pregnancy was confirmed via ultrasound examination (18 + 0 weeks gestation). Migalastat therapy and hormonal contraceptives were stopped; the patient continued to smoke during her pregnancy (20 cigarettes/day).

At 29 weeks' gestation, magnetic resonance imaging indicated normal fetal development (Figure 4). The pregnancy was uneventful, and a healthy female infant (45 cm, 2.29 kg, *GLA* WT, Table 1) was delivered via cesarean section at 37+ weeks of gestation. After delivery, ERT therapy (agalsidase alfa, home infusion) was restarted and is currently ongoing.

Because the patient had complement C3 staining in her kidney biopsy specimens (Figure 3), serologic and genetic complement analyses were performed. The complement system is an important mediator of kidney injury, and complement activation is associated with a wide variety of kidney diseases [12]. Results showed that the patient had a normal complement profile, was anti-C1q, anti-FH, and C3Nef negative, and had no signs of complement activation

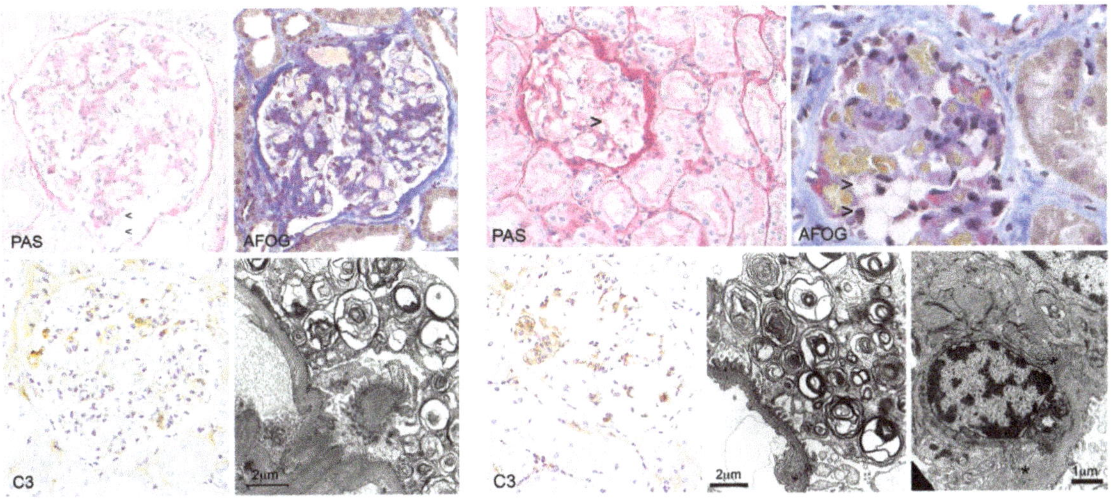

(a) (b)

FIGURE 3: Histology and transmission electron microscopy of kidney biopsy specimens obtained (a) in 2005, one month after birth of first child (second pregnancy) and (b) in 2014, during pregnancy with second child (third pregnancy). AFOG, acid fuchsin orange G; IgA, immunoglobulin A; IgG, immunoglobulin G; PAS, periodic acid-Schiff; TEM, transmission electron microscopy. (a) The first renal biopsy (2005) shows a diffuse, segmentally accentuated mesangial matrix and mesangial cell proliferation (PAS and AFOG) in >50% of the glomeruli, and segmentally obliterated capillary loops adherent to the Bowman's capsule (AFOG). There is dominant segmental C3 deposition (C3) in the absence of IgG and IgA. Podocytes show characteristic lamellar and zebroid bodies by TEM; however, the classical appearance of "foamy" podocytes was less dominant by light microscopy (PAS) due to the segmental nature of the pathological changes. (b) The second renal biopsy (2014) shows characteristic foamy macrophages (PAS and AFOG) as well as segmental mesangial matrix and mesangial cell proliferation. Dominant C3 deposits (C3) correspond to mesangial electron dense deposits (*) by TEM (right) while almost all podocytes contain lamellar and zebroid inclusion bodies (a).

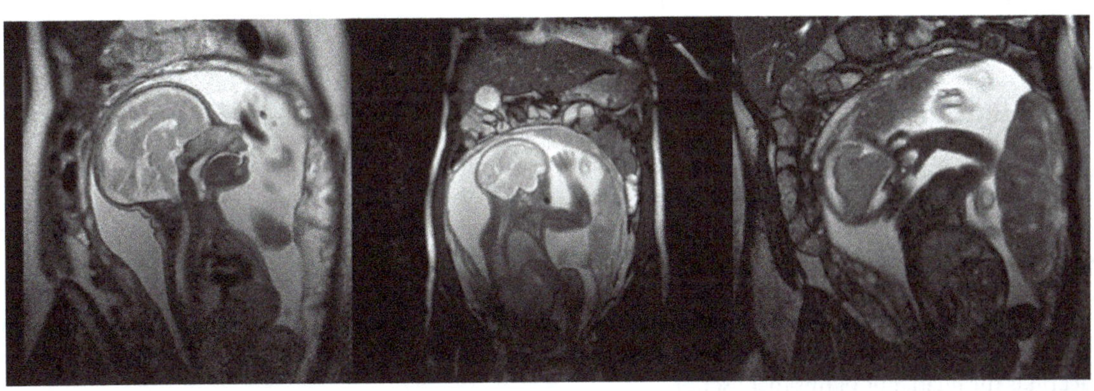

FIGURE 4: Fetal MRI (coronal plane) during pregnancy at 29 weeks' gestation. MRI, magnetic resonance imaging. Images presented with patient permission.

or consumption. DNA sequencing revealed no mutations in *CFH, CFI, CD62, C3, CFB, THBD, CFHR5*, and *ADAMTS13*; MLPA results showed no disease-causing deletions or duplications of *CFH, CFHR1, CFHR2, CFHR3*, and *CFHR5*.

3. Discussion

We report on the case of a woman with Fabry disease who had a successful pregnancy outcome after receiving migalastat for 18 weeks, with no significant negative effect on her child. Except for a birth weight (2.29 kg) that met criteria for being low for gestational age [13, 14], the pregnancy outcome in this case was normal. The specific reason for the low birth weight is unknown; however, the patient smoked during her pregnancy, which is known to be associated with low birth weight [15, 16]. To our knowledge, there is no report of an association between low birth weight and Fabry disease and normal birth weight has been reported for Fabry-complicated pregnancies [17].

Interestingly, both kidney biopsies (one obtained shortly after her second pregnancy, and one obtained during the third pregnancy) showed evidence of Fabry disease and segmental C3 staining in the glomeruli. In-depth serological and genetic analyses did not confirm a specific cause for C3 glomerulopathy. Thus, our findings may point to an inflammatory response in the kidney triggered by pregnancy and Fabry disease, resulting in heavy proteinuria during pregnancy that resolved after childbirth in both instances.

Successful pregnancy outcomes have been reported in women with Fabry disease receiving ERT with agalsidase alfa [18–20] or agalsidase beta [20–25] infusions. This is the first report of a successful pregnancy outcome with migalastat. In a separate phase 3 trial of migalastat in patients with Fabry disease [10] one woman discontinued from the study because of pregnancy after being exposed to migalastat for 34 days. The pregnancy was uneventful, and she delivered a healthy baby girl. In a rabbit embryo-fetal toxicity study, migalastat doses associated with maternal toxicity were associated with embryo-fetal death, a reduction in mean fetal weight, retarded ossification, and slightly increased incidence of minor skeletal abnormalities [9]. Therefore, migalastat therapy is not advised during pregnancy. Despite the successful pregnancy reported here, the safety of migalastat during pregnancy is still uncertain.

Consent

The patient provided written consent for her case to be published.

Disclosure

Previously presented at the 14th Annual WORLD *Symposium*™; February 5–9, 2018; San Diego, CA and Society for the Study of Inborn Errors of Metabolism Annual Symposium; September 4–7, 2018; Athens, Greece.

Authors' Contributions

Natalja Haninger-Vacariu and Gere Sunder-Plassmann drafted the manuscript. Natalja Haninger-Vacariu, Sarah El-Hadi, Udo Pauler, Marina Foretnik, Alice Schmidt, Nina Skuban, Jay A. Barth, Gere Sunder-Plassmann collected clinical data for this manuscript. Renate Kain did the histopatholgy analysis of kidney biopsies. Zoltán Prohászka did the complement-related analyses. All authors approved the final version of the manuscript. Natalja Haninger-Vacariu is the guarantor of this manuscript.

Acknowledgments

The authors thank the patient and her family. The patient was a part of the ATTRACT clinical trial which was funded by Amicus Therapeutics, Inc. Third-party medical writing assistance was provided by Lynn Brown, PhD, and Cindy Gobbel, PhD, of ApotheCom (Yardley, PA) and was supported by Amicus Therapeutics, Inc.

References

[1] S. Ishii, H. H. Chang, K. Kawasaki et al., "Mutant alpha-galactosidase a enzymes identified in Fabry disease patients with residual enzyme activity: biochemical characterization and restoration of normal intracellular processing by 1-deoxygalactonojirimycin," *Biochemical Journal*, vol. 406, no. 2, pp. 285–295, 2007.

[2] R. Schiffmann, D. A. Hughes, G. E. Linthorst et al., "Screening, diagnosis, and management of patients with Fabry disease: conclusions from a kidney disease: improving global outcomes (KDIGO) controversies conference," *Kidney International*, vol. 91, no. 2, pp. 284–293, 2017.

[3] D. P. Germain, "Fabry disease," *Orphanet Journal of Rare Diseases*, vol. 5, p. 30, 2010.

[4] R. Schiffmann and M. Ries, "Fabry disease: a disorder of childhood onset," *Pediatric Neurology*, vol. 64, pp. 10–20, 2016.

[5] C. M. Eng, D. P. Germain, M. Banikazemi et al., "Fabry disease: guidelines for the evaluation and management of multi-organ system involvement," *Genetics in Medicine*, vol. 8, no. 9, pp. 539–548, 2006.

[6] M. Biegstraaten, R. Arngrimsson, F. Barbey et al., "Recommendations for initiation and cessation of enzyme replacement therapy in patients with Fabry disease: the European Fabry Working Group consensus document," *Orphanet Journal of Rare Diseases*, vol. 10, 2015.

[7] G. Sunder-Plassmann, R. Schiffmann, and K. Nicholls, "Migalastat for the treatment of Fabry disease," *Expert Opinion on Orphan Drugs*, vol. 6, no. 5, pp. 301–309, 2018.

[8] D. A. Hughes, K. Nicholls, S. P. Shankar et al., "Oral pharmacological chaperone migalastat compared with enzyme replacement therapy in Fabry disease: 18-month results from the randomised phase III attract study," *Journal of Medical Genetics*, vol. 54, no. 4, pp. 288–296, 2017.

[9] Galafold [summary of product characteristics], *Amicus Therapeutics UK Ltd*, Amicus Therapeutics, Buckinghamshire, UK, 2017.

[10] D. P. Germain, D. A. Hughes, K. Nicholls et al., "Treatment of Fabry's disease with the pharmacologic chaperone migalastat," *New England Journal of Medicine*, vol. 375, no. 6, pp. 545–555, 2016.

[11] M. Gaggl, C. Aigner, D. Csuka et al., "Maternal and fetal outcomes of pregnancies in women with atypical hemolytic uremic syndrome," *Journal of the American Society of Nephrology*, vol. 29, no. 3, pp. 1020–1029, 2018.

[12] J. M. Thurman, "Complement in kidney disease: core curriculum 2015," *American Journal of Kidney Disease*, vol. 65, no. 1, pp. 156–168, 2015.

[13] P. A. Janssen, P. Thiessen, M. C. Klein, M. F. Whitfield, Y. C. MacNab, and S. C. Cullis-Kuhl, "Standards for the measurement of birth weight, length and head circumference at term in neonates of European, Chinese and South Asian ancestry," *Open Medicine*, vol. 1, no. 2, pp. e74–e88, 2007.

[14] J. A. Martin, B. E. Hamilton, M. J. K. Osterman, A. K. Driscoll, and P. Drake, "Births: final data for 2016," *National Vital Statistics Reports*, vol. 67, no. 1, pp. 1–55, 2018.

[15] B. D. Magee, D. Hattis, and N. M. Kivel, "Role of smoking in low birth weight," *Journal of Reproductive Medicine*, vol. 49, no. 1, pp. 23–27, 2004.

[16] P. P. Pereira, F. A. Da Mata, A. C. Figueiredo, K. R. C. de Andrade, and M. G. Pereira, "Maternal active smoking during pregnancy and low birth weight in the Americas: a systematic review and meta-analysis," *Nicotine & Tobacco Research*, vol. 19, no. 5, pp. 497–505, 2017.

[17] E. Parent, J. R. Wax, W. Smith et al., "Fabry disease complicating pregnancy," *The Journal of Maternal-Fetal & Neonatal Medicine*, vol. 23, no. 10, pp. 1253–1256, 2010.

[18] G. Kalkum, D. Macchiella, J. Reinke, H. Kölbl, and M. Beck, "Enzyme replacement therapy with agalsidase alfa in pregnant women with Fabry disease," *European Journal of Obstetrics, Gynecology, and Reproductive Biology*, vol. 144, no. 1, pp. 92–93, 2009.

[19] S. Wendt, C. Whybra, C. Kampmann, E. Teichmann, and M. Beck, "Successful pregnancy outcome in a patient with Fabry disease receiving enzyme replacement therapy with agalsidase alfa," *Journal of Inherited Metabolic Disease*, vol. 28, no. 5, pp. 787–788, 2005.

[20] C. V. Madsen, E. I. Christensen, R. Nielsen, H. Mogensen, Å. K. Rasmussen, and U. Feldt-Rasmussen, "Enzyme replacement therapy during pregnancy in Fabry patients: review of published cases of live births and a new case of a severely affected female with Fabry disease and pre-eclampsia complicating pregnancy," *Journal of Inherited Metabolic Disorders Reports*, vol. 44, pp. 93–101, 2019.

[21] B. L. Thurberg and J. M. Politei, "Histologic abnormalities of placental tissues in Fabry disease: a case report and review of the literature," *Human Pathology*, vol. 43, no. 4, pp. 610–614, 2012.

[22] E. Senocak Tasci and Z. Bicik, "Safe and successful treatment with agalsidase beta during pregnancy in fabry disease," *Iranian Journal of Kidney Diseases*, vol. 9, no. 5, pp. 406–408, 2015.

[23] J. M. Politei, "Treatment with agalsidase beta during pregnancy in Fabry disease," *Journal of Obstetric Gynaecology Research*, vol. 36, no. 2, pp. 428–429, 2010.

[24] D. P. Germain, P. Bruneval, T. C. Tran, P. Balouet, B. Richalet, and K. Benistan, "Uneventful pregnancy outcome after enzyme replacement therapy with agalsidase beta in a heterozygous female with Fabry disease: a case report," *European Journal of Medical Genetics*, vol. 53, no. 2, pp. 111–112, 2010.

[25] M. G. Bouwman, C. E. M. Hollak, M. A. van den Bergh Weerman, F. A. Wijburg, and G. E. Linthorst, "Analysis of placental tissue in fabry disease with and without enzyme replacement therapy," *Placenta*, vol. 31, no. 4, pp. 344–346, 2010.

[26] F. C. Battaglia and L. O. Lubchenco, "A practical classification of newborn infants by weight and gestational age," *The Journal of Pediatrics*, vol. 71, no. 2, pp. 159–163, 1967.

9

Aortic Dissection in a Pregnant Patient without Other Risk Factors

Priya V. Patel[1], **Raanan Alter**[2], **Recia Frenn**[1] and **Thaddeus P. Waters**[1]

[1]*Department of Obstetrics and Gynecology, Loyola University Medical Center, Maywood, IL, USA*
[2]*Department of Gynecology Oncology, University of Chicago, Chicago, IL, USA*

Correspondence should be addressed to Priya V. Patel; priya.patel@lumc.edu

Academic Editor: Irene Hoesli

Background. An aortic dissection is a life-threatening condition in which the intima of the artery tears causing separation of the intima and media. Pregnancy places women at a significantly increased risk of common vascular events including venous thromboembolism, myocardial infarction, and stroke, while also increasing the risk of rarer vascular events such as aortic dissection and aortic rupture. *Case.* A 30-year-old previously healthy multiparous woman presenting at 36 weeks of pregnancy with a Type A aortic dissection. She underwent a combined emergent cesarean delivery followed by repair of her aortic root. *Conclusions.* Aortic dissection should be high on the differential for pregnant patients presenting with the characteristic complaints and physical exam findings given the high mortality rate associated with this vascular event. *Teaching Points.* (1) This report reviews the characteristic presentation, risk factors, and physical exam findings in a patient with an aortic dissection. (2) The report includes treatment options for pregnant patients based on the classification of the dissection.

1. Introduction

An aortic dissection is a life-threatening condition in which the intima, the inner layer of the aorta, tears causing the intima and media, the middle layer, to dissect [1]. There are two main systems for classifying aortic dissections, the DeBakey system and the Stanford classification system. The DeBakey system is an anatomical description of the aortic dissection, categorizing it by where the original intimal tear is located and the extent of the dissection. The Stanford classification is divided into two groups depending on whether the ascending aorta is involved or not. Risk factors for acute aortic syndromes include hypertension, gender, age, family history, connective tissue diseases (i.e., Ehlers-Danlos syndrome and Marfans syndrome), heavy smoking, vascular inflammation, trauma, and pregnancy. The most common presenting symptom is pain, described as severe and sharp, unlike any pain experienced before. The pain occurs in over 90% of patients, with 85% noting the onset of pain to be abrupt and causing the patient to seek medical attention immediately [2]. On physical exam, patients with an aortic dissection may have a pulse deficit, new diastolic murmur, hypotension, or widened pulse pressure. Work-up typically includes 12-lead EKG, troponin, d-dimer, and cardiac imaging. EKG findings typically show nonspecific ST-T wave changes that may mimic myocardial ischemia, thought to be due to an acute decrease in perfusion of the coronary arteries [3]. Troponin levels are often only mildly elevated whereas D-dimer levels are typically markedly elevated compared to the normal elevations expected during pregnancy. Diagnosis is based on imaging with either CT, MRI, or transthoracic/transesophageal echocardiogram (TTE/TEE), which would show intimal separation with a true and false lumen [2].

The pregnant state places women at a significantly increased risk of common vascular events including venous thromboembolism, myocardial infarction, and stroke, while also increasing the risk of more uncommon vascular events such as aortic dissection and aortic rupture. These rare vascular events can often lead to death of the mother and fetus without prompt treatment [4]. The pregnant state places women at risk due to an increase in circulating blood volume and cardiac output that lead to vascular structural changes. The pathophysiology of aortic dissection in pregnancy is likely related to these known vascular and structural changes leading to degeneration of the aortic media, cystic medial necrosis, and an increased aortic diameter and compliance [5].

Clinical documentation of aortic dissection in pregnancy is limited. As such, there is a lack of clinical trials determining definitive protocols to prevent, screen, and treat pregnant patients with an aortic dissection. This case report aims to describe a patient presenting in the third trimester of pregnancy with an acute diagnosis of a Stanford Type A aortic dissection and review treatment options and outcomes.

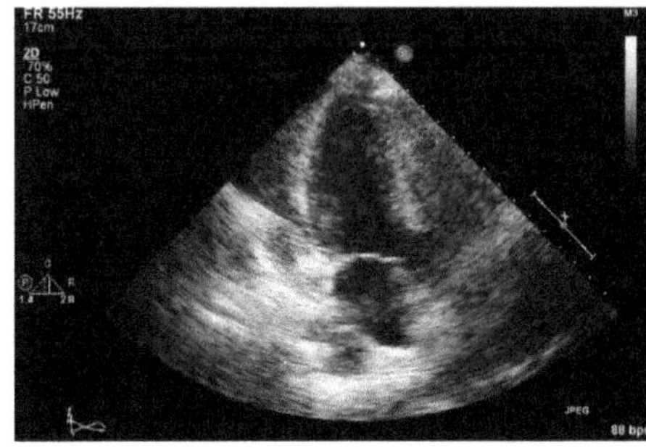

FIGURE 1: TTE of ascending aorta [6].

2. Case

The patient was a 30-year-old G2P1001 at 36 weeks and 4 days who was transferred to Loyola University Medical Center (LUMC) with a Type A aortic dissection. Her pregnancy was complicated by gestational hypertension that had been diagnosed one week prior to her initial presentation. Baseline HELLP labs (which include a CBC, CMP, and urine protein to creatinine ratio) were obtained and were normal at that time. The patient's blood type was O negative and antibody negative and she was Group B streptococcus positive; her serologies were otherwise unremarkable. She had had a prior normal spontaneous vaginal delivery at term without complications. Her past medical history and past surgical history were otherwise noncontributory. She had been taking her prenatal vitamins daily. She was a former smoker having quit one year prior; her social history was otherwise negative for alcohol or recreational drug use. The patient had a negative family history of connective tissue disease or aortic dissection.

She initially presented to an outside hospital two weeks prior to her admission to LUMC, complaining of left-sided chest pain; initial evaluation with EKG and CTPE was negative for acute coronary syndrome and pulmonary embolism and she was discharged home. Over the subsequent two weeks, her chest pain had slowly improved. On the day of her presentation to LUMC, however, her pain acutely increased, characterized as "sharp" and "tearing." At the outside hospital, CTPE was negative, though the retrospective read of her second CT identified the aortic dissection. EKG showed mild ST-depression and her troponin levels were increased to 1.75. On physical exam, the patient was tachycardic with normal blood pressures and oxygen saturation; she was found to have a new continuous aortic murmur with bounding pulses. She was sent for a TTE with the final read showing evidence of dilation of the ascending aorta (4.2cm) with a dissection flap of aorta seen in the ascending aorta and aortic arch, severe aortic regurgitation, and severe diastolic dysfunction (Figure 1).

She was transferred to our tertiary care center. On presentation to LUMC, her blood pressures were mild range and her HELLP labs and coagulation factors were normal. The fetus had a category I tracing. She was consented for cesarean delivery with repair of aortic dissection. She underwent a primary low transverse cesarean section under general anesthesia; total estimated blood loss (EBL) for this portion of the case was 1L. She was given Pitocin, misoprostol, and a B-lynch was performed for uterine atony. As there was concern for potential coagulopathy related to her aortic repair, a JP drain was left in place. She delivered a liveborn male infant with APGAR score of 9/9 and an umbilical artery pH of 7.34 with a 1+ base excess. After completing the obstetrics portion of the case, the patient underwent an emergency repair of the aortic dissection with resuspension of the aortic valve, primary repair of the left main ostial dissection, insertion of a hemishield graft, and cut-down of the left femoral artery. She was given 4L of cardioplegia, a sterile, isotonic crystalloid solution used to induce cardiac stasis and protect the myocardium during open-heart surgery, and was placed on cardiac bypass during the procedure with a pump time of 230 minutes and a cross-clamp time of 208 minutes [7]. The patient received 500cc of cell saver, 1U of platelets, 2U of FFP, 1U of cryoprecipitate, and 1U of pRBCs; total EBL for the second portion of the case was 800mL. Her postoperative course was uncomplicated, and she was discharged home on postoperative day seven with a hemoglobin of 7.4 and planning to use the copper IUD for contraception.

3. Discussion

Aortic dissection in the pregnant population is a relatively uncommon but can be catastrophic for both the mother and fetus. For Type A dissections, mortality increases by 1-3% per hour after presentation, increasing to 25% after 24 hours, 70% by 1 week, and 80% mortality by 2 weeks. Aortic dissection in pregnancy occurs more commonly in the third trimester due to the hyperdynamic state and the hormonal effect on vasculature [8]. In the nonpregnant population, a majority of cases of aortic dissection occur in patients with a previously dilated and therefore weakened aorta; however, in pregnancy, this finding may be absent [6]. Though aortic complications in pregnancy have been reported in women with Marfan syndrome, the vascular type of Ehlers-Danlos syndrome, Turner syndrome, Loeys-Dietz syndrome, and congenital aortic malformations such as bicuspid aortic valve, the majority of cases in the pregnant population occur in women without any other known risk factors [4]. Of note, the only risk factors the presented patient had were pregnancy and a prepregnancy history of tobacco use. Typical for the gravid women with a dissection, the patient presented with nonspecific chest pain. This case highlights the importance of vigilance in evaluating pregnant women with new onset cardiopulmonary symptoms that could be related to one of several life-threatening etiologies.

For Stanford Type A dissections, the mainstay of treatment is surgery whereas, for Type B dissections, treatment involves medical management. Surgical management involves excision of the intimal tear, obliteration of entry into the proximal false lumen, reconstitution of the aorta with interposition of a synthetic vascular graft, and repair or replacement of the aortic valve. Medical management involves beta-blocker administration with the goal to keep blood pressures below 120/80 and endovascular stent grafting for patients with complications related to their dissection. Complications include occlusion of a major aortic branch with end-organ ischemia and persistent severe hypertension or chest pain [7]. When surgically managing pregnant patients beyond 24 weeks' gestation with an aortic dissection, emergent cesarean delivery is recommended before the mother is placed on cardiac bypass. In patients below 24 weeks' gestation, individualized discussions are needed as the risk of fetal demise is high, and delivery does not demonstrate improvement in maternal circulation [8]. Given the high mortality rate of aortic dissections, pregnant patients with and without risk factors should be treated with a high index of suspicion when presenting with characteristic complaints and physical exam findings of aortic dissection.

Consent

Human subjects: written consent was obtained by the participant in this study.

References

[1] J. Cui, Z. Jing, and S. Zhuang, "D-dimer as a biomarker for acute aortic dissection: a systematic review and meta-analysis," *Journal of Vascular Surgery*, vol. 61, no. 5, p. 1377, 2015.

[2] J. Golembiewski and N. Bourtsos, "Cardioplegia solution," *Journal of Pharmacy Practice*, vol. 6, no. 4, pp. 182–189, 2016.

[3] K. Hirata, M. Wake, T. Takahashi, and J. Nakazato, "Electrocardiographic changes in patients with acute aortic dissection -incidence, patterns and underlying mechanisms in 280 cases," *Journal of the American College of Cardiology*, vol. 59, no. 13, p. E562, 2012.

[4] P. G. Hagan, C. A. Nienaber, E. M. Isselbacher et al., "The international registry of acute aortic dissection (IRAD): new insights into an old disease," *Journal of the American Medical Association*, vol. 283, no. 7, pp. 897–903, 2000.

[5] P. D. Patel and R. R. Arora, "Pathophysiology, diagnosis, and management of aortic dissection," *Therapeutic Advances in Cardiovascular Disease*, vol. 2, no. 6, pp. 439–468, 2008.

[6] Nawwar Al-Attar, "Acute aortic dissection," *Aortic Diseases*, pp. 55–112, 2009.

[7] J. Zhu, W. Ma, S. Peterss et al., "Aortic dissection in pregnancy: management strategy and outcomes," *The Annals of Thoracic Surgery*, vol. 103, no. 4, pp. 1199–1206, 2017.

[8] L. Kinney-Ham, H. Nguyen, R. Steele, and E. Walters, "Acute aortic dissection in third trimester pregnancy without risk factors," *Western Journal of Emergency Medicine*, vol. 12, no. 4, pp. 571–574, 2011.

10

Giant Vulvar Condylomata: Two Cases and a Review of the Literature

Funda Gungor Ugurlucan,[1] Cenk Yasa,[1] Omer Demir,[1] Ozlem Dural,[1] Ekrem Yavuz,[2] and Suleyman Engin Akhan[1]

[1]*Istanbul University Istanbul Faculty of Medicine, Department of Obstetrics and Gynecology, Turkey*
[2]*Istanbul University Istanbul Faculty of Medicine, Department of Pathology, Turkey*

Correspondence should be addressed to Funda Gungor Ugurlucan; fgungor@yahoo.com

Academic Editor: Erich Cosmi

Introduction. Giant vulvar condyloma is usually associated with the HPV subtypes 6 and 11 and is characterized by excessive growth of verrucous lesions on the genitals and/or perianal region. It may be observed in sexually inactive as well as sexually active women. Immunosuppression plays an important role in the development of the disease. *Patients and Methods.* We report two cases of giant vulvar condyloma together with the review of the literature. *Results.* One case was a 21-year old sexually inactive woman with a history of Type 1 Diabetes. Second case was a 20-year-old sexually active woman with a rapidly progressing disease and cervical dysplasia. Both cases were operated; all the condylomatous structures were resected with preservation of the anatomy and clitoral innervation and blood flow. Skin and subcuticular dehiscence was the only complication encountered in the first case. *Conclusion.* Main treatment of giant vulvar condyloma is surgical resection with maintenance of the vulvar anatomy. Preservation of especially the clitoral innervation as much as possible is very important.

1. Introduction

Genital human papilloma virus (HPV) infections are transmitted primarily through sexual contact, with a lifetime risk of 50-80% [1]. The highest rate of genital HPV infection has been identified in adults between 18 and 28 years of age [2]. Vulvar condyloma is a sexually transmitted disease caused by Human Papillomavirus (HPV). Giant vulvar condyloma, also called Buschke-Löwenstein tumor, was first described by Abraham Buschke and Loewenstein Ludwig in 1925 [3]. Giant condyloma is usually associated with the HPV subtypes 6 and 11 and is characterized by excessive growth of verrucous lesions on the genitals and/or perianal region and is considered benign with high rate of recurrence and low risk of malignant transformation [4]. Host's immunity plays an important role in the development of the disease. Main risk factors for giant condylomas include smoking, having multiple sexual partners, chronic genital infections, poor hygiene, and immune deficiencies. Surgical excision is the treatment of choice in the management of giant condylomas.

Here we present two cases with giant vulvar condylomas and their management with a review of the literature.

2. Cases

2.1. Case 1. A 22-year-old sexually inactive woman presented with a rapidly growing mass in the vulva and perianal region. The lesions appeared 3 months before presentation and developed rapidly. The patient had no sexual activity. She was a regular smoker and the medical history included Type 1 diabetes mellitus for 15 years. The serologic screening for Hepatitis B (HBsAg), Hepatitis C (Anti-HCV), Human Immunodeficiency Virus (Anti-HIV), and syphilis (VDRL) was negative. Patient had no history of sexual diseases. On physical examination, a giant mass thought of as a giant condyloma, extending from the mons pubis till the anal mucosal lining and distorting the labial and clitoral anatomy was observed [Figure 1]. Biopsy of the lesion revealed a condyloma. Under general anesthesia a Foley catheter was introduced. Partial

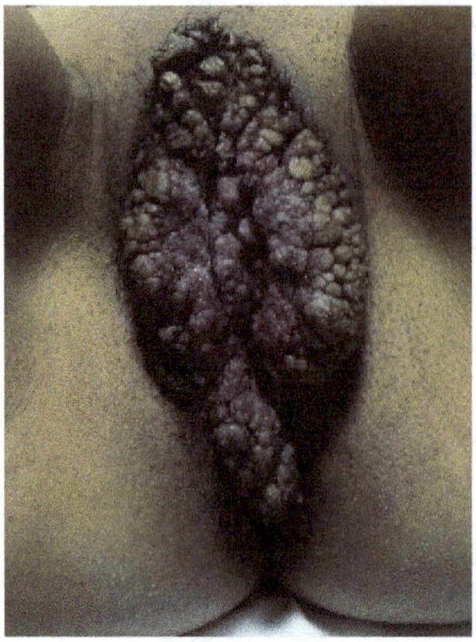

FIGURE 1: The appearance of Case 1 with distortion of labial and clitoral anatomy.

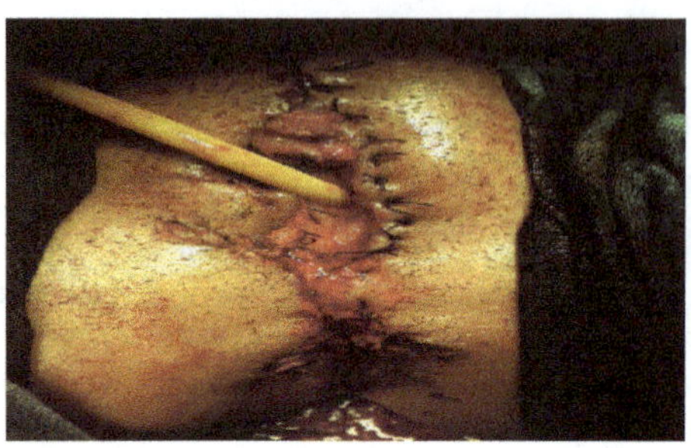

FIGURE 2: The appearance of Case 1 immediately after surgical resection.

skinning vulvectomy was performed with preservation of clitoral and labial anatomy and all condylomatous structures were removed. Incisions were sutured primarily using single mattress sutures with No: 2/0 polyglactin [Figure 2]. No complications developed during the operation. Mobility was restricted and oral antibiotics were used in the postoperative period and the Foley catheter was left in situ. On the postoperative 5th day, a 2-3 cm wound dehiscence involving the skin and subcuticular fatty tissue developed on the perineal area near the anal orifice and was treated with secondary healing using sitz baths, antibiotics, and topical creams [Figure 3]. Pathology report revealed condyloma acuminatum [Figures 4(a) and 4(b)]. No recurrences developed during one year of follow-up.

2.2. Case 2. A 20-year old sexually active woman presented with a giant vulvar mass involving the vulva and the anal area. Lesions began to develop 5 months before presentation and developed rapidly. Medical history was unremarkable. Serologic screening for Hepatitis B (HBsAg), Hepatitis C (Anti-HCV), Human Immunodeficiency Virus (Anti-HIV), and syphilis (VDRL) was negative. Patient had no history

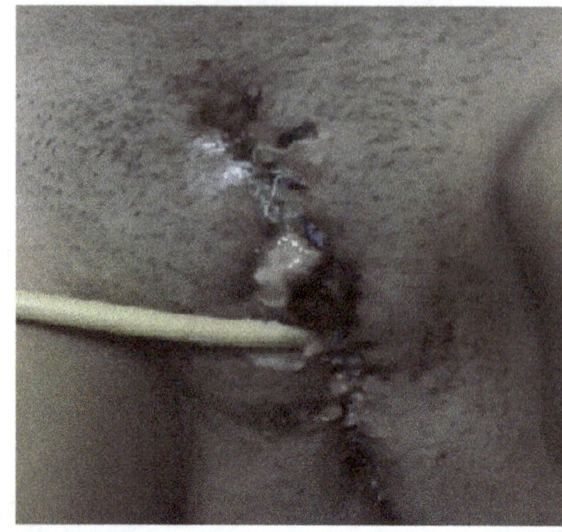

FIGURE 3: Postoperative appearance of Case 1.

of sexually transmitted diseases. Physical examination of the patient revealed condylomatous masses extending from the lower perineum to the intergluteal folds [Figure 5]. Biopsy of the lesion revealed a condyloma. PAP-smear was obtained and the result was low-grade squamous intraepithelial lesion. Colposcopy was performed and biopsy was taken from acetowhite areas which revealed cervical intraepithelial neoplasia (CIN)-II and follow-up was planned for cervical dysplasia. Under general anesthesia the condylomatous lesions were excised sharply and the condylomatous tissues around the clitoris were cauterized in order to preserve the anatomy and innervation of the clitoris. Drains were inserted in the gluteal incisions [Figure 6]. No complications developed during the postoperative period. Pathology report revealed condyloma acuminatum [Figures 7(a) and 7(b)]. No recurrences developed and the cervical dysplasia regressed during one year of follow-up.

3. Discussion

Buschke-Loewenstein tumor is a sexually transmitted disease caused by HPV subtypes 6 and 11, with benign histological features, but with excessive local growth and high recurrence rates [4]. They may rarely be associated with high-risk HPV types such as HPV type 16 [5]. Main site of appearance is the vulva in women and it is almost always preceded by condyloma acuminate [4]. The overgrowth results in hygienic problems, increases the risk of secondary infections, and distorts the genital image, which leads to social and psychological damage. Rarely giant condyloma may be associated with fistula formation. The host's immunodeficiency is important in the progression of disease; rapid progression and recurrences are usually associated with various types of immunodeficiency [6].

Rachman and Hasan reported a case of a 42-year-old woman presenting with giant vulvar condyloma diagnosed with systemic lupus erythematosus (SLE) one year ago and treated with surgical excision [7]. The patient was using methylprednisolone and mycophenolate mofetil and HPV types 6 and 11 were isolated from the vulva, vagina, and

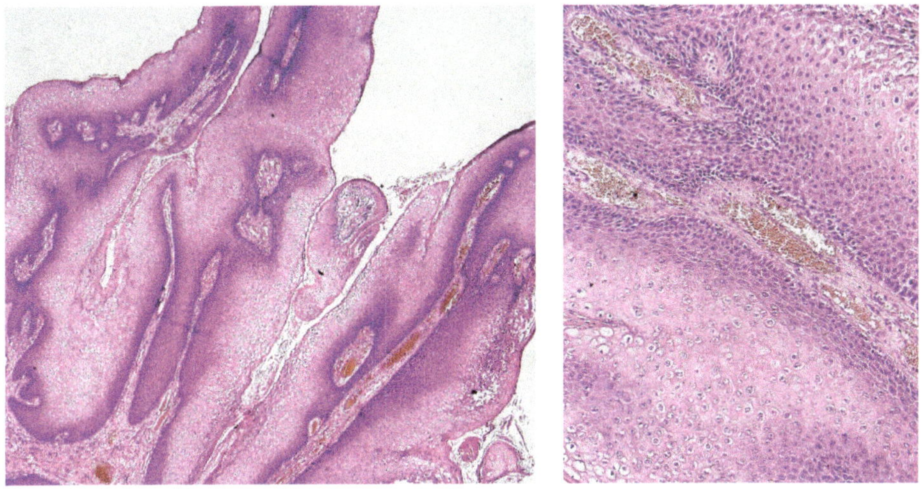

(a) (b)

FIGURE 4: Histology of giant condyloma of Case 1. (a) x4 magnification (b) x20 magnification.

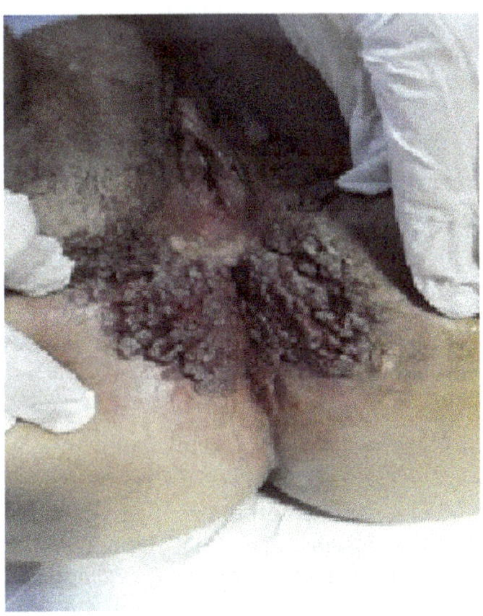

FIGURE 5: The appearance of Case 2 with main involvement of the anal region.

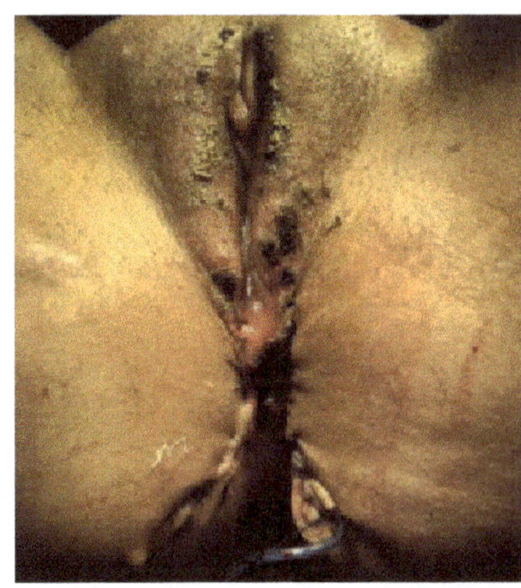

FIGURE 6: The appearance of Case 2 immediately after surgical resection.

the cervix. Lube et al. reported that 289 of 5682 patients in the pediatric rheumatology unit were diagnosed with SLE and 4 of the 289 had giant condyloma acuminata (1.4%). All patients were under corticosteroid and immunosuppressant treatment [8].

CostaPinto et al. reported a 33-year-old patient diagnosed with SLE during pregnancy presenting with giant vulvar condyloma after delivery [9]. The patient was started on corticosteroids, immunosuppressant treatment including mycophenolate mofetil after pregnancy. Topical treatment with trichloroacetic acid, imiquimod, and podophyllin were only partially effective.

Petrini et al. reported a case of a 16-year-old patient with alcohol consumption and illicit drug usage [4]. The authors linked the appearance of the disease in this young patient with associated immunosuppression. Trombetta and Place reviewed the 51 cases published in the literature and observed that the disease was more frequent among men with a male to female ratio of 2.7 [10]. They also observed that the disease was becoming more common among younger people, with a rate of 3.5 in people less than 50 years of age. Both of our cases were young and one was sexually inactive. One had type I diabetes, which is an immunosuppressive state, and was a regular smoker. On the other hand, second case had no apparent immunosuppressive predisposing factor, but she was sexually active, yet the lesion developed quite rapidly.

Main treatment of giant vulvar condylomas is surgical excision. Apart from the aesthetic appearance of giant vulvar condylomas and the difficulty of surgical treatment, it is even more important to note that vulvar verrucous carcinoma should be included in the differential diagnosis of

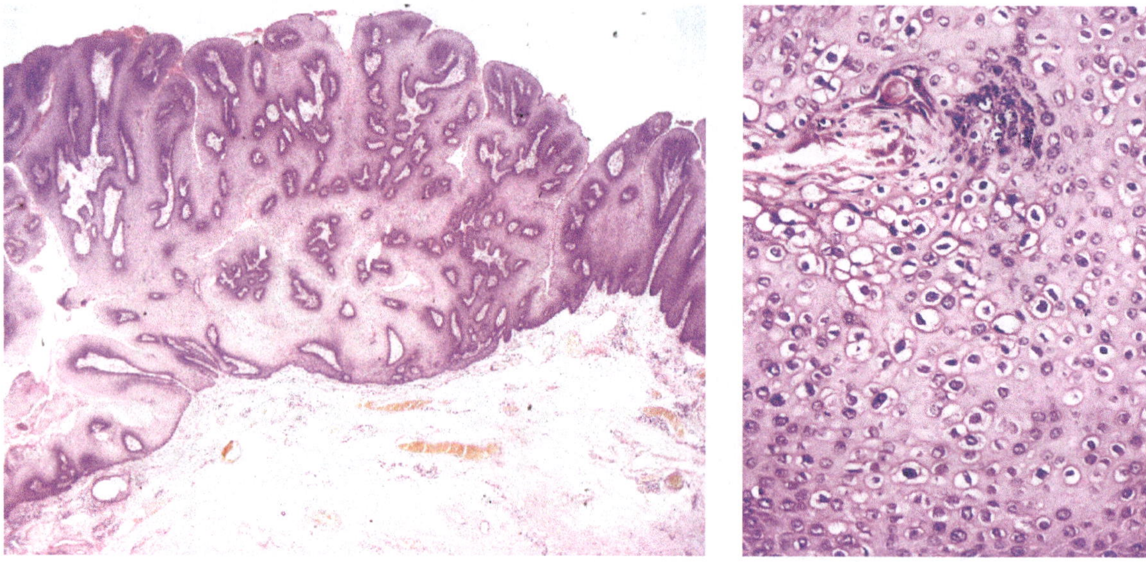

(a) (b)

FIGURE 7: The histology of giant condyloma of Case 2. (a) x2 magnification (b) x40 magnification.

giant vulvar condylomas. Zerkan et al. reported a case of giant vulvar condyloma, which was resistant to conservative treatment and operated five times. The definitive pathologic examination revealed superficial vulvar carcinoma [11]. Liu et al. described six cases of vulvar verrucous carcinoma and three of these were accidentally diagnosed as giant vulvar condylomata [12]. Authors suggested that these tumors should be distinguished from giant condyloma acuminatum and well-differentiated squamous cell carcinoma, and surgery is the most effective treatment.

In conclusion, giant vulvar condylomas, which are caused by low-risk HPV types and treated with surgery, should be distinguished from verrucous carcinoma. Local aggressively growing vulvar condylomata, are seen more often in women with immunosuppression and should be treated as soon as they are diagnosed.

Consent

Informed consent was obtained from all individual participants included in the study.

Authors' Contributions

Ugurlucan did the project development, data collection, and manuscript writing. Yasa performed data collection, manuscript writing. Demir did data collection, manuscript writing. Dural did data collection. Yavuz did data collection, manuscript writing. Akhan did project development, manuscript writing.

References

[1] K. V. Shah, P. J. Snijders, and C. J. Meijer, "International agency for research on cancer multicenter cervical cancer study group: epidemiologic classification of human papillomavirus types associated with cervical cancer," *The New England Journal of Medicine*, vol. 348, Article ID 518527, 2003.

[2] L. Koutsky, "Epidemiology of genital human papillomavirus infection," *American Journal of Medicine*, vol. 102, no. 38, 1997.

[3] C. Steffen, "The men behind the eponym - Abraham Buschke and Ludwig Lowenstein: Giant condyloma (Buschke-Loewenstein)," *American Journal of Dermatopathology*, vol. 28, no. 6, pp. 526–536, 2006.

[4] C. Petrini, P. Melli, P. Magnani et al., "Giant condyloma (buschke-loewenstein tumor) in a 16-year-old patient," *Revista Brasileira de Ginecologia e Obstetrícia/RBGO Gynecology and Obstetrics*, vol. 38, no. 09, pp. 471–476, 2016.

[5] P. S. Bhageerathy, M. Cecilia, A. Sebastian et al., "Human papilloma virus-16 causing giant condyloma acuminata," *Journal of Surgical Case Reports*, vol. 1, 2014.

[6] F. Niazy, K. Rostami, and A. R. Motabar, "Giant condyloma acuminatum of vulva frustrating treatment challenge," *World Journal of Plastic Surgery*, vol. 4, no. 2, pp. 159–162, 2015.

[7] A. Rachman and N. Hasan, "Giant condyloma acuminata in indonesian females with sle under immunosuppressant and steroid therapy," *Case Reports in Immunology*, vol. 2016, Article ID 4710979, 6 pages, 2016.

[8] G. Lube, N. E. Aikawa, M. Tacla et al., "Condyloma acuminatum by human papillomavirus infection in childhood-systemic lupus erythematosus patients," *Acta Rheumatologica Portuguesa*, vol. 39, no. 2, pp. 182–187, 2014.

[9] L. Costapinto, M. F. R. Grassi, K. Serravalle, A. C. V. Travessa, V. N. O. Olavarria, and M. B. Santiago, "Giant disseminated condylomatosis in SLE," *Lupus*, vol. 21, no. 3, pp. 332–334, 2012.

[10] L. J. Trombetta and R. J. Place, "Giant condyloma acuminatum of the anorectum: trends in epidemiology and management. report of a case and review of the literature," *Diseases of the Colon & Rectum*, vol. 44, no. 12, pp. 1878–1886, 2001.

[11] J. Zekan, D. Petrovic, S. El-Safadi, M. Banovic, D. Hulina, and Z. Hrgovic, "A surgical approach to giant condyloma (buschke-löwenstein tumour) with underlying superficial vulvar carcinoma: a case report," *Oncology Letters*, vol. 5, no. 2, pp. 541–543, 2013.

[12] G. Liu, Q. Li, X. Shang et al., "Verrucous carcinoma of the vulva: a 20 year retrospective study and literature review," *Journal of Lower Genital Tract Disease*, vol. 20, no. 1, pp. 114–118, 2016.

11

Torsion of a Large Myomatous Uterus Associated with Progressive Renal Failure and Paralytic Ileus in an 86-Year-Old Woman

Guiwen Wang, Hiroshi Ishikawa, Asuka Sato, and Makio Shozu

Department of Reproductive Medicine, Graduate School of Medicine, Chiba University, Chiba 260-8670, Japan

Correspondence should be addressed to Hiroshi Ishikawa; ishikawa@chiba-u.jp

Academic Editor: Seung-Yup Ku

Uterine torsion of a nongravid uterus is rare, and proper diagnosis is challenging. Herein, we report a case of torsion of a large myomatous uterus in an 86-year-old woman who was presented with progressive renal failure and paralytic ileus. She was presented with abdominal discomfort, loss of appetite, and oliguria. A large myomatous uterus with broad calcification was identified when she underwent surgery to repair an umbilical hernia one year before the symptoms developed. Computed tomography revealed that one year later, the myomatous uterus significantly increased in size and the calcified lesion of the fibroid was largely displaced. She was also presented with paralytic ileus, and her general condition progressively worsened. Her serum creatinine levels were increased (3.5 mg/dL) and hemoglobin levels were low (8.5 g/dL). Emergency laparotomy revealed that the uterus was rotated 360 degrees clockwise at the level of the isthmus. The uterus was discolored, appearing dark red, and accompanied by broad congestion, and the cervix was elongated. The patient's renal function and ileus recovered after a hysterectomy. In conclusion, torsion of a large myomatous uterus could become life-threatening in an oldest-old woman, and early release of the torsion is necessary to avoid serious complications.

1. Introduction

Uterine torsion, defined as rotation of the uterine body by more than 45 degrees around the long axis of the uterus, is a rare but serious condition [1]. Most of the reported cases of uterine torsion involve a gravid uterus; however, a large myomatous uterus is another potential cause for uterine torsion [2, 3]. The uterus in its normal state has little mobility, as it is firmly held by round ligaments, broad ligaments, and sacrouterine ligaments; however, a large, heavy uterus such as a gravid or myomatous uterus may rotate, exerting traction on the uterus.

The most common symptom in women with uterine torsion is abdominal pain, but the presentation is nonspecific and variable, and can include vaginal bleeding, gastrointestinal problems, and urinary discomfort [3]. In addition, the symptoms vary from mild to severe, and they have the potential to progress into a life-threatening condition.

Herein, we report a case of torsion of a large myomatous uterus in an 86-year-old woman who was presented with progressive renal dysfunction, severe anemia, and paralytic ileus.

2. Case Presentation

An 86-year-old woman (2 gravida, 2 para), who was presented with an increased pelvic mass, was referred to our facility. She had undergone surgery to repair an umbilical hernia one year previously, and a large abdominal mass with broad calcification, measuring 16 × 13 × 13.1 cm (longitudinal × transverse × anteroposterior), was identified by plain computed tomography (CT) before the hernia repair surgery. The mass was consistent with a uterus containing calcified uterine fibroids (Figure 1(a)). The patient felt the increased pelvic mass and experienced gastric discomfort related to the stomach being compressed by the mass, resulting in complete appetite loss for the previous week. She was also presented with continuous uterine bleeding and urinary discomfort. The latest CT examination showed that the myomatous uterus significantly increased in size, measuring 27 × 16.5 × 17 cm (Figure 1(b)), and the calcified lesion was largely displaced (Figures 1(c) and 1(d)).

On admission, her height was 150 cm and body weight was 60 kg. Her body temperature was 35.8°C, pulse rate was

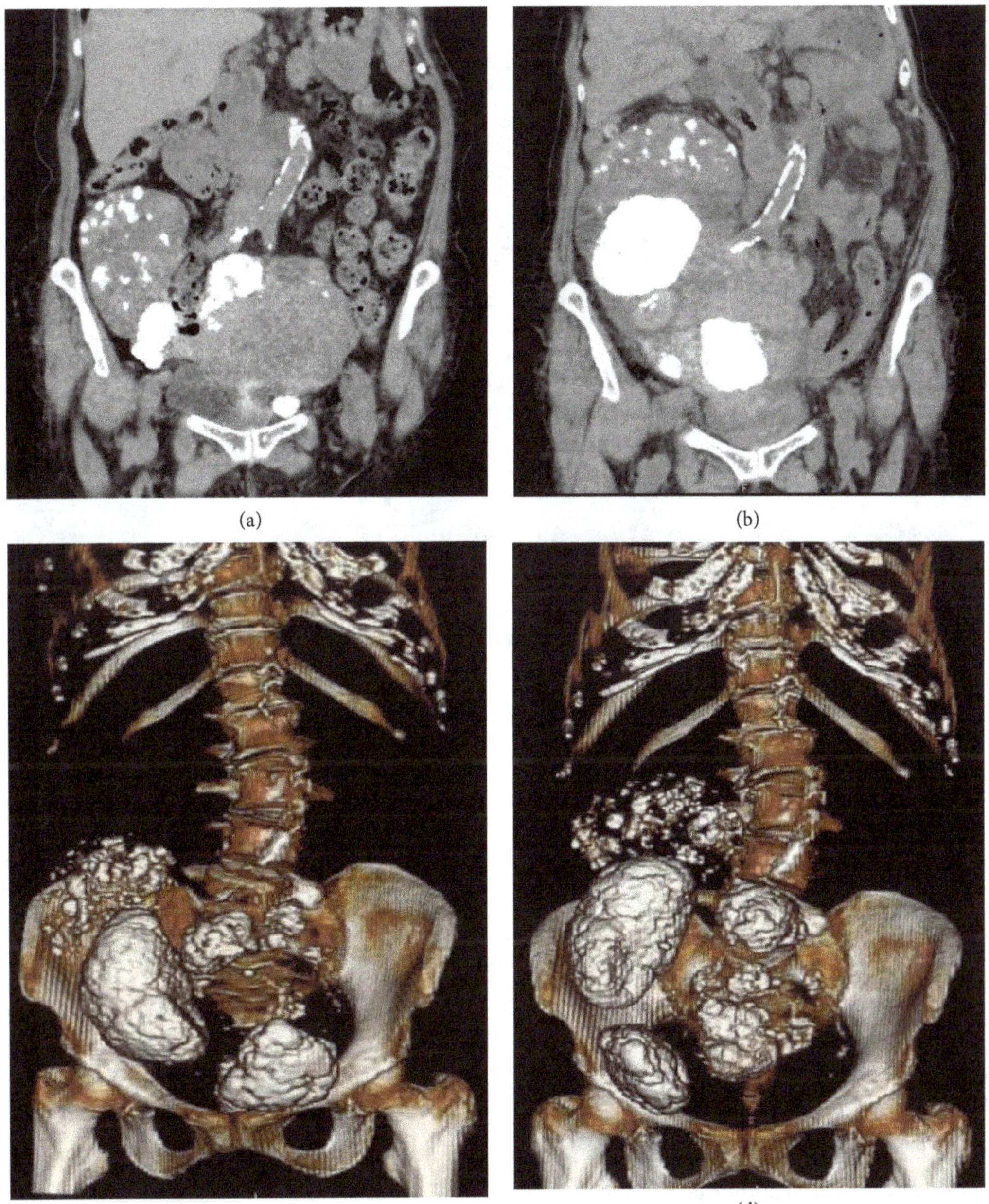

(a) (b) (c) (d)

FIGURE 1: Computed tomography (CT) findings of the myomatous uterus. (a) Coronal section of the abdomen one year before the uterine torsion. The myomatous uterus and calcified portion are observed. (b) Coronal section of the abdomen at the time of uterine torsion. The myomatous uterus significantly increased in size, and the calcified lesion was displaced. (c) Three-dimensional reconstruction images of the lower abdomen one year before the uterine torsion. (d) Three-dimensional reconstruction images of the lower abdomen at the time of uterine torsion. The calcified area inside the uterus was largely displaced.

81/min, and blood pressure was 88/40 mmHg. Although she was lucid, her Eastern Cooperative Oncology Group (ECOG) performance status was level 3, accompanied by disabling fatigue [4]. Her abdomen was distended by an irregular hard mass equivalent to 28 weeks' gestation. There was mild tenderness without rebound tenderness on the mass. On pelvic examination, the portio was normal and no vaginal bleeding was observed. Transabdominal ultrasound showed a large pelvic mass with peripheral calcification suggestive of uterine fibroids. Both ovaries were undetectable and minimal ascites was observed. Both kidneys were normal, with no dilatation of the renal pelvis and ureter. Plain CT images revealed that the uterine cervix was elongated and moved upward compared with its position one year before (Figure 2).

Blood tests showed an elevated white blood cell count (32,500/μL), low hemoglobin levels (9.9 g/dL), elevated C-reactive protein (16.4 mg/dL), and high serum creatinine (2.45 mg/dL). We initially suspected a malignant tumor arising from the uterus or ovary, such as uterine leiomyosarcoma, carcinosarcoma, or ovarian cancer, based on the patient's

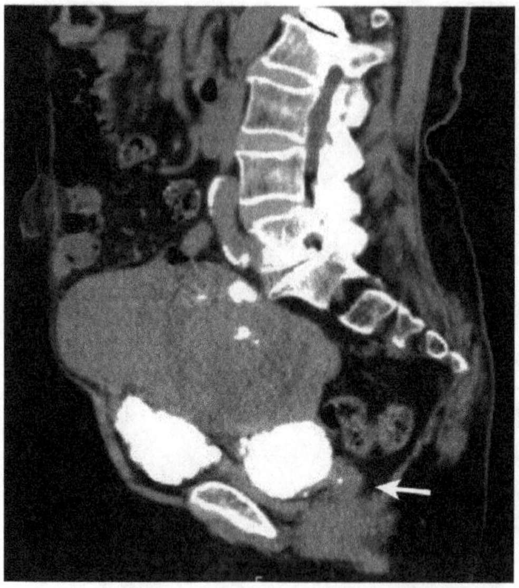

(a)

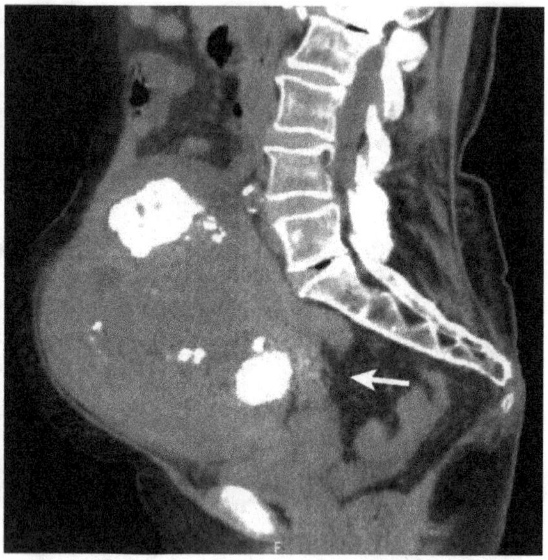

(b)

FIGURE 2: CT findings of the cervix. (a) Axial section of the lower abdomen one year before the uterine torsion. (b) Axial section of the lower abdomen at the time of uterine torsion. The cervix was elongated and moved upward compared with its position one year before (arrow).

advanced age, abnormal uterine bleeding, rapidly growing abdominal mass, and ascites. Therefore, we performed cervical cytology, endometrial cytology, and a puncture of the pouch of Douglas to assess the cytology of the ascites. The results of all cytological examinations were negative for malignancy. Transvaginal ultrasonography revealed that the endometrium was thin; therefore, we did not perform an endometrial biopsy. On the second hospital day, the patient's vital signs were stable, but her ECOG performance status fell to level 4. She was completely confined to the bed and could not carry out any self-care tasks; this change in status was accompanied by delirium. Paralytic ileus developed and her bowel was decompressed with a gastric tube. A small amount of uterine bleeding was observed, and her urine volume gradually decreased. Her hemoglobin level decreased (8.5 g/dL), and her white blood cell count (37,800/μL) and serum creatinine levels (3.5 mg/dL) were elevated. On the third hospital day, she remained in a state of delirium. Hemorrhagic fluid was collected from the pouch of Douglas by a needle aspiration. The preoperative diagnosis was degeneration and infection of the large myomatous uterus; however, the relationship between the diagnosis and the deleterious change in her general condition remained unknown. During emergency surgery, the uterus was found to be rotated 360 degrees clockwise at the level of the isthmus (Figure 3). The rotated uterus had suffered total infarction. A small amount of hemorrhagic fluid was present in the peritoneal cavity. A part of the small intestine was compressed by the uterus. We performed a total abdominal hysterectomy and bilateral salpingo-oophorectomy. The weight of the uterus was 3.8 kg. The postoperative course was uneventful, and the patient was discharged on the seventh postoperative day. Histopathology showed fibroids and extensive uterine and adnexal hemorrhagic infarcts consistent with uterine torsion.

3. Discussion

In this report we describe an 86-year-old woman who experienced torsion of a large myomatous uterus. Torsion of a nongravid uterus is extremely rare, and most of the reported cases involve a large myomatous uterus [5–8]. Onset of uterine torsion can vary from reproductive age to oldest-old age. Although the mechanisms of uterine torsion are unknown, rotation could occur after the ligaments have been stretched for many years by the heavy myomatous uterus. The uterus may rotate due to its weight, thus exerting traction on the uterus. Other conditions reported in cases of torsion of a nongravid uterus are a normal-sized uterus accompanied by a large ovarian cyst [1, 9, 10] and a uterine anomaly in combination with complete cervical agenesis [11].

The most common symptom in women with uterine torsion is acute abdominal pain, but the symptoms and their severity are variable. A similar case of uterine torsion in an oldest-old woman has been reported, wherein the patient had a large myomatous uterus, bowel symptoms, and a rapid decline in hemoglobin levels [5]. She was presented with acute abdominal pain and distention for two days, but she had no history of vomiting, urinary symptoms, vaginal bleeding, or fever. However, our current case demonstrates that uterine torsion should still be considered even in the absence of severe abdominal pain.

Although our patient only presented with slight abdominal pain, and tenderness around the myomatous uterus was also mild, she presented with progressive renal dysfunction and severe anemia. Her general condition worsened progressively to a bedridden state. The mechanism of progressive renal dysfunction due to uterine torsion remains unknown. One possibility is a postrenal obstruction caused by deviation of the ureters. Torsion results in drastic elongation of the broad

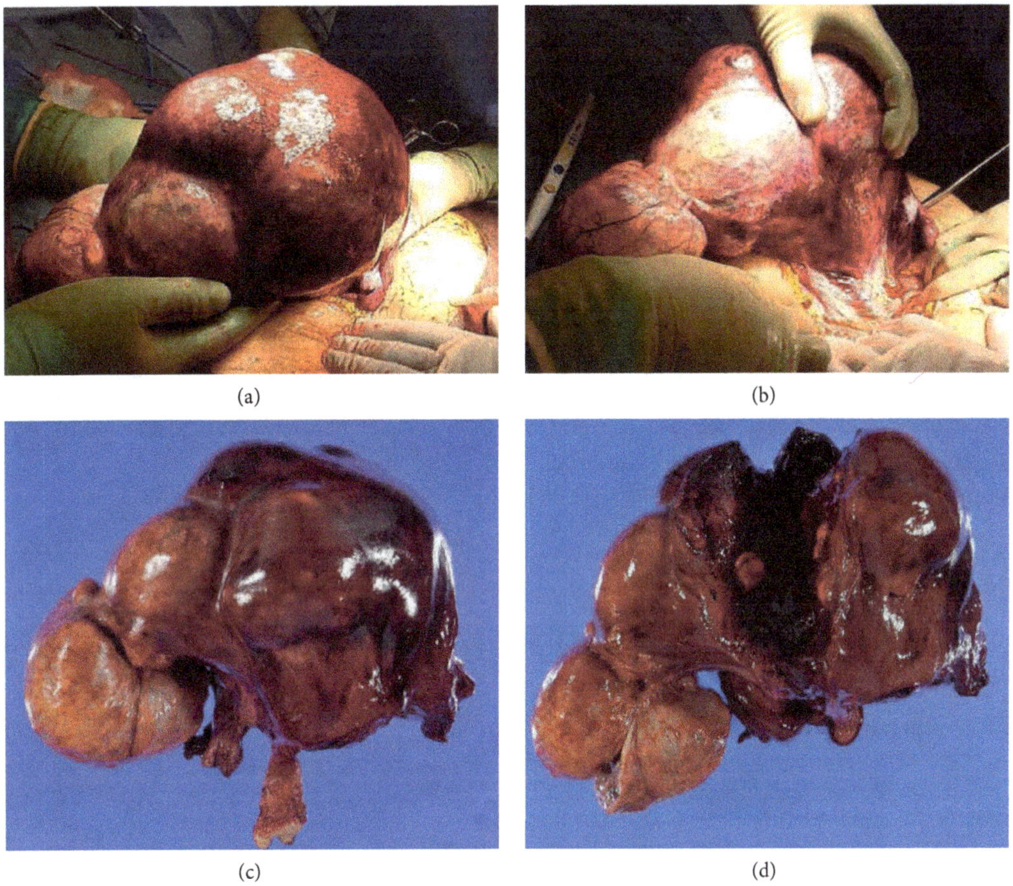

FIGURE 3: Operative findings of the twisted myomatous uterus. (a) The myomatous uterus was rotated 360 degrees clockwise on the long axis at the level of the isthmus. The uterine surface was discolored, appearing dark red because of the congestion. (b) After releasing the torsion, the uterine color turned red and the lower uterine segment was observed. (c) The resected myomatous uterus and bilateral adnexa. The surface of the uterus was dark red and the cervix was significantly elongated. (d) A cross-section of the uterus revealed the accumulation of clotting blood inside the uterus.

ligaments; this could obstruct the course of the retroperitoneal ureter at the level of the pelvic side wall. Another possibility is that severe congestion inside the rotated uterus may lead to acute cardiovascular failure accompanied by acute renal dysfunction. Progressive severe anemia is also associated with hypovolemia. Compared with reproductive-age women, oldest-old women are less adaptable during acute progressive hypovolemia.

Although preoperative diagnosis of uterine torsion is challenging because of its rarity and lack of specific symptoms, imaging findings are helpful for the diagnosis. Contrast-enhanced CT is one of the most valuable imaging methods for suspected uterine torsion. One of the characteristic findings is a whorled structure of the uterine cervix [5]. Multiplanar reformatted images are helpful for understanding the twisting of the cervix [8]. Both uterine torsion and pedunculated fibroid torsion show enhancement of the surrounding capsule of the uterine muscle layer and fibroid nodule. Unfortunately, it was impossible to perform contrast-enhanced CT for our patient because she was experiencing renal dysfunction; however, it was possible to compare the plain CT images between the onset of uterine torsion and images obtained one year previously. The notable imaging findings were that the volume of the myomatous uterus significantly increased in size and the cervix elongated and deviated upward at the onset of torsion compared with one year before. In addition, three-dimensional reconstruction of the images clearly showed substantial movement of the calcified lesion in the uterus. Given these results, we recommend CT imaging, ideally contrast-enhanced, for patients with a large, myomatous uterus after menopause to identify such changes and enable the early detection of uterine torsion. Congestion of the twisted uterus results in uterine enlargement accompanied by severe, progressive anemia. In general, uterine fibroids remain stable or decrease in size after menopause. If a myomatous uterus suddenly increases in size and the fibroid location changes after menopause, uterine torsion should be considered.

Differential diagnoses for torsion of a nongravid uterus include torsion of adnexal tumors, torsion of a pedunculated uterine fibroid, and infarction and/or degeneration of uterine fibroids. In cases of uterine torsion, a whorled structure of the uterine cervix on contrast-enhanced CT has been described. In cases of adnexal torsion, a thickened and twisted pedicle with adnexal tumors, primarily cystic tumors, has been identified. The twisted pedicle frequently contained the pedunculated, congested fallopian tubes. In cases of pedunculated subserosal uterine fibroids, most of the stalk is thin and usually undetectable by imaging. The pedunculated fibroid nodule is poorly enhanced. Magnetic resonance imaging (MRI) is useful for diagnosing the infarction and/or degeneration of uterine fibroids. Both intranodule hemorrhage and degeneration reveal high and low intensity mosaic patterns on T2-weighted images. Thus, imaging modalities such as contrast-enhanced CT and MRI can be used to properly distinguish between these conditions. It is noteworthy that torsion of a nongravid, normal-sized uterus and torsion of a large ovarian cyst have also been reported [9, 10].

4. Conclusions

Torsion of the nongravid uterus is an extremely rare condition, but it should be considered in menopausal oldest-old women with large uterine fibroids. Early release of the torsion may prevent progression to a critical condition caused by severe circulatory failure.

Consent

Written informed consent has been obtained from the patient for reporting.

Acknowledgments

This work is supported by grants-in-aid of Japan Society for the Promotion of Science.

References

[1] P. Collinet, F. Narducci, and L. Stien, "Torsion of a nongravid uterus: an unexpected complication of an ovarian cyst," *European Journal of Obstetrics, Gynecology, and Reproductive Biology*, vol. 98, no. 2, pp. 256–257, 2001.

[2] D. Wilson, A. Mahalingham, and S. Ross, "Third trimester uterine torsion: case report," *Journal of Obstetrics and Gynaecology Canada*, vol. 28, no. 6, pp. 531–535, 2006.

[3] E. H. T. Cheong, T. J. Tan, and K. M. Wong, "Torsion of a myomatous non-gravid uterus: CT findings," *Journal of Radiology Case Reports*, vol. 12, no. 4, pp. 6–14, 2018.

[4] Common Toxicity Criteria, "Version2.0," 1999, http://ctep.cancer.gov/protocolDevelopment/electronic_applications/docs/ctcv20_4-30-992.pdf.

[5] Y. Y. Jeong, H. K. Kang, J. G. Park, and H. S. Choi, "CT features of uterine torsion," *European Radiology*, vol. 13, no. 6, pp. L249–L250, 2003.

[6] W. K. Nicholson, C. C. Coulson, M. C. McCoy, and R. C. Semelka, "Pelvic magnetic resonance imaging in the evaluation of uterine torsion," *Obstetrics and Gynecology*, vol. 85, no. 5, pp. 888–890, 1995.

[7] J. D. Salvig, K. R. Petersen, and B. R. Moller, "Acute abdominal pain caused by torsion of an enlarged non-pregnant uterus," *Journal of Obstetrics and Gynaecology*, vol. 25, no. 1, pp. 81–82, 2005.

[8] D. Simms-Stewart, J. Hardie, P. Mitchell, H. Fletcher, A. Reid, and D. Shah, "Torsion in a perimenopausal non-gravid uterus with infarction and gangrene of uterus and adnexa: a proposed means of making the diagnosis clinically," *Journal of Obstetrics and Gynaecology*, vol. 32, no. 3, pp. 312–319, 2012.

[9] H. Matsumoto, T. Ohta, K. Nakahara, T. Kojimahara, and H. Kurachi, "Torsion of a nongravid uterus with a large ovarian cyst: usefulness of contrast MR image," *Gynecologic and Obstetric Investigation*, vol. 63, no. 3, pp. 163–165, 2007.

[10] F. Y. Yap, R. Radin, and H. Tchelepi, "Torsion, infarction, and rupture of a nongravid uterus: a complication of a large ovarian cyst," *Abdominal Radiology*, vol. 41, no. 12, pp. 2359–2363, 2016.

[11] K. Omurtag, D. Session, P. Brahma, A. Matlack, and C. Roberts, "Horizontal uterine torsion in the setting of complete cervical and partial vaginal agenesis: a case report," *Fertility and Sterility*, vol. 91, no. 5, pp. 1957.e13–1957.e15, 2009.

12

Enterocele Presenting as Anterior Rectal Prolapse: Resolution with Vaginal Repair

Geoffrey D. Towers, Candace Benoit, Rose Maxwell, and Jerome Yaklic

Department of Obstetrics and Gynecology, Wright State University Boonshoft School of Medicine, 128 E. Apple Street, Suite 3800 CHE, Dayton, OH 45409, USA

Correspondence should be addressed to Geoffrey D. Towers; geoffrey.towers@wright.edu

Academic Editor: Seung-Yup Ku

An enterocele is a pelvic hernia formed from the separation of endopelvic fascia, associated with the posterior or anterior vaginal fornix, and most commonly located in the posterior superior vaginal segment. Rectal prolapse is a debilitating condition in which the mucosa of the rectum protrudes circumferentially from the anus. Surgical repair is the recommended treatment for rectal prolapse, and though there are many different surgical options, there is no consensus on which approach is best. We present a case of anterior rectal prolapse due to enterocele which was treated by correction of enterocele with a vaginal approach and propose some clinical features and diagnostic techniques that may distinguish this entity from traditional rectal prolapse.

1. Introduction

An enterocele is a pelvic hernia formed from the separation of endopelvic fascia, associated with the posterior or anterior vaginal fornix, and most commonly located in the posterior superior vaginal segment [1]. As a true hernia, an enterocele may contain abdominal contents and is often found concurrently with other pelvic floor defects. It is estimated that up to 3% of females in the United States suffer from some type of vaginal prolapse [2], usually presenting with complaints of a vaginal bulge or pressure. In contrast, rectal prolapse occurs when anal mucosal or rectal tissue protrudes circumferentially through the anal orifice and is typically a continuum starting with internal intussusception and progressing to eventual full-thickness procedentia. This complete concentric prolapse is uncommon, present in less than 0.5% of the population [3], and occurs more frequently in females and the elderly. Symptoms are variable and can include physical bulge, defecatory dysfunction, stool abnormalities, pain, and bleeding [4]. It is common for patients with rectal prolapse to have other coexisting pelvic floor disorders. Quality of life is universally negatively impacted [5]. Rectal prolapse is diagnosed clinically based on history and physical examination findings, with surgical repair as the treatment of choice [4]. A myriad of surgical procedures is available to treat rectal prolapse, with open abdominal, perineal, and endoscopic approaches both with and without graft augmentation [4]. Although a vaginal approach to rectal prolapse repair is not typically described, a single case was reported in 2017 by Devakumar et al. in which successful repair of anterior rectal prolapse was accomplished with a vaginal approach, including enterocele repair with Moschowitz culdoplasty [6]. We present a similar case of anterior rectal prolapse also surgically corrected with vaginal reconstructive surgery. Written informed consent for publication of this case was obtained from our patient.

2. Case Presentation

An 84-year-old postmenopausal white female (gravida 3, para 2) was referred to our urogynecology clinic for evaluation and treatment of a persistent rectal bulge (Figure 1) (Video 1). She had noticed this bulge for over 10 years and initially thought that it was a hemorrhoid. She had been evaluated by a colorectal surgeon 10 years prior to presentation who recommended an abdominal resection rectopexy. The patient elected to not pursue surgery at that time. She described a bulge at the anus with the size of a lemon which

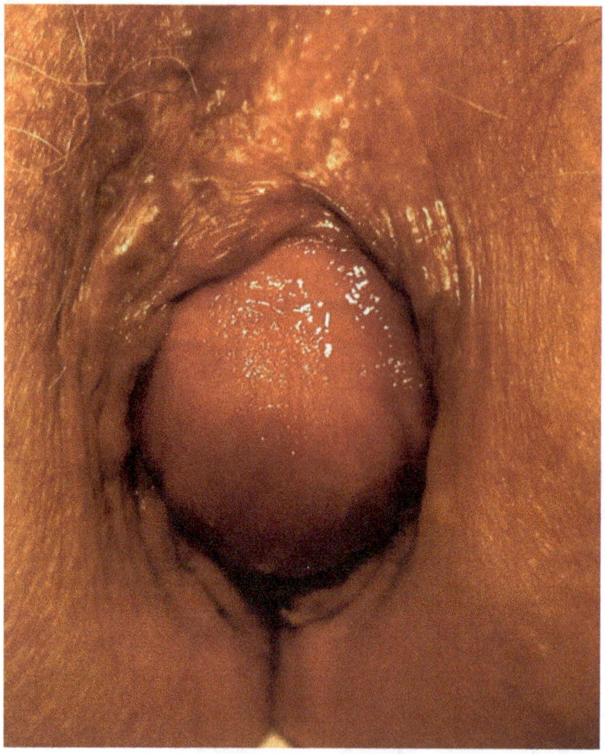

Figure 1: 84-year-old female with isolated anterior rectal prolapse due to enterocele. Note the smooth surface with lack of concentric folds.

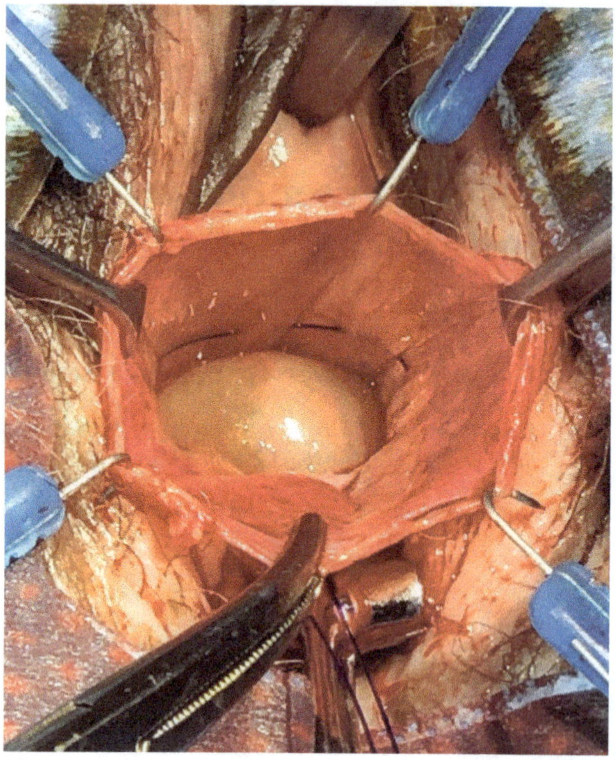

Figure 2: Purse-string repair of enterocele using delayed absorbable monofilament suture.

worsened with physical activity and reported accidental leakage of bowel contents consisting of pellet-formed stool. She was sometimes unable to differentiate between the bulge and stool. She reported significant adverse impact on her quality of life, including impairment of her ability to mow her lawn or to exercise. Additionally, she reported anal laxity, constipation, and occasional bright red blood per rectum. She denied any urinary symptoms or vaginal prolapse.

Pelvic exam revealed an atrophic vagina with no significant anterior or posterior vaginal wall prolapse. Her cervix was absent surgically, and her pelvic organ prolapse quantification was as follows: GH 2, PB 2, Aa -3, Ba -3, Ap -3, Bp -3, C -7, D n/a, and TVL 7. Rectal exam showed normal perianal skin and sphincter tone. With Valsalva, she demonstrated significant anterior rectal wall prolapse with palpable contents consistent with small bowel enterocele in the rectovaginal space. Prolapse was approximately 6 cm in size with the anterior rectal wall extending outside the anal verge and no evidence of posterior or circumferential rectal prolapse. Endoanal ultrasound showed normal levators, intact external anal sphincter circumferentially, and attenuation of the internal anal sphincter. There were no discernible masses, but the patient was unable to produce her rectal prolapse with the ultrasound transducer in place. Transperineal ultrasound was used to dynamically evaluate the perineal and rectal anatomy and demonstrated a large enterocele prolapsing between the vagina and the rectum with apparent fat or small bowel contents. Prolapse at the anterior rectal wall was directly associated with this enterocele. Defecography and dynamic MRI were not available at our facility.

The patient was evaluated by a colorectal surgeon for opinion on treatment plans. This surgeon indicated that a rectopexy would be acceptable, but it would be reasonable to attempt to repair the enterocele first to see if her symptoms would resolve and to potentially spare the patient from a more morbid procedure. The patient indicated a desire to proceed with an attempt at repair with the vaginal approach.

The patient was admitted to the hospital and anesthetized for surgery. A vertical posterior vaginal incision was made, extending into the perineal body. The vaginal epithelium was separated from the underlying endopelvic fascia, and dissection was performed superiorly and laterally to the level of the ischial spines and levator ani. A large enterocele was identified, opened, ligated with two purse-string sutures of delayed absorbable monofilament suture, and then excised (Figures 2 and 3). A suture capturing device was used to pass a polypropylene suture through the levator tendon immediately distal to the ischial spine bilaterally, following which these sutures were attached superiorly and laterally to the rectovaginal septum completing the iliococcygeus suspension in a tension-free manner (Figures 4 and 5). Small site-specific rectovaginal septal defects were repaired. The vaginal epithelium was then closed, and the perineal body was reconstructed.

Postoperatively, the patient recovered well and was discharged home on the first postoperative day with complete resolution of her rectal prolapse symptoms. She was seen at 1 month and 3 months postoperatively and by 3 months had resumed her normal activities of daily living with complete symptom resolution and normal defecation without incontinence.

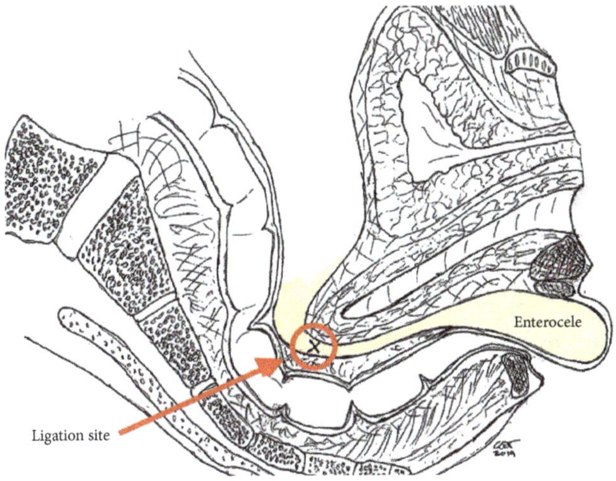

FIGURE 3: Location of the repair site for rectal enterocele.

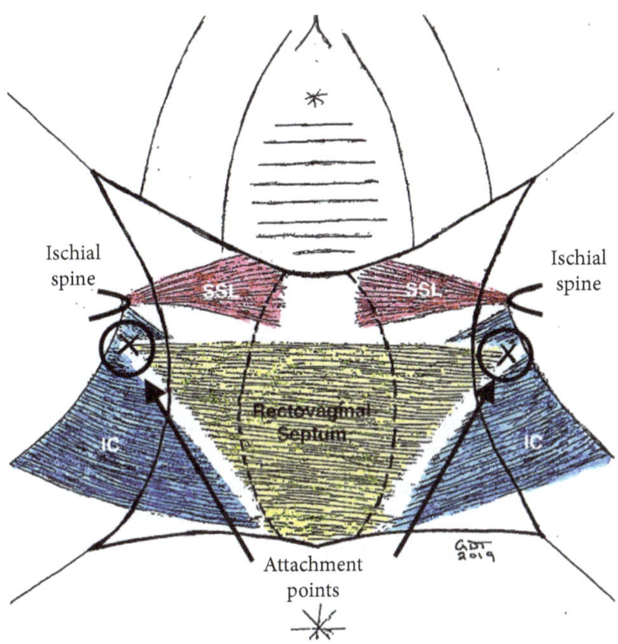

FIGURE 4: Fixation location for iliococcygeus suspension sutures. A finger is placed on the ischial spine and a suture capturing device used to place a delayed absorbable or permanent suture into the iliococcygeus tendon at the marked location. IC = iliococcygeus muscle; SSL = sacrospinous ligament.

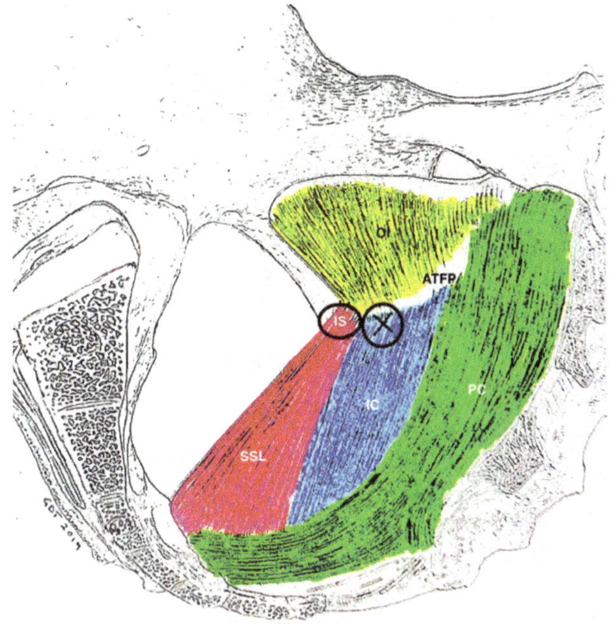

FIGURE 5: Location of placement of fixation suture for iliococcygeus suspension. Suspension in this case was necessary due to inferior/posterior prolapse of the rectovaginal septum associated with the rectal enterocele. IS = ischial spine; PC = pubococcygeus; IC = iliococcygeus; SSL = sacrospinous ligament; ATFP = arcus tendineus fasciae pelvis; OI = obturator internus.

3. Discussion

Rectal prolapse is a challenging and debilitating disease, with significant negative impact on sufferers. A significant number of surgical procedures (>100) are available to apply in these cases, and there is no consensus on which procedure is best [7]. Current practice is to tailor the treatment to the individual patient, accounting for medical comorbidities and patient desires with careful surgical planning [4], and to involve experts in the pelvic floor for surgical reconstruction should other pelvic floor defects be identified [7]. Most rectal prolapse literature, however, addresses full-thickness rectal prolapse specifically, and there is very little which addresses isolated anterior rectal prolapse. Indeed, ours is a case substantially like that reported by Devakumar et al. in 2017, where isolated anterior rectal prolapse was treated with repair of enterocele using a vaginal approach [6], and is only the second such case reported in the literature. In their case, treatment of the enterocele was with a Moschowitz culdoplasty and mesh vaginal suspension, while we were able to close the defect with purse-string ligation of the enterocele and suture suspension of the posterior vaginal wall. It is possible that any of the described enterocele repair techniques would be effective in a similar setting, depending on the individual patient.

As noted in Devakumar's discussion, Moschowitz proposed in 1912 that rectal prolapse could be the result of a deep pouch of Douglas which would allow pressure on the anterior rectal wall to cause the rectum to evert outside the anus [6, 8], and certainly this mechanism appears to be applicable in these two cases. The question remains, however, whether rectal prolapse initiated by this mechanism would progress to full-thickness circumferential prolapse or whether isolated anterior rectal prolapse in the setting of enterocele is a separately identifiable condition that justifies a different surgical approach.

It is important to note that there are likely significant differences between these two cases and traditional circumferential rectal prolapse. It is possible that these are unique clinical entities. In looking at the images in Devakumar's case and in our case (Figure 1) (Video 1), it can be easily seen that rectal presentation of an enterocele differs clinically from full-thickness rectal prolapse that results from intussusception (Figure 6) (Video 2). Note particularly that the concentric rings seen in traditional rectal prolapse are absent

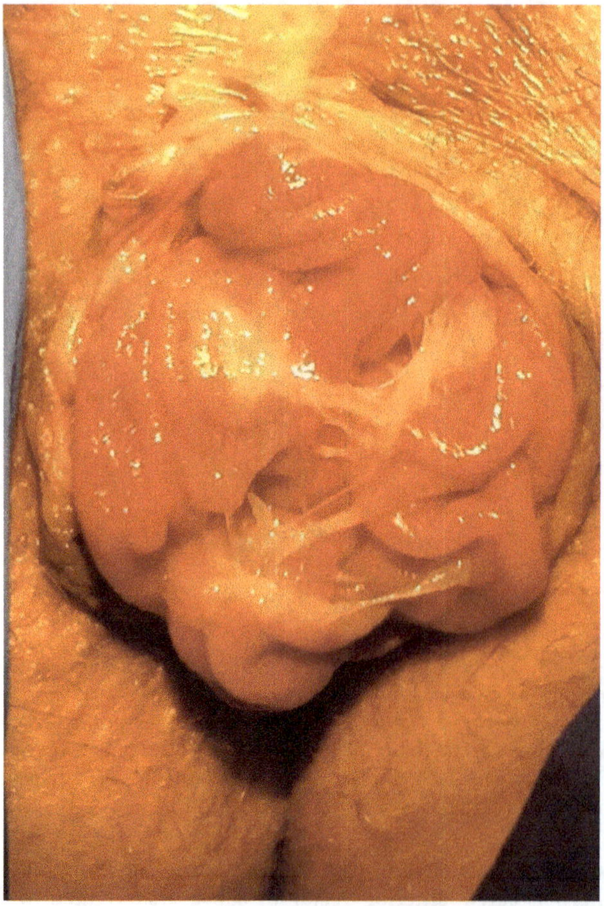

FIGURE 6: A different patient with full-thickness rectal prolapse due to intussusception. Note the concentric mucosal folds.

in these cases, suggesting lack of full-thickness prolapse and a difference in the mechanism (herniation of enterocele rather than intussusception). In our case, bowel contents of the enterocele could be easily palpated, and the diagnosis was supported by transperineal ultrasound imaging. Though defecography and dynamic MRI were not available to us and though such imaging could be useful if the diagnosis were in doubt, we did not feel they were necessary in this case.

4. Conclusion

Enterocele presenting as anterior rectal prolapse appears to be a rare condition, but one that may be amenable to a vaginal approach to treatment rather than traditional rectal prolapse repair. Careful physical examination is crucial. As a key physical exam finding, absence of circumferential mucosal folds and isolated anterior prolapse may herald the presence of an enterocele and should prompt an appropriate evaluation. There are no studies or case series describing the ideal approach for surgical correction of this rare presentation, and as in the case of any rectal prolapse, careful individualized evaluation and planning are warranted. Further research into the mechanism of rectal prolapse and the role of enterocele is needed. In this case, a vaginal surgical approach resulted in excellent results, at least in the short term, and allowed the avoidance of potentially more invasive and morbid procedures.

Supplementary Materials

Supplementary 1. Video Clip 1: subject patient with enterocele causing anterior rectal prolapse.

Supplementary 2. Video Clip 2: comparison patient with full-thickness circumferential rectal prolapse.

References

[1] C. Zimmerman, "Vaginal hysterectomy," in *TeLinde's Operative Gynecology*, J. A. Rock and H. W. Jones, Eds., p. 715, Wolters Kluwer, Philadelphia, PA, USA, 11th edition, 2015.

[2] I. Nygaard, M. D. Barber, K. L. Burgio et al., "Prevalence of symptomatic pelvic floor disorders in US women," *JAMA*, vol. 300, no. 11, pp. 1311–1316, 2008.

[3] M. Kairaluoma and I. Kellokumpu, "Epidemiologic aspects of complete rectal prolapse," *Scandinavian Journal of Surgery*, vol. 94, no. 3, pp. 207–210, 2005.

[4] L. Bordeianou, C. W. Hicks, A. M. Kaiser, K. Alavi, R. Sudan, and P. E. Wise, "Rectal prolapse: an overview of clinical features, diagnosis, and patient-specific management strategies," *Journal of Gastrointestinal Surgery*, vol. 18, no. 5, pp. 1059–1069, 2014.

[5] L. Bordeianou, T. Rockwood, N. Baxter, A. Lowry, A. Mellgren, and S. Parker, "Does incontinence severity correlate with quality of life? Prospective analysis of 502 consecutive patients," *Colorectal Disease*, vol. 10, no. 3, pp. 273–279, 2008.

[6] H. Devakumar, N. Chandrasekaran, A. Alas, L. Martin, G. W. Davila, and E. Hurtado, "Resolution of rectal prolapse by vaginal reconstruction," *Female Pelvic Medicine & Reconstructive Surgery*, vol. 23, no. 1, pp. e4–e7, 2017.

[7] S. A. Vogler, "Rectal prolapse," *Diseases of the Colon and Rectum*, vol. 60, no. 11, pp. 1132–1135, 2017.

[8] A. V. Moschcowitz, "Alexis Victor Moschcowitz 1865-1937," *Diseases of the Colon & Rectum*, vol. 26, no. 8, pp. 553–565, 1983.

13

A Rare Case of Watery Vaginal Discharge due to Caesarean Scar Dehiscence following Brace Suture and Balloon Tamponade for the Management of Postpartum Hemorrhage

Krystal Koh,[1] **Devendra Kanagalingam**,[2] **and Rajeswari Kathirvel**[3]

[1]*Department of Obstetrics and Gynecology, KK Women's and Children's Hospital, Singapore*
[2]*Department of Obstetrics and Gynecology, Singapore General Hospital, Singapore*
[3]*Department of Obstetrics and Gynecology, KK Women's and Children's Hospital, Lee Kong Chian School of Medicine, Duke NUS Medical School and Yong Loo Lin School of Medicine, Singapore*

Correspondence should be addressed to Krystal Koh; krystalgermaine@gmail.com

Academic Editor: Yossef Ezra

A woman in her early twenties with dichorionic diamniotic twins underwent emergency caesarean section (CS) for failed induction of labor for discordant growth at 37 weeks. Her CS was complicated by atonic postpartum hemorrhage (PPH) requiring uterotonics, B-lynch suture, and Bakri balloon. She presented on the 5th postoperative day (POD) with fever and wound pain and collapsed due to desaturation. Investigations confirmed ascites on computed tomography (CT) of her abdomen and cardiomyopathy on echocardiogram. She was readmitted on the 22nd POD with watery vaginal discharge. CT abdomen revealed a dehisced CS scar and loculated ascites. Her discharge settled after three weeks with antibiotics and drainage of the ascites. A CT scan 3 months later showed reduction of the peritoneal collection. Caesarean scar dehiscence should be considered for patients presenting with ascites and vaginal discharge after a CS, particularly in the presence of risk factors such as infection or anemia.

1. Introduction

Intra-abdominal infection (IAI) and peritonitis are known complications of caesarean section (CS). Endomyometritis, uterine incisional necrosis and dehiscence, and perioperative bladder and/or bowel injury are possible causes [1]. Uterine dehiscence occurs in 0.06 to 3.8% of caesarean cases [2]. Risk factors include diabetes, emergency surgery, infection, suture technique, hematoma on the uterine incision line, and retrovesical hematoma [3]. While peritonitis often presents as abdominal pain and fever, the presence of vaginal discharge should raise suspicion of uterine dehiscence or a vesicovaginal fistula. We present an unusual case of watery vaginal discharge in a young woman post-CS that was complicated by postpartum hemorrhage (PPH) managed with brace suture and balloon tamponade.

2. Case Presentation

A woman in her early twenties with dichorionic diamniotic twins, antenatally noted to have iron deficiency anemia, underwent an emergency caesarean section (CS) following failed induction of labor for discordant growth of twins at 37 weeks gestation. Her CS was complicated by atonic PPH of 1.2 liters (L) that was managed by uterotonics, B-lynch suture, and insertion of a Bakri balloon. Postoperatively, her hematocrit was 20.3% and hemoglobin was 6.4 g/dL, from a preoperative hematocrit and hemoglobin of 29.7% and 9.0 g/dL, respectively. She received 4 units of packed cell transfusion postoperatively followed by oral hematinics and was discharged on the 3rd POD in a stable condition with a hematocrit of 24.6% and hemoglobin of 8 g/dL.

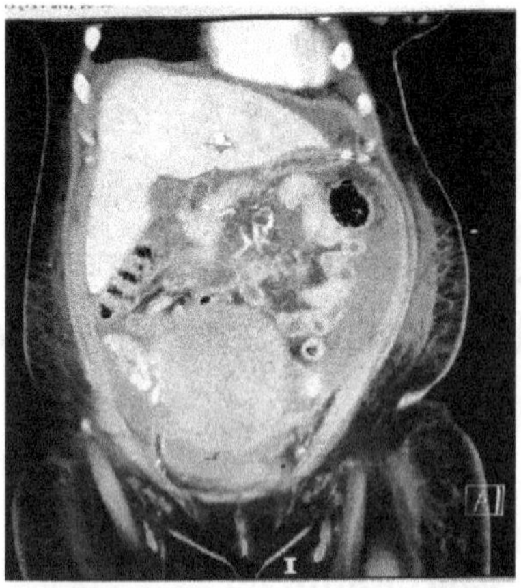

Figure 1: CT abdomen and pelvis showing ascites out of keeping with recent caesarean section.

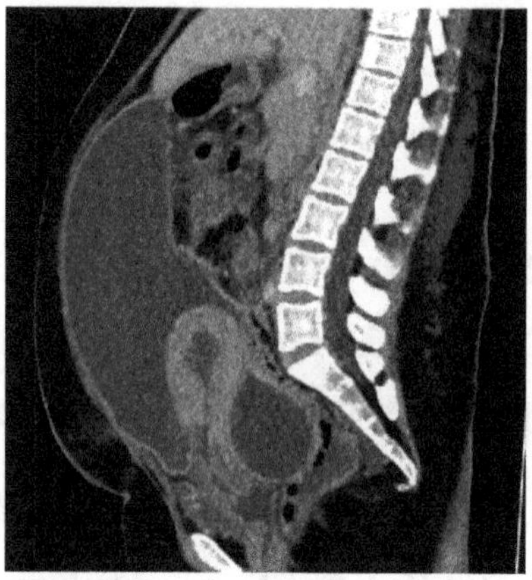

Figure 2: Initial CT findings of a dehisced CS scar and increase in size of the loculated ascites.

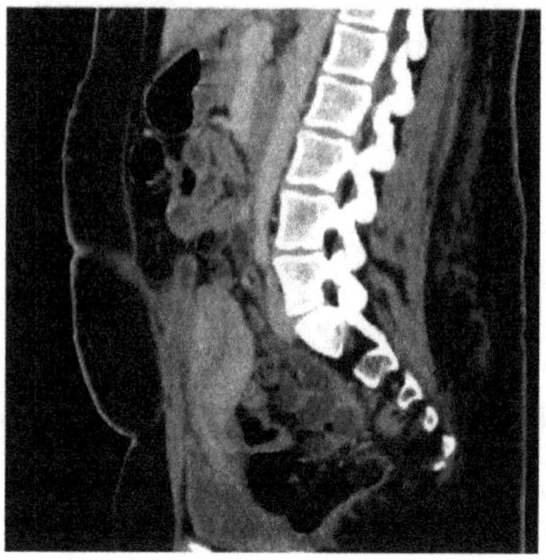

Figure 3: Follow-up CT scan showing reduction of the abdominal fluid collection after drainage and antibiotics 3 months after drainage (4 months postoperatively).

She was readmitted on the 5th POD with fever, wound site pain, and blood pressure of 144/89 mm of Hg. On readmission, her hemoglobin was 7.8 g/dL with hematocrit of 24.5%, total white cell count was normal at 8.29×10^9/L, and urinalysis showed a predominance of white cells. She was treated empirically for urinary tract infection and given oral labetalol for her hypertension. She collapsed the next day on the ward due to desaturation (SpO_2 85% on nonrebreather mask) associated with hypertension of 191/70 mm of Hg and tachycardia of 180 to 190 beats per minute (bpm). She was stabilized in the intensive care unit (ICU) with endotracheal intubation, adenosine for supraventricular tachycardia, and intravenous magnesium sulfate for presumed preeclampsia, followed by noradrenaline for subsequent hypotension due to septic shock. Initial differentials included preeclampsia, pulmonary embolism, type 2 myocardial infarction, and pneumonia complicated by septic shock. She was thereafter thoroughly investigated, and the positive findings were that of a cardiomyopathy confirmed by echocardiography with a left ventricular ejection fraction of 25 to 30% and global hypokinesia, ascites confirmed by computed tomography (CT) of her abdomen and pelvis (Figure 1), and positive blood cultures for *Bacteroides fragilis*. Her cardiomyopathy was thought to be precipitated by anemia and *Bacteroides fragilis* bacteremia from a likely pelvic source. She was transferred to a coronary care unit and recovered clinically with supportive treatment for cardiomyopathy and broad spectrum antibiotics. She received a total of 7 days of intravenous (IV) piperacillin/tazobactam and 9 days of metronidazole, oralized to amoxicillin/clavulanic acid for 2 weeks on discharge. She was started on perindopril, bisoprolol, spironolactone, and ivabradine for optimization of her cardiac function. She was discharged on the 16th POD in a stable condition.

She was readmitted on the 22nd POD with copious amounts of watery vaginal discharge. The initial impression was that of a vesicovaginal fistula. A CT scan of the abdomen and pelvis ruled out a urinary tract injury but confirmed a dehisced CS scar and loculated ascites with the possibility of superimposed infection. The ascites increased in size from the previous CT scan (Figure 2). She was treated with antibiotics, and the ascites was drained abdominally under ultrasound guidance. She received 13 days of IV ceftriaxone and metronidazole, oralized to ciprofloxacin and metronidazole for another 2 weeks. A total of 850 mL of hemoserous fluid was drained from the abdomen within 24 hours of the drain insertion. The total fluid drainage over 13 days was 3560 mL. Ascitic fluid cultures yielded no bacterial or fungal growth. Vaginal swab and vaginal discharge cultures revealed mixed flora.

Interval scans showed a marked reduction in the fluid collection, and she was discharged two weeks later on the 36th POD. Her vaginal discharge eventually settled after three weeks. After discharge, she was reviewed in the outpatient clinic, and interval ultrasound scans of the pelvis one and two months later and a CT scan three months later showed further reduction of the pelvic collection with only a sliver of fluid in the lower abdomen at the fourth month postoperatively (Figure 3). She was thereafter discharged from the gynecology clinic. She was also seen in the cardiology outpatient clinic two months after discharge and was stable. Unfortunately, she defaulted on subsequent cardiology follow-up visits for a repeat echocardiogram.

A summary of the patient's clinical course is shown in Figure 4.

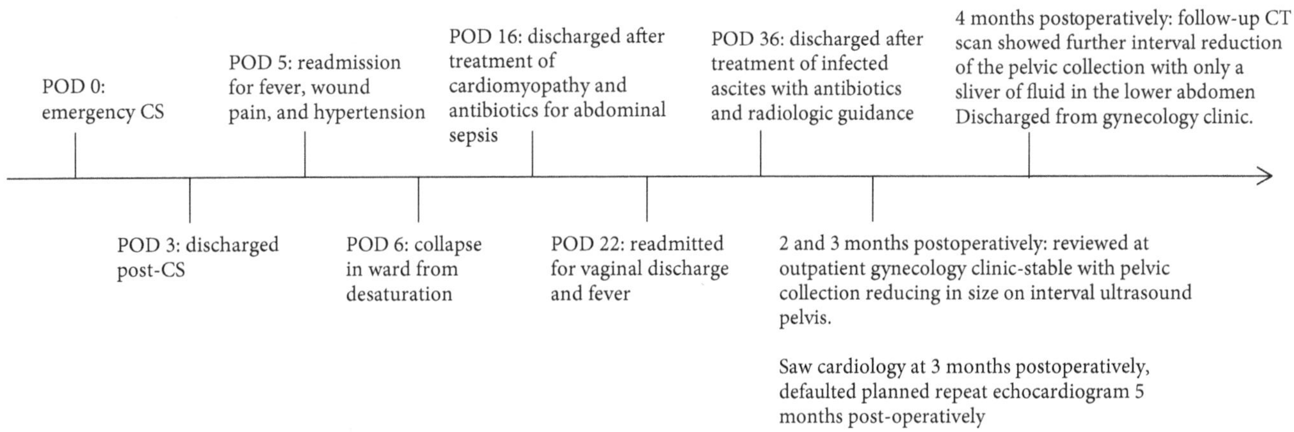

FIGURE 4: Timeline of patient's course.

3. Discussion

This patient had vaginal discharge due to leaking of inflammatory exudate following IAI through the dehisced CS wound. It is rather unusual to see ascitic fluid draining through the dehisced CS scar into the vagina. Plausible pathophysiologies include uterine endomyometritis predisposing to uterine scar dehiscence leading to secondary peritonitis and ascites, primary peritonitis predisposing to dehiscence of the uterine scar and drainage of ascites through the vagina, and inflammatory ascites as a result of discharge of lochia into the abdominal cavity via the dehisced uterine wound, with resultant negative ascitic fluid culture.

Our patient required concurrent use of brace suture and balloon tamponade (sometimes called the "uterine sandwich" technique) [4] to manage her postpartum hemorrhage. Sepsis following this could have contributed to the uterine dehiscence that in turn could have led to peritonitis. Cardiomyopathy and anemia compromising perfusion could have been additional risk factors for uterine dehiscence in this patient. Other predisposing factors for peritonitis include immunocompromise, genital infection [5], and inadvertent bladder and/or bowel injury. These were not seen in this case. Uterine necrosis following the "uterine sandwich" technique has been described [6, 7] and could also have led to dehiscence; however, this was thought to be less likely as she was clinically well at the time of second admission to our hospital.

Cases of postcaesarean peritonitis in the literature describe uncommon infective organisms including *Candida* [8] and *Streptococcus pneumoniae* [9], along with noninfective etiologies such as reactive [10] and vernix caseosa [11] peritonitis. Similar cases of uterine dehiscence complicated by peritonitis have varied clinical presentations including fever, abdominal pain, distension, vaginal discharge, wound infection [12], and PPH [13]. These features manifested from anywhere between the first POD to two months postoperatively. Our patient similarly presented with fever and wound site pain on the 5th POD and watery vaginal discharge with fever on the 22nd POD.

A broad range of differential diagnoses was considered for each of the presenting complaints for this patient in view of nonspecific features at presentation. On initial presentation when she presented on the 5th POD with fever, wound site pain, and headache with a temperature of 38.3 degrees Celsius and blood pressure of 144/89 mm of Hg, the initial differentials included fever secondary to urinary tract infection and possible preeclampsia. Following her collapse on 6th POD due to desaturation, hypertension, and tachycardia, further investigations revealed raised serum troponin T, and a chest X-ray and CT pulmonary angiogram showed bilateral lower lobe consolidation with diffuse patchy ground glass opacities of both lungs, and CT of the abdomen and pelvis revealed ascites that were more than what would have been expected with the recent caesarean section. She also subsequently developed hypotension with systolic blood pressure dropping to a nadir of 70 mm of Hg with a temperature of 38 degrees Celsius, attributed to septic shock. Differentials at this point were acute pulmonary oedema secondary to cardiomyopathy and sepsis from respiratory, urinary, and abdominal sources. Postpartum endometritis, infected intra-abdominal collection, urinary tract infection, and pelvic septic thrombophlebitis were considered as a possible source for pelvic sepsis, and vesicovaginal fistula was considered as a differential for the watery vaginal discharge when she was readmitted on the 22nd POD.

Stepwise investigations are crucial in such cases and should include serum inflammatory markers, microbiology (blood culture, urine culture, ascitic fluid culture, vaginal swab, and vaginal fluid culture), and serial ultrasound and CT scans, which were performed on this patient.

Management options for uterine dehiscence include conservative treatment with antibiotics and drainage. However, in the presence of infection, laparotomy with either repair of the uterine defect or hysterectomy should be considered [1, 3, 14]. Fortunately, our patient settled with conservative management with antibiotics and drainage.

As there are varied etiologies and unusual presentations of intra-abdominal infection postcaesarean, there should be a high index of suspicion for uterine dehiscence and bladder or bowel injury with any postoperative fluid accumulation or abnormal vaginal discharge postoperatively.

This case also demonstrates multiple complications occurring simultaneously in the postpartum period including PPH, cardiomyopathy precipitated by anemia and sepsis, and uterine dehiscence. Optimal management by a multidisciplinary team consisting of obstetricians, anesthetists, cardiologists, respiratory medicine, and infectious disease specialists eventually led to a good outcome.

Consent

Patient consent was not obtained as the patient defaulted on subsequent follow-up and returned to India. Attempt to contact the patient was unsuccessful. All details are anonymous with no patient identifiers.

Authors' Contributions

The guaranteeing author is Dr. Rajeswari Kathirvel, and K. Koh summarized the case records and wrote the paper. D. Kanagalingam and R. Kathirvel managed the case, supervised, and contributed to writing the paper. All authors commented on the final paper and have approved the final version.

References

[1] F. G. Cunningham, K. Leveno, S. Bloom, J. Hauth, D. Rouse, and C. Spong, *Williams Obstetrics*, McGraw-Hill Medical, New York, 23rd edition, 2010.

[2] A. H. Shaamash, A. G. M. Ahmed, M. M. Abdel Latef, and S. A. Abdullah, "Routine postpartum ultrasonography in the prediction of puerperal uterine complications," *International Journal of Gynecology & Obstetrics*, vol. 98, no. 2, pp. 93–99, 2007.

[3] A. S. El-Agwany, "Conservative management of infected postpartum uterine dehiscence after cesarean section," *Journal of Medical Ultrasound*, vol. 26, no. 1, pp. 59–61, 2018.

[4] W. L. Nelson and J. M. O'Brien, "The uterine sandwich for persistent uterine atony: combining the B-lynch compression suture and an intrauterine Bakri balloon," *American Journal of Obstetrics and Gynecology*, vol. 196, no. 5, pp. e9–e10, 2007.

[5] D. C. Plummer, S. M. Garland, and G. L. Gilbert, "Bacteraemia and pelvic infection in women due to Ureaplasma urealyticum and Mycoplasma hominis," *The Medical Journal of Australia*, vol. 146, no. 3, pp. 135–137, 1987.

[6] E. J. Treloar, R. S. Anderson, H. S. Andrews, and J. L. Bailey, "Uterine necrosis following B-lynch suture for primary postpartum haemorrhage," *BJOG: An International Journal of Obstetrics & Gynaecology*, vol. 113, no. 4, pp. 486–488, 2006.

[7] A. G. Gottlieb, S. Pandipati, K. M. Davis, and R. S. Gibbs, "Uterine necrosis: a complication of uterine compression sutures," *Obstetrics and Gynecology*, vol. 112, 2, Part 2, pp. 429–431, 2008.

[8] M. Rottenstreich, F. Khatib, and R. Rotem, "Post cesarean candida peritonitis," *European Journal of Obstetrics, Gynecology, and Reproductive Biology*, vol. 229, pp. 203-204, 2018.

[9] G. Kourounis, Y. Panayiotou, P. P. Tabet, B. D. W. Richards, A. Petrou, and M. Loizou, "A case of pneumococcal peritonitis after caesarean section in a healthy woman," *Case Reports in Surgery*, vol. 2015, Article ID 350573, 3 pages, 2015.

[10] A. Gado, H. Badawi, and A. Karim, "An unusual case of peritonitis following a caesarean delivery," *Alexandria Journal of Medicine*, vol. 54, no. 4, pp. 369–371, 2018.

[11] A. Chambers, A. Patil, R. Alves, J. Hopkins, J. Armstrong, and R. Lawrence, "Delayed presentation of vernix caseosa peritonitis," *Annals of the Royal College of Surgeons of England*, vol. 94, no. 8, pp. 548–551, 2012.

[12] K. K. Bharatam, P. K. Sivaraja, N. J. Abineshwar et al., "The tip of the iceberg: post caesarean wound dehiscence presenting as abdominal wound sepsis," *International Journal of Surgery Case Reports*, vol. 9, pp. 69–71, 2015.

[13] T. Baba, M. Morishita, M. Nagata, Y. Yamakawa, and M. Mizunuma, "Delayed postpartum hemorrhage due to cesarean scar dehiscence," *Archives of Gynecology and Obstetrics*, vol. 272, no. 1, pp. 82-83, 2005.

[14] M. E. Rivlin, C. S. Carroll Sr., and J. C. Morrison, "Infectious necrosis with dehiscence of the uterine repair complicating cesarean delivery: a review," *Obstetrical & Gynecological Survey*, vol. 59, no. 12, pp. 833–837, 2004.

14

A Case of Markedly Elevated Isolated Alkaline Phosphatase in the Third Trimester of Pregnancy

Courtney T. Connolly[1] **Olivia Grubman,**[1] **Zainab Al-Ibraheemi,**[1] **and Tatyana Kushner**[1,2]

[1]*Department of Obstetrics, Gynecology and Reproductive Science, Icahn School of Medicine at Mount Sinai, New York City, USA*
[2]*Department of Medicine and Liver Disease, Icahn School of Medicine at Mount Sinai, New York City, USA*

Correspondence should be addressed to Courtney T. Connolly; courtney.connolly@icahn.mssm.edu

Academic Editor: Giuseppe Gullo

Background. Alkaline phosphatase (ALP) is an enzyme produced by the liver, small intestine, bone, and kidneys as well as the placenta during pregnancy. ALP levels may increase up to twice the normal limit during pregnancy secondary to placental release and fetal bone growth. Rare case reports of extremely elevated levels of ALP during pregnancy have demonstrated possible association with adverse pregnancy outcomes. *Case.* The patient is a 36-year-old G2P1001 who was found to have extremely elevated ALP levels during pregnancy after presenting with bilateral lower leg swelling and rash after receiving the Pfizer COVID-19 vaccine. She subsequently developed intrahepatic cholestasis of pregnancy and preeclampsia. ALP peaked at 2,601 U/L immediately prior to delivery at 36 weeks 1 day. She was followed postpartum, and her ALP levels had nearly normalized by 15 weeks postpartum. *Conclusion.* Our case demonstrates a rare report of an extremely elevated level of ALP in the setting of multiple adverse pregnancy outcomes, including preterm delivery, preeclampsia without severe features, and intrahepatic cholestasis of pregnancy.

1. Introduction

Alkaline phosphatase (ALP) is an enzyme produced by various tissues, including the liver, small intestine, bones, kidneys, and placenta during pregnancy. It is not uncommon to see elevations in ALP during pregnancy, and by the 15th to 26th weeks of pregnancy, term placental ALP isozymes can be detected in the maternal serum [1]. These isozymes are likely produced by syncytiotrophoblasts in the placenta and are theorized to play a role in transport across cell membranes and metabolism [1, 2]. ALP increases with increasing gestational age, with contributions likely from both placental isoenzymes. ALP peaks in the third trimester and usually reaches levels double that of a nonpregnant individual but normalizes postpartum [2–5]. However, it is important to exclude other causes of elevated ALP out of proportion to what is expected when detected during pregnancy, including malignancy, drugs, and bone, renal, and hepatic diseases.

Few cases of extremely elevated levels of ALP have been reported in the literature, and ALP has been associated with adverse outcomes including low birth weight [6, 7], intrauterine growth restriction [8], preterm delivery [9, 10], and hypertensive disorders of pregnancy [11]. It has been thought that ALP may be a marker of uteroplacental vascular disease [12].

We describe a case of extremely elevated ALP detected during a pregnancy complicated by preterm delivery, intrahepatic cholestasis of pregnancy, and preeclampsia. There were no adverse fetal effects. ALP levels returned to near baseline by 15 weeks postpartum.

2. Case Presentation

A 36-year-old gravida 2 para 1001 at 29 weeks 6 days, dated by a 14-week ultrasound inconsistent with her last menstrual period, re-presented to the high-risk obstetrics clinic where she was previously followed for type 1 diabetes for evaluation of a new finding of abnormally elevated alkaline phosphatase. She had been seen in the Emergency Department (ED) two days prior where she reported the development of bilateral ankle rash, pain, leg swelling, and subjective fever 1 day after receiving the Pfizer COVID-19 vaccine. She denied chills, chest pain, dyspnea, myalgias, abdominal pain, and exposure to irritating substances or new clothing in the area of her rash. There were no symptoms, focal signs of infection, or recent travel to suggest exposure to the Zika virus. Her medical history was significant for bipolar disorder, prior cholecystectomy, hypothyroidism stable on levothyroxine 50 mcg daily, and type 1 diabetes mellitus complicated by suboptimal glucose control in the current pregnancy and two prior hospital admissions for diabetic ketoacidosis, most recently 4 years ago.

On presentation to the ED, she was afebrile, and vital signs were stable. Physical exam revealed 1+ bilateral pitting edema and a nonblanching confluent erythematous rash on the medial and posterior of the lower extremities. Abdominal exam was unremarkable aside from gravid uterus, and the rash was not warm to the touch.

Bilateral lower extremity Doppler ultrasound was negative for deep venous thrombosis. Basic labs were ordered as part of her work-up, and a comprehensive metabolic panel was notable for alkaline phosphatase (ALP) of 1,327 U/L and albumin of 2.5 g/dL. AST, ALT, total protein, and total and direct bilirubin were within normal limits. There was no leukocytosis, anemia, or thrombocytopenia. Her last ALP measured at 16 weeks 4 days was 258, demonstrating significant interval change.

Given her benign abdominal exam and labs not suggestive of an active infection, she was discharged with close outpatient follow-up. She was seen two days later in the obstetrics high-risk clinic, where she was noted to be clinically stable. She was then referred to the hepatology practice for further evaluation and was seen at 31 weeks 6 days. On further history, she reported no use of acetaminophen or nonsteroidal anti-inflammatory drugs, alcohol, intravenous drug, herbal supplements, and antibiotics and denied recent travel. Family history was positive for Hepatitis C infection in her brother, most likely acquired secondary to intravenous drug use. She was immune to Hepatitis B. She noted pruritus and continued to endorse bilateral pedal edema with improvement in the rash.

Further work-up at that time was significant for ALP now elevated to 1,937 U/L, albumin of 2.3 g/dL, total bile acids elevated at 22 μmol/L, and ceruloplasmin of 63.4 mg/dL. Mitochondrial (M2) antibody, Hepatitis A IgM, and Hepatitis E IgM were negative. GGT was normal. Complete blood count with differential, ALT, AST, total and direct bilirubin, and serum alpha-1-antitrypsin were within normal limits. Hepatitis C RNA was not detected. Liver ultrasound showed normal size at 16.0 cm, normal contour, mildly increased echogenicity, extrahepatic common bile duct 0.2 cm, and a surgically absent gallbladder, compatible with nonspecific hepatic parenchymal disease.

She was diagnosed with intrahepatic cholestasis of pregnancy with plan for induction of labor at 37 weeks and was started on ursodiol 300 mg TID. She was evaluated again at 34 weeks 6 days by the high-risk obstetrics and liver medicine teams, reporting continued pruritus refractory to topical treatments and ursodiol. Follow-up labs revealed bile acids of 35 μmol/L, albumin of 2.2 g/dL, and ALP of 2,069 IU/L. Alkaline phosphatase isoenzymes were liver fraction of 59%, bone fraction of 40%, and intestinal fraction of 1%. Placental fraction was not able to be quantified by the specific laboratory processing the specimen.

She presented to Labor and Delivery triage at 35 weeks 2 days with mild range blood pressures, elevated urine protein/creatinine ratio of 824 mgTP/gCr, and otherwise normal labs, which was consistent with the diagnosis of preeclampsia without severe features. She re-presented at 35 weeks 4 days in latent labor. She delivered a liveborn female weighing 3,020 grams via normal spontaneous vaginal delivery, and Apgar scores were 8 and 8. Placental pathology demonstrated a 625-gram placenta with mild intervillous fibrin deposition. On pathology, the fetal membranes had mild focal acute chronic inflammation. No special stains were performed.

Her ALP peaked at 2,601 U/L (approximately 22 times the upper limit of normal) (ALP trend demonstrated in Figure 1), the final measurement before delivery at 35 weeks 5 days. By postpartum day 2, ALP was 2,019 U/L, and she was discharged in stable condition. She was seen again on postpartum day five for preeclampsia postpartum monitoring, and ALP had decreased to 1,483 U/L. At her six-week postpartum visit, ALP was 300 U/L, and by 15 weeks postpartum, it was 156 U/L.

3. Discussion

Our case report is one of few in the literature that describes an extremely elevated level of ALP discovered incidentally during pregnancy that was later complicated by intrahepatic cholestasis of pregnancy, preterm delivery, and preeclampsia. In our case, the patient delivered at 36 weeks 1 day, and alkaline phosphatase levels had nearly normalized by 15 weeks postpartum.

A review of previous case reports demonstrates an association between elevated ALP and adverse pregnancy outcomes. Specifically, several patient cases documented an association with mild hypertension or other hypertensive disorder of pregnancy [2, 13, 14]. A case control study by Rajagambeeram et al. further supported this finding and showed that total serum ALP and placental (heat stable) ALP were significantly elevated in women with hypertensive disorders of pregnancy versus controls [11]. Other cases reported associations with preterm delivery [8, 14], preterm premature rupture of membranes [15], gestational diabetes [14, 16, 17], and intrauterine growth restriction [8]. One case report interestingly noted thrombocytopenia in the mother with extremely elevated placental isoenzymes, and upon further investigation was found to have several relatives with elevated baseline ALP suggesting a possible genetic link [18]. In addition, while the majority of cases of this extreme elevation in ALP have been associated with adverse pregnancy outcomes or pregnancy complications, it is important to note that there were also several case reports of elevated ALP in an otherwise uncomplicated pregnancy [19, 20].

Our case aligns with several of the associations suggested by previous reports, specifically preterm delivery and

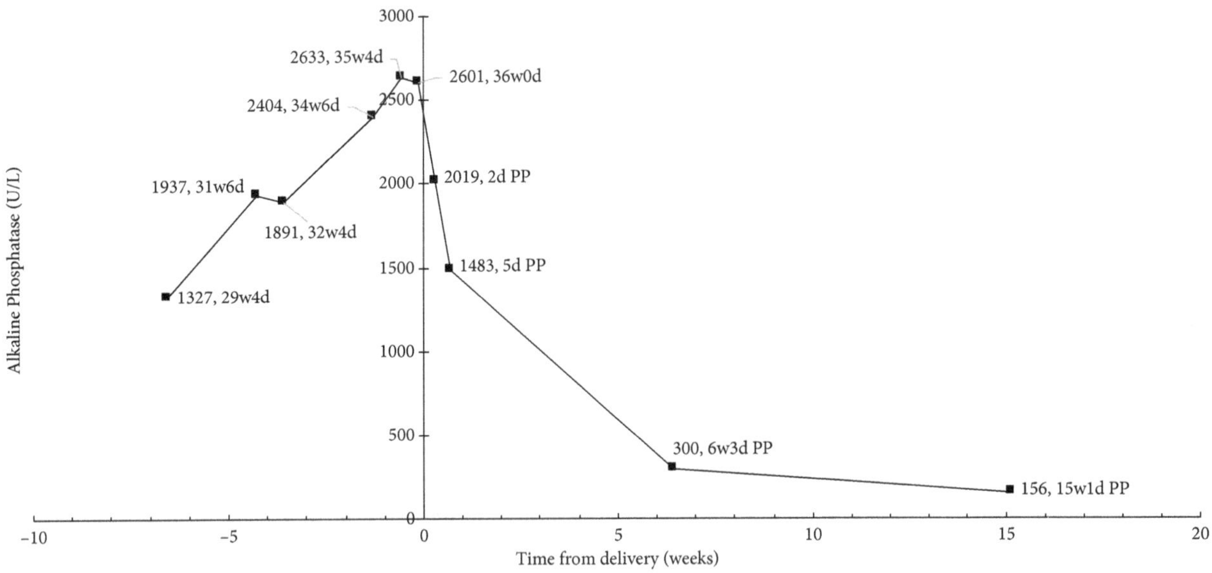

Figure 1: Total alkaline phosphatase levels over time relative to delivery at 36 weeks 1 day. PP: postpartum.

hypertensive disorder of pregnancy. However, our case was unique in that we report an association that developed after administration of a vaccination and the presence of elevated bile acids suggesting a diagnosis of intrahepatic cholestasis of pregnancy. While a rise in ALP may occur with intrahepatic cholestasis of pregnancy, an increase of 22x the upper limit of normal range is unusually high. Interestingly, *in vitro fertilization* has also been found to be associated with cholestasis of pregnancy, but there is no current evidence suggesting that extreme elevations in alkaline phosphatase are associated with assisted reproductive technology.

The vast majority of reported cases, if able to speciate the isoenzymes, found placental isoenzyme to be the predominant fraction [2, 13–16, 18–20]. There was a rare case of elevation in the bone isoenzyme in a patient who was discovered to have an elevated ALP of 1525 U/L at the onset of labor induction despite high-normal ALP earlier in pregnancy with rapid progression to 2561 U/L 95 minutes later [17].

Most cases of elevated alkaline phosphatase resolved within six to 12 weeks postpartum [2, 8, 15–20]. However, one case took up to 18 weeks to resolve, which appears to be more consistent with the timeline of our patient's course [13] (Figure 1). This may be partially explained by the relatively longer half-life of placental isoenzymes of ALP (approximately 7 days) versus liver and bone isoenzymes (1-3 days) [19].

Finally, it is important to emphasize that other causes of elevated ALP must be excluded. Drug-induced liver injury secondary to the COVID-19 vaccination was considered in our patient's case. However, the onset of lab abnormalities in temporal relation to the vaccination does not suggest an immunologic reaction, and this is not an established adverse effect of the COVID-19 vaccine. In cases of elevated ALP levels, it should be determined early on whether it is of isolated hepatic origin, bone, or placental origin. A concurrent elevation in GGT likely indicates that the ALP is hepatic in origin, and appropriate work-up with further labs and ultrasound imaging should be performed to investigate for intrahepatic causes (e.g., primary biliary cholangitis, primary sclerosing cholangitis (PSC), viral hepatitis, and sarcoidosis) and extrahepatic causes (e.g., PSC, bile duct strictures, and stones). An elevated bone fraction of ALP indicates increased bone turnover, which can be attributed to diseases such as osteosarcoma and metastatic cancer as well as hyperparathyroidism, Paget disease, osteomalacia, and others. Our patient had a normal gamma-glutamyl transpeptidase as well as normal liver, bone, and intestinal fractions of ALP but an overall elevation in total ALP. While we could not fractionate the placental isoenzyme, we presume that it is possible the placental isoenzyme may have been elevated in our patient's case. Of note, the placental ALP isoenzyme is heat labile and migrates with the bone fraction. For future cases, we suggest sending these samples to a laboratory that is capable of processing all isoenzyme types and specifically quantifying the placental isozyme. There is a Regan isoenzyme that is a placental-type isoenzyme and has been associated with ovarian serous cystadenocarcinoma, lung cancer, and seminoma [13]. Our team requested placental pathology results to investigate whether there were any placental factors that contributed to such a high release of alkaline phosphatase. We believe there may be an association between placental pathology, preeclampsia, and alkaline phosphatase. However, we cannot prove this with our case report and suggest further studies to investigate.

In conclusion, we report a case of incidentally diagnosed markedly elevated ALP in a pregnancy complicated by intrahepatic cholestasis of pregnancy, preterm delivery, and preeclampsia without severe features. Our case report adds to the growing body of literature that suggests elevated ALP levels may be a harbinger of adverse pregnancy outcomes and highlights the importance of fractionating the isoenzymes and continuing close follow-up during pregnancy and postpartum. However, future large studies are needed to establish ALP as a marker of a placental pathology or high-risk pregnancy.

Consent

Written informed consent was obtained from the patient.

References

[1] A. Boronkai, N. G. Than, R. Magenheim et al., "Extremely high maternal alkaline phosphatase serum concentration with syncytiotrophoblastic origin," *Journal of Clinical Pathology*, vol. 58, no. 1, pp. 72–76, 2005.

[2] B. Ferro, I. Marques, J. Paixão, and M. D. C. Almeida, "Incidental finding of extreme elevation of serum alkaline phosphatase in pregnancy," *Cureus*, vol. 13, no. 8, article e17211, 2021.

[3] A. Safarova, Ö. Bige, E. Doğan, and C. Kaymaz, "Origin and significance of extremely elevated serum alkaline phosphatase activity during normal pregnancy," *Journal of Clinical Obstetrics & Gynecology*, vol. 17, no. 5, pp. 405–408, 2007.

[4] A. Larsson, M. Palm, L. O. Hansson, and O. Axelsson, "Reference values for clinical chemistry tests during normal pregnancy," *BJOG : An International Journal of Obstetrics and Gynaecology*, vol. 115, no. 7, pp. 874–881, 2008.

[5] P. Jamjute, A. Ahmad, T. Ghosh, and P. Banfield, "Liver function test and pregnancy," *The Journal of Maternal-Fetal & Neonatal Medicine*, vol. 22, no. 3, pp. 274–283, 2009.

[6] R. G. Best, R. E. Meyer, and C. F. Shipley, "Maternal serum placental alkaline phosphatase as a marker for low birth weight: results of a pilot study," *Southern Medical Journal*, vol. 84, no. 6, pp. 740–742, 1991.

[7] D. J. Brock and L. Barron, "Measurement of placental alkaline phosphatase in maternal plasma as an indicator of subsequent low birthweight outcome," *British Journal of Obstetrics and Gynaecology*, vol. 95, no. 1, pp. 79–83, 1988.

[8] S. McErlean and C. King, "Does an abnormally elevated maternal alkaline phosphatase pose problems for the fetus," *BMJ Case Reports*, vol. 12, no. 4, p. e229109, 2019.

[9] R. E. Meyer, S. J. Thompson, C. L. Addy, C. Z. Garrison, and R. G. Best, "Maternal serum placental alkaline phosphatase level and risk for preterm delivery," *American Journal of Obstetrics and Gynecology*, vol. 173, no. 1, pp. 181–186, 1995.

[10] A. H. Moawad, R. L. Goldenberg, B. Mercer et al., "The preterm prediction study: the value of serum alkaline phosphatase, alpha-fetoprotein, plasma corticotropin-releasing hormone, and other serum markers for the prediction of spontaneous preterm birth," *American Journal of Obstetrics and Gynecology*, vol. 186, no. 5, pp. 990–996, 2002.

[11] R. Rajagambeeram, S. Abu Raghavan, S. Ghosh, S. Basu, R. Ramasamy, and S. B. Murugaiyan, "Diagnostic utility of heat stable alkaline phosphatase in hypertensive disorders of pregnancy," *Journal of Clinical and Diagnostic Research*, vol. 8, no. 11, pp. Cc10–CC13, 2014.

[12] C. J. Davis, J. Booth, J. Summerfield, E. J. Lazda, and L. Regan, "Grossly elevated placental derived alkaline phosphatase in pregnancy as a marker for uteroplacental vascular disease," *Journal of Obstetrics and Gynaecology*, vol. 19, no. 5, pp. 533-534, 1999.

[13] V. Vongthavaravat, M. M. Nurnberger, N. Balodimos, H. Blanchette, and R. S. Koff, "Isolated elevation of serum alkaline phosphatase level in an uncomplicated pregnancy: a case report," *American Journal of Obstetrics and Gynecology*, vol. 183, no. 2, pp. 505-506, 2000.

[14] R. Wilkof-Segev, M. Hallak, and R. Gabbay-Benziv, "Extremely high levels of alkaline phosphatase and pregnancy outcome: case series and review of the literature," *Journal of Perinatal Medicine*, vol. 49, no. 2, pp. 191–194, 2021.

[15] A. Bashiri, O. Katz, E. Maor, E. Sheiner, I. Pack, and M. Mazor, "Positive placental staining for alkaline phosphatase corresponding with extreme elevation of serum alkaline phosphatase during pregnancy," *Archives of Gynecology and Obstetrics*, vol. 275, no. 3, pp. 211–214, 2007.

[16] S. Lozo, A. Atabeygi, and M. Healey, "Extreme elevation of alkaline phosphatase in a pregnancy complicated by gestational diabetes and infant with neonatal alloimmune thrombocytopenia," *Case Reports in Obstetrics and Gynecology*, vol. 2016, 4896483 pages, 2016.

[17] A. E. Heazell, J. K. Judge, and N. R. Bhatti, "A case of isolated peripartum elevation of alkaline phosphatase in pregnancy complicated by gestational diabetes," *The Journal of Maternal-Fetal & Neonatal Medicine*, vol. 19, no. 5, pp. 311–313, 2006.

[18] J. Wojcicka-Bentyn, K. Czajkowski, J. Sienko, M. Grymowicz, and M. Bros, "Extremely elevated activity of serum alkaline phosphatase in gestational diabetes: a case report," *American Journal of Obstetrics and Gynecology*, vol. 190, no. 2, pp. 566-567, 2004.

[19] H. Celik, M. Tosun, M. B. Cetinkaya, A. Bektab, and E. Malatyalýodlu, "Markedly elevated serum alkaline phosphatase level in an uncomplicated pregnancy," *The Journal of Maternal-Fetal & Neonatal Medicine*, vol. 22, no. 8, pp. 705–707, 2009.

[20] Z. Stanley, K. Vignes, and M. Marcum, "Extreme elevations of alkaline phosphatase in pregnancy: a case report," *Case Reports in Women's Health*, vol. 27, article e00214, 2020.

Pregnancy in Noncommunicating Rudimentary Horn of Unicornuate Uterus: A Case Report and Review of the Literature

Melese Gezahegn Tesemma

Arsi University, College of Health Science, Department of Obstetrics & Gynecology, Asella, Ethiopia

Correspondence should be addressed to Melese Gezahegn Tesemma; get.melese@gmail.com

Academic Editor: Erich Cosmi

Pregnancy implanted in the rudimentary horn of unicornuate uterus is very rare with an incidence of 1 in 75,000 to 1 in 150,000 pregnancies. Both prerupture and postrupture diagnosis of ectopic pregnancy in the rudimentary horn of a unicornuate uterus is difficult. Here is a case of a 21-year-old gravida 5 para 3 abortion 1 mother presented with abdominal pain of 2 days duration following a falling accident. The patient was severely anemic and was in hypovolemic shock at the time of presentation. She had diffused lower abdominal tenderness with hemoperitonium. After clinical and ultrasound evaluation, emergency laparotomy was decided for preop diagnosis of ruptured cornual ectopic pregnancy to rule out uterine rupture at gestational age of 16 weeks. Intraoperatively, ruptured ectopic pregnancy in noncommunicating rudimentary horn was diagnosed. Resection of rudimentary horn and ipsilateral salpingectomy was done. She was transfused with 5 units of compatible blood. It is better to increase awareness about pregnancy occurring in this rare uterine anomaly, so as to have a high index of suspicion as early detection before it gets ruptured is difficult.

1. Introduction

A unicornuate uterus with a rudimentary horn results from incomplete development of one of the Müllerian ducts and an incomplete fusion with the contralateral side [1–3]. The incidence of pregnancy occurring in a rudimentary horn of the unicornuate uterus is very rare ranging from 1 in 75,000 to 150,000 pregnancies. Usually the diagnosis is difficult and sometimes missed as the majority of the cases present on emergency with hemoperitonium [2, 4, 5]. About 85% of rudimentary uterine horns are noncommunicating in type [1, 5]. Ectopic pregnancy in this extremely rare anomaly ends up with rupture during all trimesters of pregnancy. Diagnosis of ectopic pregnancy in rudimentary horn is difficult, especially in a woman with a prior vaginal delivery. Thus a high index of suspicion is needed as in the majority of cases it is detected after it gets ruptured [3, 6]. Ectopic pregnancy in the rudimentary horn of unicornuate uterus is associated with life threatening complications, one of which is uterine rupture with a 50% risk [4, 5]. Here, I report a case of ectopic pregnancy in the rudimentary horn of a unicornuate uterus at gestational age of 16 weeks.

2. Case Report

A 21-year-old gravida 5 para 3 (all alive) abortion 1 mother with a pregnancy of 4 months was presented with severe lower abdominal pain of 2 days duration following a falling accident on her abdomen 5 days ago. She had easy fatigability, vertigo, and light headedness since two days after the accident, but had no vaginal bleeding, fever, headache, chills, and vaginal discharge and she did not feel fetal movement yet. She had no antenatal care follow up. She was referred from a nearby primary hospital to the Jimma university medical center with diagnosis of septic shock secondary to septic abortion where she was admitted and given antibiotics. Medical abortion was tried, but failed at the primary hospital. She had no personal or familial history of hypertension and diabetes. She had no history of chronic pelvic pain. She had no history of ectopic pregnancy, but had one history of spontaneous abortion which occurred at the 4th month. Prior to this accident, she had no history of abdominal pain, bloating, and epigastric pain.

On physical examination, she was acutely sick looking, agitated, and confused in appearance. Her vital signs were as follows: Blood Pressure: 70/30 mmHg, PR: 148 bpm, RR: 24 br/m,

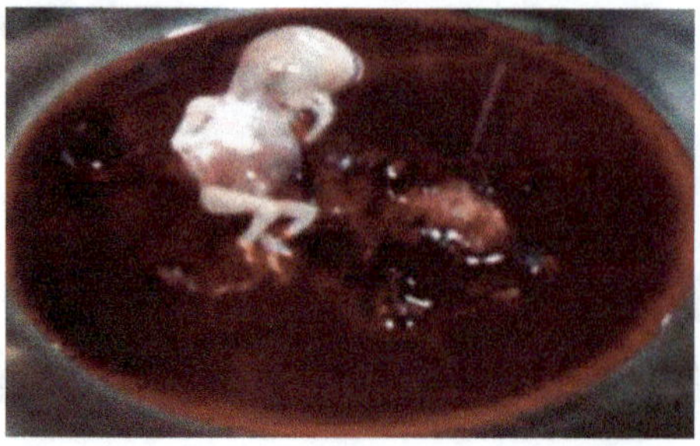

FIGURE 1: Dead male fetus and placenta removed from the peritoneal cavity.

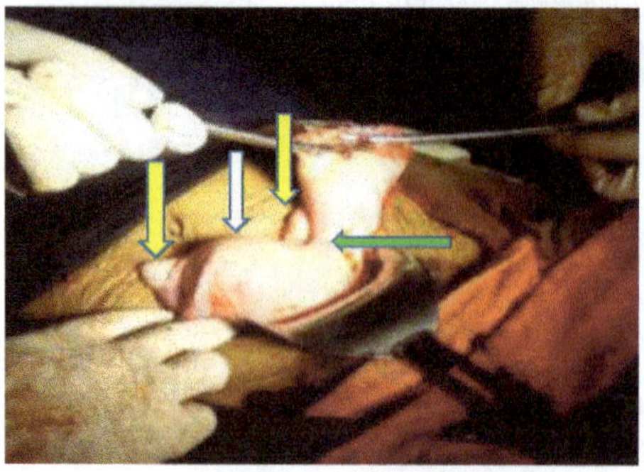

FIGURE 2: Uni-cornuate uterus (white arrow) with left side rudimentary horn (green arrow) attached to uterine body by dense fibro-muscular tissue. Ovaries are bilaterally visible (yellow arrows).

T^0: 37.5. Her conjunctiva was paper white and had dry tongue and buccal mucosa. Chest was clear and resonant. S3 gallop was heard. On the abdomen there was diffuse lower abdominal tenderness and guarding with positive signs of fluid collection. On pelvic examination cervix was closed with no blood on the examining finger, but, had a right adnexal tenderness.

On ultrasound exam, empty uterus was seen. A collapsed fetus with no cardiac activity having femur length measurement corresponding to 16 weeks and placenta measuring 4 cm × 5 cm looks attached to the left cornual part of the uterus was seen. There was significant free fluid in cul-de-sac and paracolic gutter. Otherwise liver and both kidneys were grossly normal. With impression of hypovolemic shock secondary to acute blood loss secondary to ruptured cornual ectopic pregnancy to rule out uterine rupture and severe anemia. The patient was resuscitated with 3 liters of intravenous crystalloids while preparing for an emergency laparotomy. She was investigated for blood group and Rh (A+) and complete blood count. Hematocrit was 6%, RBC count was only 0.7 million, platelet count was 52,000, WBC count was 11,000, and neutrophils was 85%. Four units of cross-matched blood were prepared before taking to the operation theatre.

Intraoperatively there was about 2500 ml hemoperitonium, ruptured left side rudimentary horn ectopic pregnancy, dead male fetus weighing about 300 gm (Figure 1), and the placenta partly attached to the cavity of the rudimentary horn. The unicornuate uterus with a normal ovary and tube was seen. The rudimentary horn had a cavity which was noncommunicating with the unicornuate uterine cavity and it was attached to the unicornuate uterus by fibrous tissue. The left round ligament and the ovary are directly attached to the rudimentary horn rather than the unicornuate uterus.

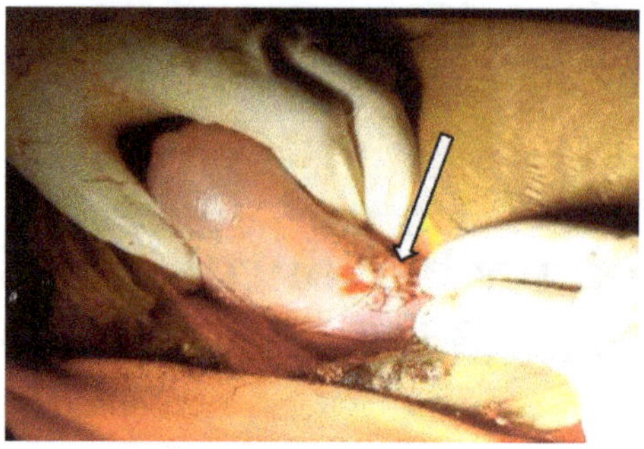

FIGURE 3: Stump (arrow) of the resected rudimentary horn after resection done.

Hemoperitonium was sucked out, the fetus and the placenta was removed. The round ligament and the utero ovarian ligament of the horn was clamped, cut, and ligated. The ruptured rudimentary horn was clamped and resected at its base and left side salpingectomy was done (Figure 2). The base was ligated to secure hemostasis and finally the stump was checked for any bleeding. (Figure 3). At the end, the abdominal cavity was mopped and closed in layers. The patient was transfused with 2 units of compatible blood intraoperatively and the other two on the immediate post-op day. Intraoperatively, a diagnosis of ruptured ectopic pregnancy in noncommunicating rudimentary horn of unicornuate uterus was made.

After being transfused with a total of 5 units of blood post-op, hematocrit increased to 30%, and symptoms of anemia improved. Post-operative condition was smooth and was finally discharged on the 6th post-op day after providing contraception and with an advice to continue her ferrous sulfate and to come early for an ultrasound evaluation in subsequent pregnancies to prevent the recurrence risk of ectopic pregnancy.

3. Discussion

Mechanism of pregnancy occurrence in the noncommunicating rudimentary horn is assumed to be by transperitoneal migration of either the fertilized ovum or the spermatozoon from the contralateral tube [2, 7, 8]. Despite the rarity and its diagnostic challenge, such type of ectopic pregnancy is associated with severe fetal-maternal morbidities [7, 8]. This was true in our case where the diagnosis of rudimentary horn ectopic pregnancy in unicornuate was missed before laparotomy and the patient presented with hypovolemic shock and severe anemia necessitating massive transfusion. Thus creating awareness on this clinical presentation is very important so as to increase the rate of early diagnosis before rupture and prevent catastrophic adverse maternal outcomes [8, 9]. The natural fate of ectopic pregnancy in rudimentary horn is usually rupture during the last two trimesters due to underdevelopment, variable thickness, and poor distensibility of myometrium and dysfunctional endometrium. As a result very few (10%) of these pregnancies reach full term out of which only 2% of the fetuses can survive [10].

Although antenatal diagnosis of pregnancy in rudimentary horn is still tricky, advanced first trimester scanning may provide a clue for early diagnosis [4, 9]. But only few cases of rudimentary horn pregnancy were diagnosed in early trimester prior to rupture so far [8, 11]. Whenever ultrasound finding remains inconclusive one may consider magnetic resonance imaging due to its high soft tissue definition and confirmatory information [8–10]. Even though the sensitivity of ultrasonography to diagnose pregnancy in rudimentary horn is only 26–30% [3, 6], it would be helpful to use the three sonographic criterias suggested by Tsafrir and his associates for the diagnosis of rudimentary horn pregnancy [8].

Placement of a Foley catheter into the uterine cavity with filled balloon and performing a transabdominal ultrasound scan can conclusively exclude an intrauterine pregnancy as it is shown in one case report [11]. Foley catheter was also used to see whether the horn is communicating with the uterine cavity [10]. In our case, although the presence of extra uterine pregnancy was confirmed before laparotomy the fact that she sustained a falling accident and the presence of a fetus outside the uterine cavity increased our doubt of uterine rupture.

Resection of the rudimentary horn and the ipsilateral fallopian tube by either laparotomy or laparoscopy is the mainstay of the management of rudimentary horn ectopic pregnancy [1, 4, 8]. In our case, we resected the rudimentary horn with its fallopian tube by laparotomy. It is recommended not to postpone surgery once the diagnosis of a unruptured ectopic pregnancy in rudimentary horn is made as the timing of rupture depends on the thickness of the horn musculature and once it ruptures it leads to catastrophic complications [9]. Patients with unicornuate uterus with a rudimentary horn should be investigated for urinary anomalies; as imaging in some patients revealed an absent kidney on the ipsilateral side [7]. In our case, both kidneys were grossly normal on ultrasound. On discharge the patients should be advised on future risk of ectopic pregnancy and preterm birth related to this anomaly as it was addressed in our case [7].

4. Conclusion

There is a need for increased awareness of this rare anomaly and having a high index of suspicion, especially in developing countries where the possibility of early detection before rupture is difficult.

Acknowledgments

I thank the client for giving me the consent for publication. My heartfelt thank also goes to those who were involved in the management of this patient.

References

[1] P. I. Okonta, H. Abedi, C. Ajuyah, and L. Omo-Aghoja, "Pregnancy in a noncommunicating rudimentary horn of a unicornuate uterus: a case report," *Cases Journal*, vol. 3, no. 1, p. 6624, 2009.

[2] A. Tufail and H. A. Hashmi, "Ruptured ectopic pregnancy in rudimentary horn of the uterus," *Journal of the College of Physicians and Surgeons—Pakistan*, vol. 17, no. 2, pp. 105–106, 2007.

[3] D. V. Kanagal and L. C. Hanumanalu, "Ruptured rudimentary horn pregnancy at 25 weeks with previous vaginal delivery: a case report," *Case Reports in Obstetrics and Gynecology*, vol. 2012, Article ID 985076, 4 pages, 2012.

[4] Y. J. Lai, C. H. Lin, W. C. Hou, K. S. Hwang, M. H. Yu, and H. Y. Su, "Pregnancy in a noncommunicating rudimentary horn of a unicornuate uterus: prerupture diagnosis and management," *Taiwanese Journal of Obstetrics & Gynecology*, vol. 55, no. 4, pp. 604–606, 2016.

[5] G. G. Nahum, "Rudimentary uterine horn pregnancy the 20th-century worldwide experience of 588 cases," *The Journal of Reproductive Medicine*, vol. 47, no. 2, pp. 151–163, 2002.

[6] S. Thakur, A. Sood, and C. Sharma, "Ruptured noncommunicating rudimentary horn pregnancy at 19 weeks with previous cesarean delivery: a case report," *Case Reports in Obstetrics and Gynecology*, vol. 2012, Article ID 308476, 4 pages, 2012.

[7] E. Gonçalves, J. P. Prata, S. Ferreira et al., "An unexpected near term pregnancy in a rudimentary uterine horn," *Case Reports in Obstetrics and Gynecology*, vol. 2013, Article ID 307828, 4 pages, 2013.

[8] A. Tsafrir, N. Rojansky, H. Y. Sela, J. M. Gomori, and M. Nadjari, "Rudimentary horn pregnancy: first-trimester prerupture sonographic diagnosis and confirmation by magnetic resonance imaging," *Journal of Ultrasound in Medicine*, vol. 24, no. 2, pp. 219–223, 2005.

[9] V. Gaikwad, R. Gite, H. G. Deshpande, A. Pingle, and M. Puri, "Rudimentary horn pregnancy-prerupture diagnosis and management," *Medical Journal of Obstetrics & Gynecology*, vol. 2, no. 3, p. 1042, 2014.

[10] L. Della Corte, A. Fabozzi, P. Giampaolino et al., "A case of 20-week abortion in a rare communicating rudimentary horn of a misinterpreted unicornuate uterus, incorrectly diagnosed as bicornuate: a serious hazard!" *European Journal of Obstetrics & Gynecology and Reproductive Biology*, vol. 235, pp. 133–135, 2019.

[11] K. A. Buntugu, "Rudimentary horn pregnancy: pre-rupture diagnosis and management," *Ghana Medical Journal*, vol. 42, no. 2, 2009.

16

Appearances are Deceptive: Two Case Reports in Teenagers on the Conservative Laparoscopic Surgery for Adnexal Torsion with Apparent Infarction

A. Jayawardane[1] **M. Patabendige**[2] **and C. Gunathilaka**[3]

[1]*Obstetrics and Gynaecology, Faculty of Medicine, University of Colombo, Colombo, Sri Lanka*
[2]*Obstetrician and Gynaecologist, Base Hospital, Mahaoya, Sri Lanka*
[3]*National Hospital of Sri Lanka, Colombo, Sri Lanka*

Correspondence should be addressed to M. Patabendige; mpatabendige@gmail.com

Academic Editor: Maria Grazia Porpora

Introduction. Torsion of the ovary, tube, or both is estimated to be responsible for 2-7% of all gynaecological emergencies. Oophorectomy is commonly performed for adnexal torsion with a possible negative impact on fertility in women of reproductive age. *Case Presentations.* We report two cases of teenage girls presented with adnexal torsion describing their laparoscopy features. Detorsion without additional surgical intervention could save their ovaries. *Discussion.* Detorsion is a more conservative surgical approach that should be considered in all younger women with ovarian torsion.

1. Introduction

Ovarian torsion refers to the full or partial twisting of the ovary around its suspensory structures, leading to the compromised blood supply to the ovary. The resultant ischemia can cause tissue necrosis with a potential loss of the affected ovary permanently. Oophorectomy was the standard treatment for many decades due to the presumed risk of thrombosis, infection, peritonitis, and reperfusion injury following untwisting of the twisted ovary [1]. The presence of adnexal cysts may result in torsion of the adnexa, with a similar mechanism leading to ischaemia and necrosis. It is estimated that 2.7% to 7.4% of all gynaecological emergencies are due to torsion [2] [3].

This paper summarises similar case reports of two, young girls presenting with adnexal torsion where the visual inspection was highly suggestive of nonviable ischaemic necrosis of the tissues. However, proceeding to conservative laparoscopic surgery resulted in a successful outcome.

2. Case Presentations

2.1. Case: 1. A 15-year-old, previously healthy, Sri Lankan, Muslim ethnic girl presented with severe lower abdominal pain of two days duration. The pain was gradually getting worse. Her menarche was four years ago, and she had regular periods with no dysmenorrhoea. On direct inquiry, she has had three similar episodes during the last six months, but less severe in intensity. On examination, the abdomen was tender, mainly in the left iliac fossa. Urine human chorionic gonadotrophin was negative. Ultrasound revealed a 12 cm complex pelvic mass. The overall picture was suggestive of a twisted ovarian cyst with features of surrounding oedema.

She underwent laparoscopy with consent for the removal of the affected ovary. At laparoscopy, an adnexal twisting due to a left ovarian cyst was confirmed. The left tube was grossly edematous. Both ovary and the tube appeared congested, dark blue-black in colour, and gross appearance suggestive of nonviable tissues. Adnexa was untwisted and ovarian cystectomy was done. At the end of surgery (one hour), significant improvement of appearance and perfusion was noted. Her recovery was uncomplicated with low molecular weight heparin and early mobilisation. The extracted cyst wall was compatible with a benign serous cystadenoma.

Three months later, an ultrasound scan on day-15 revealed a corpus luteum in the left ovary. Figure 1 shows the sequential changes in the ovarian and tubal tissues.

2.2. Case: 2. A 13-year-old, previously healthy, Sri Lankan, Sinhala ethnic girl presented with worsening lower abdominal pain of 36 hours duration. Her menarche was one year ago. She was uncertain in her last period. On examination, she had severe right-sided lower abdominal tenderness. Urine human chorionic gonadotrophin was negative. An ultrasound scan revealed a large 6 cm complex right adnexal cyst with possible surrounding oedema.

At laparoscopy, a twisted para-ovarian cyst and fallopian tube were noted. There was significant tissue edema and the fallopian tube distal to the torsion was dark blue-black in colour and appeared nonviable. Right ovary was not involved in the torsion. Left adnexa was normal. The fallopian tube was untwisted, and removal of cyst was carried out. At the end of surgery (45 minutes), significant reperfusion was noted in the fallopian tube. The patient had an uncomplicated recovery. Cyst wall histology revealed a benign serous cyst with foci of haemorrhage. Figure 2 shows the sequential changes in the right fallopian tube.

3. Discussion

3.1. Pathophysiology of Adnexal Torsion. Adnexal torsion is an uncommon gynaecological emergency presenting with worsening lower abdominal/pelvic pain [4]. Some women describe previous self-limiting similar pain episodes, usually attributed to partial torsion followed by spontaneous detorsion. Persistent torsion leads to tissue congestion due to impeded venous drainage followed by ischaemia as arterial blood supply is compromised leading to tissue necrosis. Early identification and intervention are important to prevent permanent tissue damage and toxaemia.

3.2. Challenges in Diagnosis. In our experience, high-resolution transvaginal ultrasound (used trans-rectally if the patient is before coitarche) is an extremely useful tool available at the clinic setting. We use colour Doppler to assess limitations on the blood flow due to torsion. We aim for a presentation-to-surgery time of less than 6 hours, which is usually feasible. Diagnosis is challenging but early diagnosis and treatment can prevent catastrophic complications [5]. Although Doppler may reveal limitations on blood flow, there are no definitive tests to confirm tissue viability before surgery. Traditionally, one depends on a visual assessment of viability by the surgeon for decision making.

Laparoscopic cystectomy during torsion in a case of complex cyst might pose a potential concern due to possible oncologic problems. However, the age-adjusted incidence of ovarian malignancy is very rare, 1.072 per 100,000 per year in girls aged 10–19 years [6]. In addition, we are applying the International Ovarian Tumor Analysis (IOTA) classification (B rules and M rules) in every ovarian mass which has a higher sensitivity and specificity to rule out a malignant one [7]. There was no indication to go for magnetic resonance imaging, and a postsurgical histology report was sought as early as possible.

3.3. Surgical Management. Preexisting adnexal cysts and ovarian hyperstimulation are considered to increase the risk of torsion. Torsion may happen in all age groups, but is more common in the younger, reproductive-age females [4]. Complications attributed to torsion and tissue necrosis include increased risk of thrombosis, infection, peritonitis, and reperfusion injury [4]. Removal of the affected adnexa was the traditional standard practice for several decades worldwide [1, 8]. However, oophorectomy in a young woman carries significant implications for future fertility. Despite some reports of successful cases of conservative management, surgical management was the norm for the past few decades [1, 8–10]. The concerns of this mode of treatment are fertility and loss of ovarian tissue at a younger age [11]. Recent two reviews on adnexal torsion have emphasized the importance of conservative management among adolescents [4, 11].

3.4. Conservative Management. As the edematous, ischemic, distorted adnexal tissue is extremely friable, laparoscopic detorsion is a delicate, time-consuming process. The slow process is likely to be beneficial as gradual detorsion is thought to be protective in reducing reperfusion injury of the ischaemic adnexa [12]. Most of these girls have benign tumours hence conservative management is a good option [8]. A recent consensus on conservative management has arisen giving rise to promising results [13–15]. A recent large population-based study of around 20,000 ovarian torsions demonstrated that conservative management may not be associated with increased perioperative complications, and the application of conservative options has increased from 18.9% to 25.1% between 2001 and 2015 [14].

The present account consisting of images provides a novel insight and supports conservative management. Both patients recovered with no peri-operative and postoperative complications. An immediate change in colour was obvious at laparoscopy in both cases. There is a paucity of robust data on the long-term follow-up of conservatively managed adnexal torsion. However, some recent reports showed that long-term outcomes were good [9, 14]. Case: 2 was followed up until three months and revealed a corpus luteum indicating complete recovery of the affected ovary. In case 2, there were no complaints at 6 months follow-up postsurgery. Therefore, these two teenage girls benefited from conservative treatment rather than radical surgery even when the adnexa appeared to be necrotic [5].

A study discussing long-term follow-up experience of conservative management has mentioned successfully managed two similar cases. The first patient has normally delivered her baby, and the other one is in her seventh month of pregnancy [16]. Another retrospective case-control study ($n = 33$) has compared laparoscopic surgical versus conservative

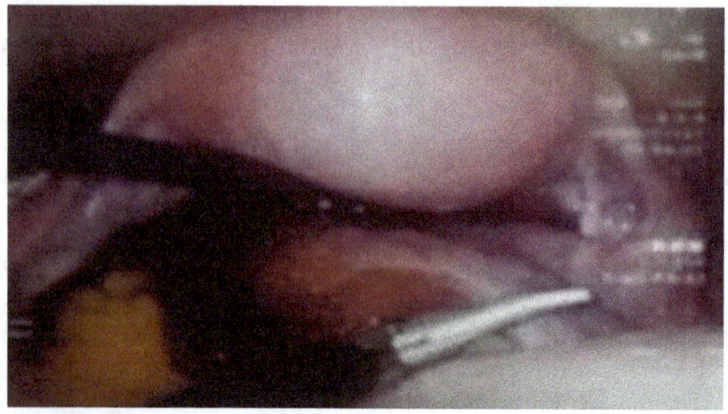

(a)

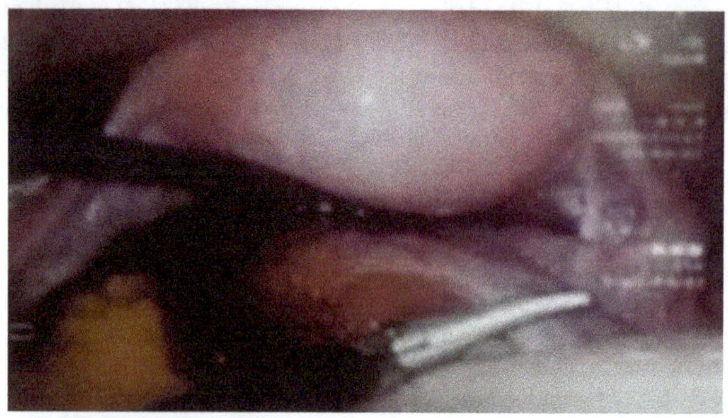

(b)

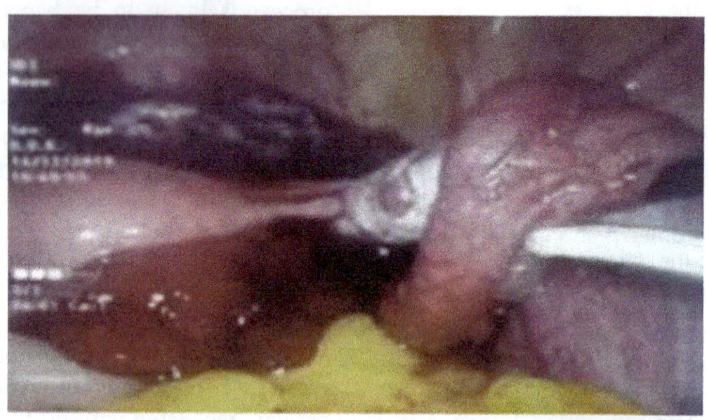

(c)

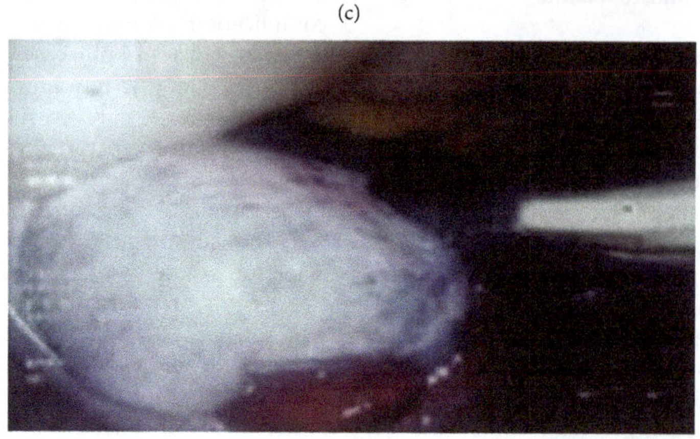

(d)

Figure 1: Sequential changes in the ovarian and tubal tissues in the teenager related to the case 1.

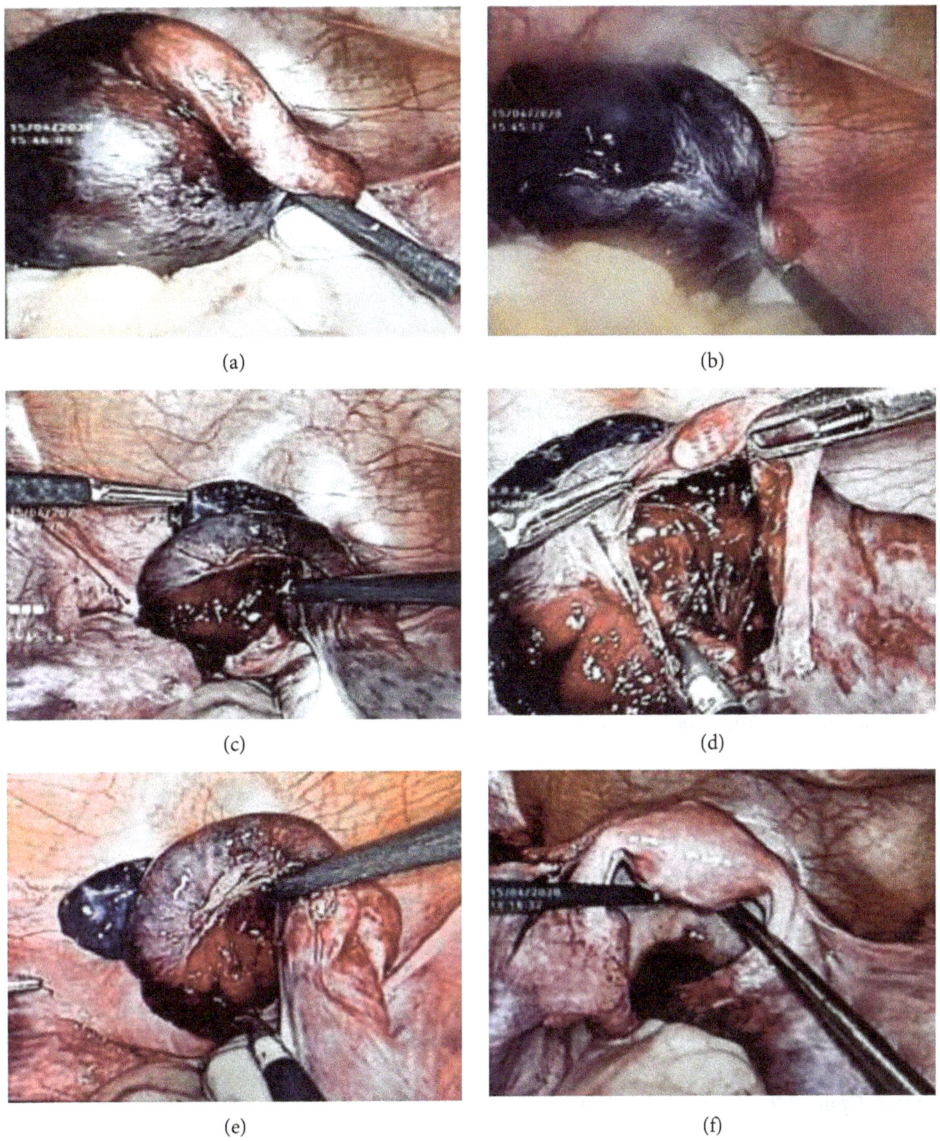

FIGURE 2: Sequential changes in the ovarian and tubal tissues in the teenager related to the case 2.

organ-sparing management [17]. In this study, the mean age was 34.9 years (range 14-68 years) [17]. Out of 33, 17 cases had "conservative" management of which only two had only detorsion alone. Their objective was to evaluate the effectiveness of laparoscopic surgery for adnexal torsion reducing the need for a laparotomy. Therefore, short-term outcomes of conservative management have not been clearly mentioned.

3.5. Drawbacks of Conservative Management. Potential drawbacks of the conservative option are possibility of adhesion around the tube and ovary, tubal occlusion, and procedure-related complications such as laparoscopy [15]. One case reported in 1995 reported a case of conservative management of an ovarian torsion leading to adnexal necrosis in two days after detorsion [18]. A three-year follow-up study by Fujishita et al. has reported 14 cases of conservative management of adnexal torsion with a good outcome, and only two cases [2/14] have been reported having significant tubal adhesions leading to tubal occlusion in second-look laparoscopy [15]. The second case discussed here is at risk of developing such long-term complications.

4. Conclusion

Prompt intervention to preserve ovarian function should be laparoscopic wherever possible. Detorsion should be the treatment of choice in young girls and women of reproductive age whose families are not complete, regardless of the colour and appearance of the ovary at the time of surgery. The two cases presented could be an interesting starting point for larger studies on conservative treatment in young patients with adnexal torsion.

Authors' Contributions

All authors contributed equally.

References

[1] D. H. Nichols and P. J. Julian, "Torsion of the adnexa," *Clinical obstetrics and gynecology*, vol. 28, no. 2, pp. 375–380, 1985.

[2] S. O. Anteby, J. G. Schenker, and W. Z. Polishuk, "The value of laparoscopy in acute pelvic pain," *Annals of Surgery*, vol. 181, no. 4, pp. 484–486, 1975.

[3] L. T. Hibbard, "Adnexal torsion," *American journal of obstetrics and gynecology*, vol. 152, no. 4, pp. 456–461, 1985.

[4] E. Damigos, J. Johns, and J. Ross, "An update on the diagnosis and management of ovarian torsion," *The Obstetrician and Gynaecologist*, vol. 14, no. 4, pp. 229–236, 2012.

[5] C. Huchon and A. Fauconnier, "Adnexal torsion: a literature review," *European Journal of Obstetrics & Gynecology and Reproductive Biology*, vol. 150, no. 1, pp. 8–12, 2010.

[6] S. H. Heo, J. W. Kim, S. S. Shin et al., "Review of ovarian tumors in children and adolescents: radiologic-pathologic correlation," *Radiographics*, vol. 34, no. 7, pp. 2039–2055, 2014.

[7] N. Nunes, G. Ambler, X. Foo, J. Naftalin, M. Widschwendter, and D. Jurkovic, "Use of IOTA simple rules for diagnosis of ovarian cancer: meta-analysis," *Ultrasound in Obstetrics & Gynecology*, vol. 44, no. 5, pp. 503–514, 2014.

[8] S. E. Dolgin, E. R. Kokoska, M. S. Keller, and T. R. Weber, "Acute ovarian torsion in children," *American Journal of Surgery*, vol. 183, no. 1, pp. 95-96, 2002.

[9] G. Oelsner, D. Bider, M. Goldenberg, D. Admon, and S. Mashiach, "Long-term follow-up of the twisted ischemic adnexa managed by detorsion," *Fertil Steril*, vol. 60, no. 6, pp. 976–979, 1993.

[10] A. Göçmen, M. Karaca, and A. Sari, "Conservative laparoscopic approach to adnexal torsion," *Archives of Gynecology and Obstetrics*, vol. 277, no. 6, pp. 535–538, 2008.

[11] C. Spinelli, J. Piscioneri, and S. Strambi, "Adnexal torsion in adolescents," *Current Opinion in Obstetrics & Gynecology*, vol. 27, no. 5, pp. 320–325, 2015.

[12] S. Ozkisacik, M. Yazici, H. Gursoy, and N. Culhaci, "Does gradual detorsion protect the ovary against ischemia-reperfusion injury in rats?," *Pediatric Surgery International*, vol. 30, no. 4, pp. 437–440, 2014.

[13] B. H. Al Wattar and Y. Afifi, "Untwist and keep: appraising evidence for conservative management of ovarian torsion," *BJOG: an international journal of obstetrics and gynaecology*, vol. 127, no. 8, p. 966, 2020.

[14] R. S. Mandelbaum, M. B. Smith, C. J. Violette et al., "Conservative surgery for ovarian torsion in young women: perioperative complications and national trends," *BJOG: An International Journal of Obstetrics & Gynaecology*, vol. 127, no. 8, pp. 957–965, 2020.

[15] A. Fujishita, H. Araki, S. Yoshida et al., "Outcome of conservative laparoscopic surgery for adnexal torsion through one-stage or two-stage operation," *The Journal of Obstetrics and Gynaecology Research*, vol. 41, no. 3, pp. 411–417, 2015.

[16] K. Chu, Q. Zhang, N. Sun, H. Ding, and W. Li, "Conservative laparoscopic management of adnexal torsion based on a 17-year follow-up experience," *The Journal of International Medical Research*, vol. 46, no. 4, pp. 1685–1689, 2018.

[17] I. Alkatout, L. Mettler, M. Anlauf, W. Jonat, C. Eckmann-Scholz, and T. Schollmeyer, "Management of adnexal torsion by laparoscopic approach," *Gynecological Surgery*, vol. 9, no. 4, pp. 405–409, 2012.

[18] R. A. Pryor, H. P. Wiczyk, and D. L. O'Shea, "Adnexal infarction after conservative surgical management of torsion of a hyperstimulated ovary," *Fertil Steril*, vol. 63, no. 6, pp. 1344–1346, 1995.

A Case of Pregnancy Complicated with Evans Syndrome with Sequential Development of Autoimmune Warm Antibody Hemolytic Anemia and Idiopathic Thrombocytopenic Purpura

Haruka Suzuki, Koji Yamanoi, Jumpei Ogura, Takahiro Hirayama, Koji Yasumoto, Shimpei Shitanaka, Yoshihide Inayama, Mie Sakai, Tsutomu Ohara, and Koh Suginami

Department of Obstetrics and Gynecology, Toyooka Public Hospital, 1094, Tobera, Toyooka City, Hyogo 6680065, Japan

Correspondence should be addressed to Koji Yamanoi; kojiymni@kuhp.kyoto-u.ac.jp

Academic Editor: Kyousuke Takeuchi

The simultaneous or sequential development of autoimmune hemolytic anemia (AIHA) and idiopathic thrombocytopenic purpura (ITP) is known as Evans syndrome. We experienced a case of Evans syndrome that developed AIHA during pregnancy and ITP long after delivery. The patient was a 35-year-old pregnant woman (gravida 2, para 1). A routine blood test at 28 weeks of gestation revealed moderate macrocytic anemia. Her haptoglobin level was markedly low, and a direct antiglobulin test (DAT) was positive. Based on these results, AIHA was considered. A healthy female newborn with bodyweight 3575 g was vaginally delivered uneventfully. After delivery, the DAT remained positive, but anemia did not develop. At 203 days after delivery, ITP was detected. Because AIHA and ITP developed sequentially, she was diagnosed with Evans syndrome. When AIHA occurs during pregnancy, long-term follow-up is needed because ITP can develop sequentially.

1. Introduction

In a pregnant woman, the hemoglobin concentration and hematocrit decrease as a result of marked plasma augmentation. Moderate or severe anemia may, however, cause fetal growth restriction or premature birth [1, 2]. Thus, it is important to identify and properly manage the cause of anemia. Hemolytic anemia is one cause of moderate or severe anemia. Autoimmune hemolytic anemia (AIHA) is a type of hemolytic anemia.

AIHA is characterized by the development of anti-erythrocyte autoantibodies and the destruction of erythrocytes, which causes moderate or severe anemia [3, 4]. In some AIHA cases, idiopathic thrombocytopenic purpura (ITP) can develop simultaneously or sequentially, which is known as Evans syndrome [5, 6]. Because Evans syndrome is a rare disease, little is known about the relationship between pregnancy and Evans syndrome.

Here we report a case of pregnancy complicated with Evans syndrome. In this case, AIHA developed during pregnancy and ITP developed long after delivery. This is the first report of a case of AIHA and ITP developing sequentially at very different times.

2. Case Presentation

A 35-year-old woman, impregnated via intracytoplasmic sperm injection (ICSI), visited our hospital at 9 weeks of gestation. She had a history of one pregnancy with a normal delivery. The patient also had a history of asthma and no history of blood cell transfusion or medication except for the use of the antibiotic cephem during ICSI to prevent infection. A blood test administered at her first visit revealed that she was D-antigen-positive and irregular antibody-negative and her hemoglobin concentration was 14.4 g/dl.

At 28 weeks of gestation, a blood test revealed acute macrocytic anemia (hemoglobin concentration, 7.9 g/dl; mean corpuscular volume, 108.1 fl; and mean corpuscular hemoglobin, 35.3 pg; Table 1(a)). A detailed examination was performed to determine the reason for these results

TABLE 1: Blood test results (reference ranges are shown).

(a) Total blood count and urine test data when anemia developed at 28 weeks of gestation

WBC	8.2 x10^3	(4.0-9.0 x10^3)	/ul
RBC	2.73 x10^6	(3.80-4.80 x 10^6)	/ul
Hb	7.9	(11.0-15.0)	g/dl
PLT	19.7 x 10^4	(12-35 x 10^4)	/ul
MCV	108.1	(83.0-99.0)	fl
MCH	35.3	(28.4-34.6)	pg
Reticulocyte	20 x 10^4	(3-10 x 10^4)	/ul
	73.4	(5.0-20.0)	‰
Urine hemoglobin	negative		

(b) Detailed blood test results at 29 weeks of gestation

AST	17	(8-30)	IU/l
ALT	10	(5-35)	IU/l
Creatinine	0.51	(0.30-0.90)	mg/dl
LDH	312	(106-211)	IU/l
LDH 1	40	(21-31)	%
LDH 2	37	(28-35)	%
LDH 3	15	(21-26)	%
LDH 4	4	(7-14)	%
LDH 5	4	(5-13)	%
UA	4.3	(2.5-7.0)	mg/dl
Total Bilirubin	0.8	(0.2-1.0)	mg/dl
C3	100	(65-135)	mg/dl
C4	29	(13-35)	mg/dl
Antinuclear antibody	negative		
Fe	100	(55-180)	ug/dl
Ferritin	40.3	(5-152)	ng/ml
UIBC	290	(130-320)	ug/dl
Haptoglobin	10>		mg/dl
Direct Coombs	positive		
Indirect Coombs	negative		
IgG	757	(870-1700)	mg/dl
IgA	160	(100-410)	mg/dl
IgM	70	(35-220)	mg/dl
Cold agglutinin reaction	128	(<256)	titer

(Table 1(b)). Hemolysis, elevated liver enzymes, low platelet count (HELLP) syndrome; hemolytic uremic syndrome (HUS); and thrombotic thrombocytopenic purpura (TTP) were unlikely. Systemic lupus erythematosus is reported as a disease that causes anemia [7] but was also unlikely because a test for anti-nuclear antibody was negative. Her C3, C4, and erythrocyte-binding IgG, IgA, and IgM levels were also normal. We then suspected the presence of hemolytic anemia and performed several additional examinations.

As shown in Table 1, an increase of reticulocyte and lactate dehydrogenase (LDH) and a marked decrease of haptoglobin (<10 mg/dl) were found. We further examined the LDH fractions and found that LDH1 and LDH2 were markedly increased. Her urine was negative for hemoglobin. These results strongly suggested the presence of hemolysis. In addition, the direct antiglobulin test (DAT) was positive for anti-IgG and negative for anti-C3d. The indirect antiglobulin test was negative. There was no corresponding medical history or symptoms of infection that could have contributed to the observed hemolytic anemia. A blood test for cold agglutinins was negative. Hill et al. have reported that they can diagnose AIHA when there is evidence of hemolytic anemia, the DAT is positive for IgG, and there is no evidence of an alternative cause of hemolytic anemia when the DAT is positive [8]. Accordingly, warm AIHA was diagnosed as the cause of anemia in this case.

Maternal blood was regularly tested. We had started iron preparation from onset of anemia empirically, and her hemoglobin level recovered to 10.1 g/dl by 31 weeks of gestation (Figure 1(a)). Although her iron level in the blood

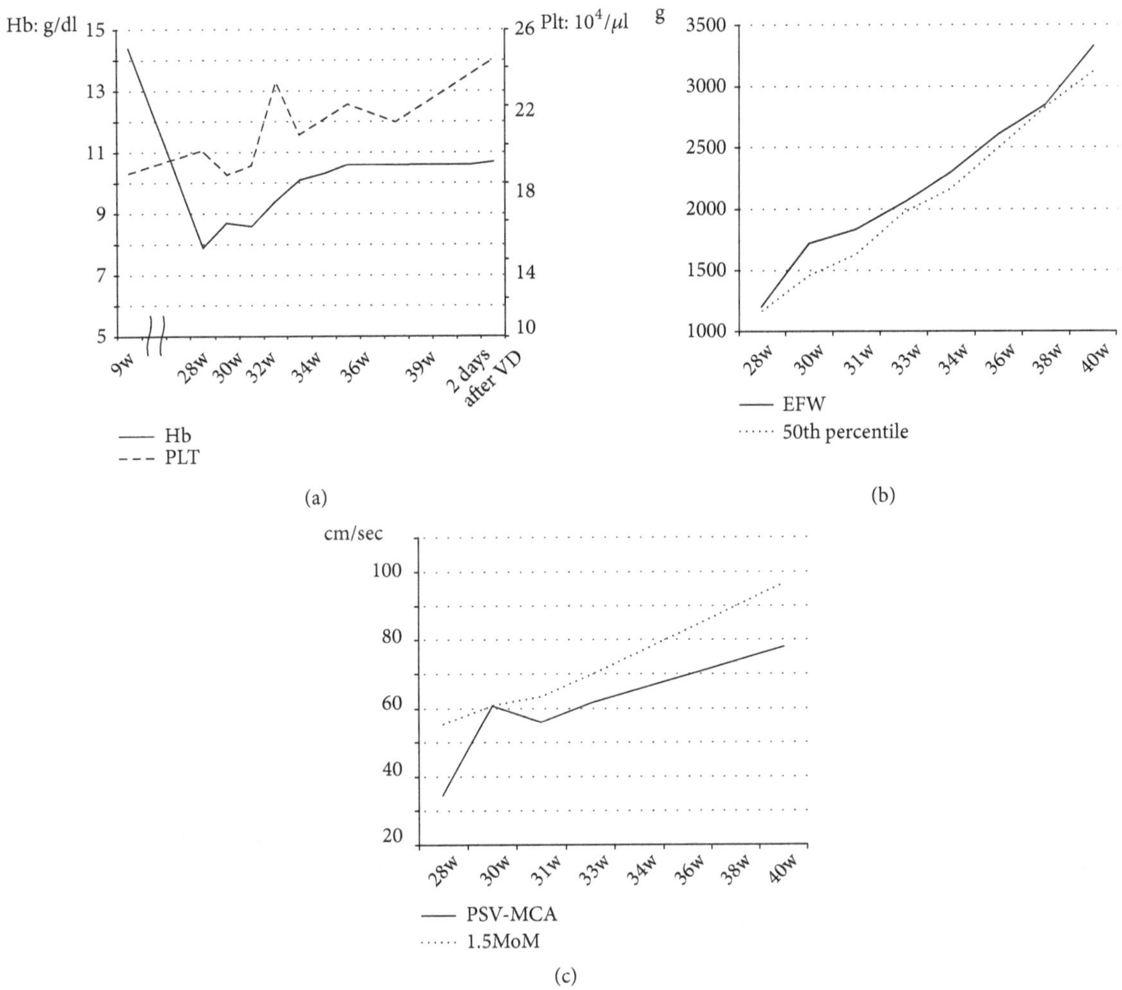

FIGURE 1: Clinical data during pregnancy and delivery. (a) Transition of hemoglobin concentration and platelet count from an early stage of pregnancy to delivery. Solid line, hemoglobin; dotted line, platelets. (b) Transition of fetal estimated weight (EFW). Solid line, EFW; dotted line, 50th percentile. (c) Transition of middle cerebral artery peak systolic velocity (MCA-PSV). Solid line, PSV-MCA; dotted line; 1.5 MoM.

was normal, we assumed that iron deficiency might have coexisted and kept iron supplementation. The DAT remained positive at 30 and 34 weeks of gestation. Fetal estimated weight and middle cerebral artery peak systolic velocity (MCA-PSV) were assessed every 2 weeks via ultrasound examination to monitor effects of the anemia (Figures 1(b) and 1(c)), and these factors remained in the normal range.

Labor started spontaneously at 40+1 weeks of gestation, and a normal female newborn was delivered. Her Apgar score was 9/9 (1/5 min), and her body weight was 3575 g. The total bleeding amount was 330 g, and the duration of labor was 380 minutes. No notable event occurred during delivery or the postpartum period. On the days following delivery, the patient's hemoglobin concentration was 10.7 g/dl. The neonatal hemoglobin concentration was 13.6 g/dl. At 2 days of age, the newborn was treated with 24-hour phototherapy because of neonatal jaundice. Both the mother and neonate were discharged on postdelivery day 5.

After discharge, the patient's DAT and hemoglobin concentrations were regularly assessed on an outpatient basis. Her DAT remained positive at 32, 95, and 203 days after delivery. Her hemoglobin level and blood platelet count were normal at 100 days after delivery. From approximately 150 days after delivery, the patient frequently observed nose bleeding and subcutaneous hemorrhage. A blood test at 203 days revealed an extremely low platelet count at 8000/μl (Table 2). The patient was admitted to the Department of Hematology, and bone marrow aspiration was performed. The form of megakaryocytes was normal, and no malignant cells were detected. A diagnosis of ITP was made. Because

TABLE 2: Total blood count data when thrombocytopenia developed at 203 days after delivery (reference ranges are shown).

WBC	5.4 x10^3	(4.0-9.0 x10^3)	/ul
Hb	14.3	(11.0-15.0)	g/dl
PLT	0.8 x10^4	(12-35 x10^4)	/ul
MCV	82.4	(83.0-99.0)	fl
MCH	28.0	(28.4-34.6)	pg
Direct Coombs	positive		

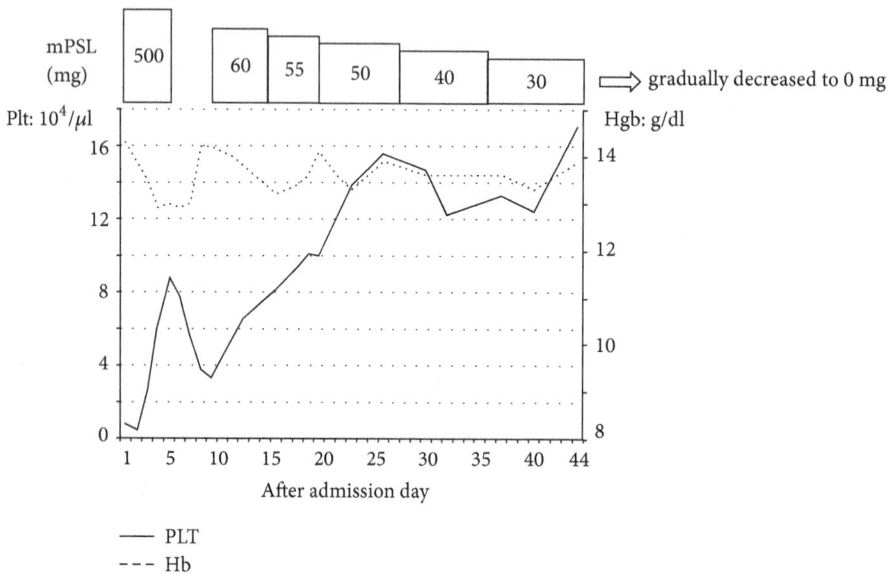

FIGURE 2: Transition of hemoglobin concentration and platelet count after development of idiopathic thrombocytopenic purpura (ITP) and subsequent treatment with corticosteroids. Solid line, platelets; dotted line, hemoglobin. The treatment procedure is also shown.

it occurred after the development of AIHA, Evans syndrome was considered.

Treatment with corticosteroids was initiated (3 days of methylprednisolone 500 mg) on the day after hospitalization, and the patient's platelet count recovered to 88,000/μl. Notably, after completion of the corticosteroids treatment, the platelet count decreased again, and oral administration of prednisolone 60 mg was initiated. Progress was satisfactory, and the prednisolone dosage was gradually decreased to 0 mg (Figure 2).

At 1 year after completing corticosteroid treatment, hemoglobin and platelet counts remained in the normal range.

3. Discussion

We presented a pregnancy complicated with Evans syndrome, which was first diagnosed as AIHA during the third trimester of pregnancy. AIHA is occasionally accompanied by ITP (0.8-3.7%), a condition known as Evans syndrome [6]. Thus far, there are few reports that refer to the relationship between Evans syndrome and pregnancy. In most cases of pregnancy complicated with Evans syndrome, anemia and thrombocytopenia occur during pregnancy or shortly after delivery [5, 9]. We could not find any reports of the development of ITP long after delivery. In the present case, we closely followed up and observed the development of ITP at 203 days after delivery. The onset of anemia and thrombocytopenia occurred at extremely different times. Although the mechanism is unclear, it should be considered that ITP can develop long after the onset of AIHA and delivery. Close and long-term follow-up is recommended when AIHA is diagnosed during pregnancy.

The two most common causes of anemia during pregnancy and the puerperium are iron deficiency and acute blood loss. Other causes include inflammation, malignancy, megaloblastic anemia, and acquired hemolytic anemia. In our case, acute blood loss, megaloblastic anemia, and malignant diseases were unlikely. Blood tests showed an increase of reticulocytes and LDH levels and a decrease of the haptoglobin level. As a result, an acquired hemolytic disease was suspected because the patient had no history of congenital hemolytic anemia.

Hemolysis occurs under many conditions, such as HELLP syndrome, acute fatty liver of pregnancy (AFLP), HUS, and TTP [3], or as a result of medication. In our case, the blood test results and medication history did not correspond to HELLP syndrome, AFLP, HUS, TTP, or drug-induced hemolysis. Furthermore, the DAT for anti-IgG was positive, indicating the likelihood of AIHA according to a diagnostic approach shown in a previous review [8]. AIHA is a disease characterized by the development of anti-erythrocyte autoantibodies and the destruction of erythrocytes. This disease is classified as warm (65%), cold (30%), and mixed (5%) type [10]. The main clinical features of AIHA are acute anemia, hemolysis, and a positive DAT result.

The presence of RBC autoantibodies is not consistently associated with hemolytic anemia. Silent RBC autoantibodies have been detected in healthy blood donors, pregnant women, and patients with autoimmune disorders. Among 60 cases of silent AIHA, five cases occurred in pregnant women, and this disease had no effect on the course of pregnancy, fetal development, or health of the newborns [11]. Hoppe et al. reported that autoimmunization against RBCs increases during pregnancy [12]. Issaragrisil et al. reported 14 cases of pregnancy-associated AIHA, with 10 of the 14 cases being women who became pregnant during the AIHA remission period, and the AIHA worsened during pregnancy [7].

In the present case, the detection of silent AIHA was uncertain, but early in pregnancy, the blood count was normal, and anemia occurred at 28 weeks of gestation. Although the exact mechanism remains unknown, this report and previous reports suggest that AIHA develops or worsens during pregnancy. Wikman et al. suggest that cytokines such as interleukin-8 may reflect antibody activation [13]. Cytokine activity markedly changes during pregnancy, and thus, pregnancy may induce antibody reactions. Further studies are required to reveal the mechanism behind the relationship between AIHA and pregnancy.

Issaragrisil et al. reported several cases of AIHA in pregnant women and noted that, in most cases, patients require treatment with corticosteroids or termination [7]. Lauzikiene et al. reported a case of resistance to corticosteroid treatment that required termination [3]. In our case, the hemoglobin level recovered and did not require corticosteroid treatment.

As warm autoantibody is an IgG antibody, it passes through the placenta and may cause fetal hemolytic anemia. Chaplin et al. reported four stillbirths and one neonatal death among 19 cases reviewed [14]. Lawe et al. reported a case that required four exchange transfusions for neonatal hyperbilirubinemia [15]. In the present case, we performed repeated ultrasonography to evaluate fetal growth and MCA-PSV, and we carefully followed up the fetal condition. The pregnancy and delivery were completed uneventfully, and the patient and her baby were uneventfully discharged from the hospital.

In conclusion, we experienced a case of Evans syndrome diagnosed from acute anemia at 28 weeks of pregnancy. In the case of acute anemia during pregnancy, a thorough investigation of the cause is important. When AIHA is diagnosed during pregnancy, close and careful observation is essential because it can worsen both the fetal and the maternal condition. In addition, close follow-up via repeated blood tests after delivery is recommended because it enables an early diagnosis of ITP.

Disclosure

The present affiliation is Department of Dermatology, Cutaneous Biology Research Center, Massachusetts General Hospital.

Acknowledgments

We thank Dr. Yoshiyuki Onda, the hematologist of our hospital, for his excellent comments and suggestions to this case.

References

[1] A. G. Ronnenberg, R. J. Wood, X. Wang et al., "Preconception hemoglobin and ferritin concentrations are associated with pregnancy outcome in a prospective cohort of Chinese women," *Journal of Nutrition*, vol. 134, no. 10, pp. 2586–2591, 2004.

[2] A. Mishra, N. Dave, and K. Viradiya, "Fatal anaphylactic reaction to iron sucrose in pregnancy," *Indian Journal of Pharmacology*, vol. 45, no. 1, pp. 93-94, 2013.

[3] D. Laužikiene, D. Ramašauskaite, T. Luža, and R. Lenkutiene, "Pregnancy Induced Autoimmune Warm Antibodies Hemolytic Anemia: A Case Report," *Geburtshilfe und Frauenheilkunde*, vol. 75, no. 11, pp. 1167–1171, 2015.

[4] B. Garvey, "Rituximab in the treatment of autoimmune haematological disorders," *British Journal of Haematology*, vol. 141, no. 2, pp. 149–169, 2008.

[5] V. Phupong, W. Sareepapong, and P. Witoonpanich, "Evans syndrome and pregnancy: A case report," *BJOG: An International Journal of Obstetrics & Gynaecology*, vol. 111, no. 3, pp. 274–276, 2004.

[6] J. C. Jaime-Pérez, L. N. Guerra-Leal, O. N. López-Razo, N. Méndez-Ramírez, and D. Gómez-Almaguer, "Experience with Evans syndrome in an academic referral center," *Revista Brasileira de Hematologia e Hemoterapia*, vol. 37, no. 4, pp. 230–235, 2015.

[7] S. Issaragrisil and M. Kruatrachue, "An Association of Pregnancy and Autoimmune Haemolytic Anaemia," *European Journal of Haematology*, vol. 31, no. 1, pp. 63–68, 1983.

[8] Q. A. Hill, R. Stamps, E. Massey, J. D. Grainger, D. Provan, and A. Hill, "The diagnosis and management of primary autoimmune haemolytic anaemia," *British Journal of Haematology*, vol. 176, no. 3, pp. 395–411, 2017.

[9] E. Lefkou, C. Nelson-Piercy, and B. J. Hunt, "Evans' syndrome in pregnancy: A systematic literature review and two new cases," *European Journal of Obstetrics & Gynecology and Reproductive Biology*, vol. 149, no. 1, pp. 10–17, 2010.

[10] P. Rai, G. Sharma, D. Singh, and J. Garg, "Rare presentation of mixed autoimmune hemolytic anemia in children: Report of 2 cases," *Journal of Laboratory Physicians*, vol. 9, no. 4, pp. 332–336, 2017.

[11] F. R. Mauro, F. Trastulli, C. Alessandri et al., "Clinical relevance of silent red blood cell autoantibodies," *Haematologica*, vol. 102, no. 12, pp. e473–e475, 2017.

[12] B. Hoppe, W. Stibbe, A. Bielefeld, A. Pruss, and A. Salama, "Increased RBC autoantibody production in pregnancy," *Transfusion*, vol. 41, no. 12, pp. 1559–1561, 2001.

[13] A. Wikman, U. Axdorph, G. Gryfelt, L. Gustafsson, M. Björkholm, and J. Lundahl, "Characterization of red cell autoantibodies in consecutive DAT-positive patients with relation to in vivo haemolysis," *Annals of Hematology*, vol. 84, no. 3, pp. 150–158, 2005.

[14] H. Chaplin Jr., R. Cohen, G. Bloomberg, H. J. Kaplan, J. A. Moore, and I. Dorner, "Pregnancy and Idiopathic Autoimmune Haemolytic Anaemia: A Prospective Study during 6 Months Gestation and 3 Months Post-Partum," *British Journal of Haematology*, vol. 24, no. 2, pp. 219–229, 1973.

[15] J. E. Lawe, "Successful exchange transfusion of an infant for AIHA developing late in mother's pregnancy," *Transfusion*, vol. 22, no. 1, pp. 66–68, 1982.

18

Pregnancy Outcome and Postnatal Chromosome Analysis of the Cord Blood and Chorionic Villi in Two Cases after Intrauterine Transfer of Mosaic Aneuploid Blastocysts

Yuki Ito,[1] Taizan Kamide,[1] Kosuke Taniguchi,[2] Taisuke Sato,[1,2] Michihiro Yamamura,[1,2] Akiko Konishi,[1] Ken Takahashi,[1,2] Hiroshi Kishi,[1] Kenichiro Hata,[2] Osamu Samura,[1] and Aikou Okamoto[1]

[1]*Department of Obstetrics and Gynaecology, The Jikei University School of Medicine, 3-25-8, Nishi-Shinbashi, Minato-ku, Tokyo, Japan 105-8461*

[2]*Department of Maternal-Fetal Biology, National Research Institute for Child Health and Development, 2-10-1, Okura, Setagaya-ku, Tokyo 157-8535, Japan*

Correspondence should be addressed to Osamu Samura; osamusamura@gmail.com and Aikou Okamoto; aikou7000@gmail.com

Academic Editor: Giovanni Monni

The long-term prognosis and genetic mechanism of pregnancy after intrauterine mosaic aneuploid blastocyst transfer remain unknown. We report the case of two babies after the aforementioned procedure and chromosomal analysis of their cord blood and chorionic villi. *Case Report 1.* A 41-year-old primipara, with two previous spontaneous abortions, was pregnant after intrauterine transfer of a blastocyst carrying 40% mosaicism of long-arm monosomy of chromosome 5. The amniocentesis results were 46,XX. A cesarean section was performed at 39 weeks. The female infant was 3,315 g at birth. *Case Report 2.* A 44-year-old primipara, with two spontaneous abortions, was pregnant after intrauterine transfer of a blastocyst carrying 40% mosaicism of long-arm monosomy of chromosome 9 and monosomy of chromosome 14. After genetic counselling, she decided not to undergo amniocentesis. No abnormalities were found by ultrasound. A cesarean section was performed at 38 weeks. The male infant was 3,340 g at birth. Chromosome analyses of postnatal cord blood and chorionic villi were performed using SNP arrays. The cord blood and chorionic villi showed no chromosomal structural abnormalities or mosaicism. For both, no disorders were observed at 10 months of age. We experienced the birth of babies after intrauterine transfer of mosaic aneuploid blastocysts.

1. Introduction

In preimplantation genetic testing for aneuploidy (PGT-A), approximately five cells are taken from the trophectoderm (TE) of the blastocyst. After whole genome amplification, next-generation sequencing (NGS) or array comparative genomic hybridization (aCGH) can be used to diagnose aneuploidy. Frequently, mosaic embryos are detected by PGT-A test results [1]. The transfer of euploid embryos is the first priority in preimplantation diagnosis, but the transfer of mosaic embryos may be considered if euploid embryos cannot be obtained [2].

The clinical results after the transfer of mosaic embryos are less favourable than those after the transfer of euploid embryos, with an implantation rate of approximately 40%–50% and an ongoing pregnancy rate of approximately 30%–40% [3]. In addition, the higher the mosaic ratio, the lower the pregnancy rate, the higher the miscarriage rate, and the lower the ongoing pregnancy rate.

There are reports of live births following mosaic embryo transfer. Victor et al. reported 21 live births after mosaic embryo transfer, 14 of which underwent amniocentesis: 11 with a normal karyotype, 2 with microdeletions, and 1 with a balanced translocation [4]. When mosaic embryos are

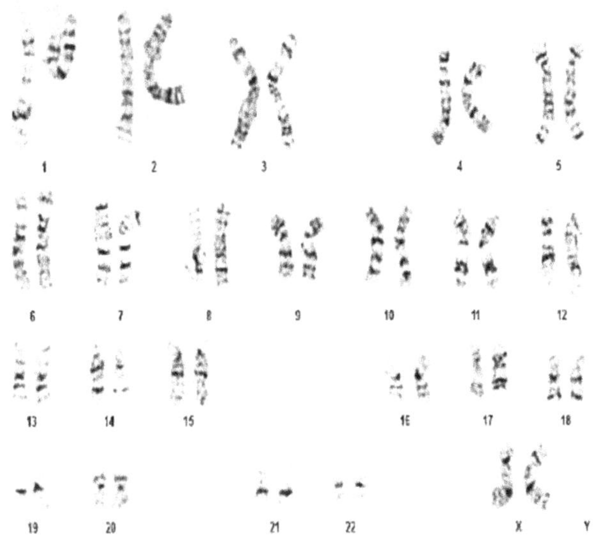

FIGURE 1: Normal female karyotype obtained after amniocentesis at 17 weeks and 1 d of pregnancy in Case 1.

TABLE 1: Summary of Cases 1 and 2.

	Age at egg retrieval (years)	Age at embryo transplantation (years)	PGT-A		Amniocentesis	Postnatal chromosomal analysis	
			Chromosomal constitution	Mosaic percentage (%)		Placenta	Cord blood
Case 1	40	41	Monosomy 5q (aCGH)	40	46,XX (G-banding)	46,XX (SNP array)	46,XX (SNP array)
Case 2	43	44	Monosomy 9q (NGS)	40	Not performed	46,XX (SNP array)	46,XX (SNP array)
			Monosomy 14 (NGS)	40			

PGT-A = preimplantation genetic testing for aneuploidy; aCGH = array comparative genomic hybridization; NGS = next-generation sequencing; SNP = single-nucleotide polymorphism.

transferred, there is a possibility of confined placental mosaicism, true foetal mosaicism with mosaicism in the foetus, or uniparental disomy (UPD)/loss of heterozygosity (LOH). Therefore, chromosome analysis of both the foetus and placenta in cases of pregnancies after mosaic embryo transfer is important.

We report the postnatal chromosome analysis of the cord blood and chorionic villi of two babies following mosaic embryo transfer.

2. Case Presentation of Cases

2.1. Case 1. A primipara had two previous spontaneous abortions. At the age of 40 years and 3 months, she had her eggs retrieved. TE biopsies were carried out on 3 blastocysts for PGT-A. aCGH revealed one mosaic embryo and no euploid embryo. Although she continued egg retrievals, she could not obtain a euploid embryo. At the age of 41 years and 5 months, she became pregnant after intrauterine blastocyst transfer with 40% mosaicism of the entire long-arm monosomy of chromosome 5 at an in vitro fertilization (IVF) clinic. She had no previous medical history. There was no family history of congenital disorder or genetic disorder. The couple were nonconsanguineous. The patient was referred to our hospital at 11 weeks of pregnancy. At 15 weeks of pregnancy, genetic counselling was provided to the couple. After counselling, she requested amniocentesis, which was performed at 17 weeks and 1 day of pregnancy. The amniocentesis (G-banding) results were 46,XX (15 cells) (Figure 1) (Table 1). Foetal screening ultrasonography at 20 and 30 weeks' gestation did not reveal any abnormalities. She underwent a cesarean section due to labour arrest at 39 weeks and 3 d of gestation. The female infant had a weight of 3,315 g, an Apgar score of 8/9 (1 min/5 min), and no evident abnormalities at birth. The size of the main placenta (placenta 1) was $18 \times 17 \times 1.5\,\text{cm}^3$ with a $7 \times 5 \times 1.5\,\text{cm}^3$ succenturiate placenta (placenta 2). No motor and intellectual disorders were observed at 10 months of age. Height and weight were appropriate for age.

2.2. Case 2. A primipara had two previous spontaneous abortions. At the age of 43 years and 8 months, she had her eggs retrieved at an IVF clinic. TE biopsies were carried out on one blastocyst for PGT-A. NGS revealed one mosaic embryo. At the age of 44 years and 1 month, she became pregnant after intrauterine blastocyst transfer with 40%

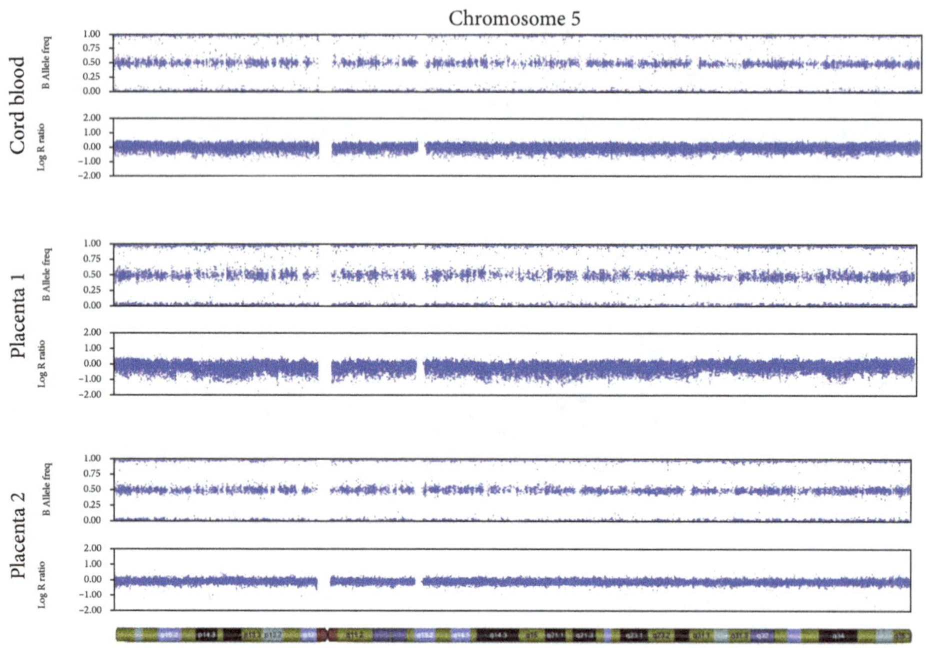

(a)

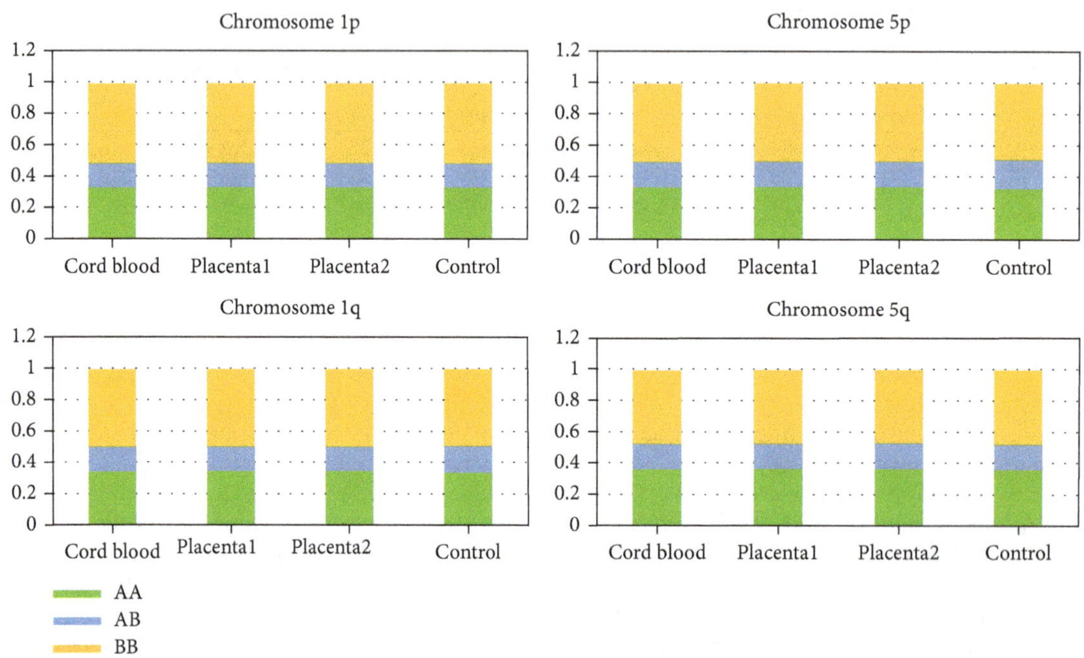

(b)

Figure 2: (a) Results of single-nucleotide polymorphism array analysis of the umbilical cord blood, main placenta (placenta 1), and succenturiate placenta (placenta 2) in Case 1: the B allele frequency indicates the frequency of B allele. The logR ratio indicates the copy number. No monosomy mosaicism or loss of heterozygosity was observed on the long arm of chromosome 5. (b) Proportion of single-nucleotide polymorphisms (AA, AB, and BB). There was no increase in the percentage of AA and BB compared to the control sample (peripheral blood of an adult woman with no previous medical history) analysed in the same panel. Chromosome 5 had similar polymorphism ratios compared to chromosome 1.

mosaicism of long-arm monosomy of chromosome 9 and monosomy of chromosome 14. She had a history of myomectomy at the age of 39 years. There was no family history of congenital disorder or genetic disorder. The couple were nonconsanguineous. The patient was referred to our hospital at 10 weeks of pregnancy. At 12 weeks of pregnancy, genetic counselling was provided to the couple. She strongly desired to continue the pregnancy and hoped that amniocentesis would not be performed if ultrasonography did not show an abnormal foetal morphology (Table 1). Foetal screening ultrasonography at 12, 20, and 30 weeks' gestation did not reveal any abnormalities. A cesarean section was performed

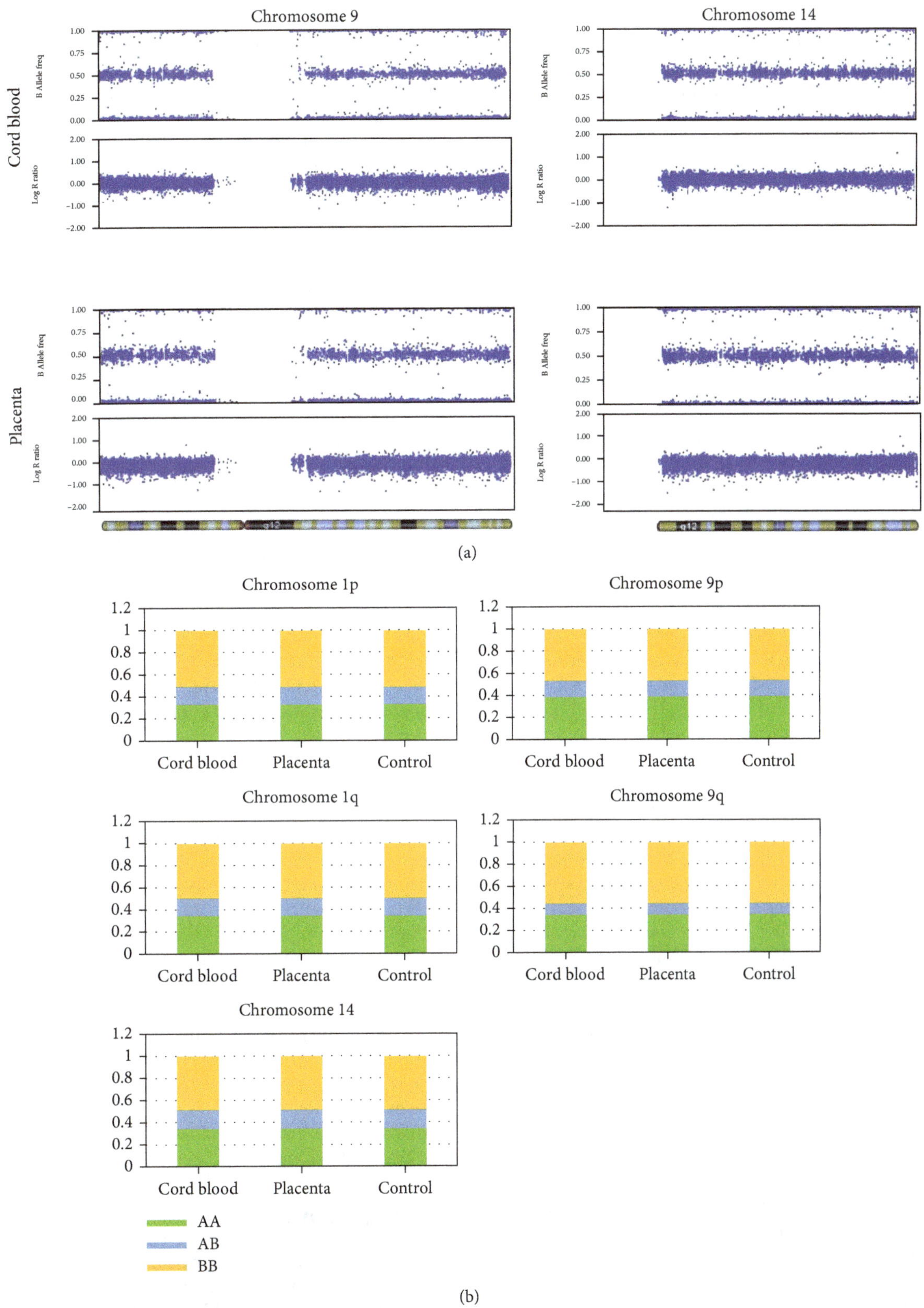

FIGURE 3: (a) Results of single-nucleotide polymorphism array analysis of the umbilical cord blood and placenta in Case 2: no monosomy mosaicism or loss of heterozygosity was observed on the long arm of chromosome 9 and chromosome 14. (b) Proportion of single-nucleotide polymorphisms (AA, AB, and BB) in Case 2. There was no increase in the percentage of AA and BB compared to that in the control sample (peripheral blood of an adult woman with no previous medical history) analysed in the same panel. Chromosomes 9 and 14 had similar polymorphism ratios compared to chromosome 1.

at 38 weeks and 3 d. The female infant had a weight of 3,340 g, an Apgar score of 8/9 (1 min/5 min), and no evident abnormalities at birth. The placenta showed no gross abnormalities. No motor and intellectual disorders were observed 1 year after birth.

2.3. Genome-Wide Single-Nucleotide Polymorphism Array. DNA was extracted from the umbilical cord blood sample and from the chorionic villi sample (Case 1: placentas 1 and 2, Case 2: placenta) as previously described [5]. Genome-wide single-nucleotide polymorphism (SNP) array analysis of the DNA samples was performed using the Infinium Asian Screening Array-24 v1.0 BeadChip (Illumina, San Diego, CA, USA) according to the manufacturer's protocols. The SNP arrays were scanned using the Illumina iScan system, and the data were analysed with KaryoStudio (version 1.4, Illumina, San Diego, CA, USA) using the default cnvPartition algorithm settings (version 3.0.7). Each SNP is sorted into A allele and B allele according to Illumina's protocol (Illumina, San Diego, CA, USA). The B allele frequency indicates the ratio of B allele. The logR ratio indicates the copy number. No decrease in the logR ratio was observed in the long arm of chromosome 5 of Case 1 and the long arm of chromosome 9 or chromosome 14 of Case 2. There was no mosaicism or LOH in B allele frequency (Figures 2 and 3). The proportion of SNP (AA, AB, and BB) was calculated, but there was no increase in the percentage of AA and BB compared to that in the control sample (peripheral blood of an adult woman with no previous medical history) analysed in the same panel. The proportion of SNP of chromosome 5 of Case 1 and chromosome 9 or chromosome 14 of Case 2 was comparable to that of chromosome 1. These chromosomes had similar polymorphism ratios compared to chromosome 1 (Figures 2 and 3). Thus, it was concluded that no mosaicism could be detected by the SNP array in both cases. There were no findings of structural abnormalities in other chromosomes.

This study was approved by the Institutional Review Boards (IRBs) of the National Center for Child Health and Development and the Jikei University School of Medicine (IRB number: 234 and IRB number: 27-060 (7945), respectively). Written informed consent was obtained from all subjects for the publication of this case report and the accompanying images.

3. Discussion

Chromosome analysis of cord blood and chorionic villi of two babies obtained after mosaic embryo transfer showed no abnormalities in the chromosome structure or mosaicism.

SNP arrays have the advantages of analysing a large number of cells simultaneously, cells in all cell cycles, and specimens without culturing cells [6]. UPD/LOH can also be detected in SNP arrays. There are reports showing the SNP array being more sensitive than aCGH and able to detect more than 5% of mosaicism [6, 7].

Partial deletion of the long arm of chromosome 5 has been reported to cause foetal growth restriction, duodenal obstruction, and cardiac disease [8]. Long-arm monosomy of chromosome 9 indicates foetal mortality. Partial deletion of the long arm of chromosome 9 has been reported to cause foetal hydrops, severe developmental delay, cardiac disease, and respiratory failure [9]. Partial deletion of the long arm of chromosome 14 has been associated with holoprosencephaly, microcephaly, and facial malformations [10]. There was no abnormality found in both infants.

Chromosome analysis of the entire placental tissue was difficult, which is a limitation of this study. However, as far as we could analyse, in both Cases 1 and 2, the SNP array results were normal, and there were no findings of LOH for whole chromosomes. These results can be attributed to two possibilities. First, once fertilization occurs normally, the monosomy mosaic appears during somatic cell division but decreases or disappears during development. Embryos with segmental mosaicism have the same miscarriage rate and live birth rate as the control group with a normal karyotype, because segment abnormal cells lacking centromeres cannot attach to the spindle during mitosis and do not proliferate during cell division [1]. Second is the presence of false positives during PGT-A analysis [11].

Mosaic embryos may be false positives for PGT-A analysis, or aneuploid cells may disappear during cell division. However, when mosaic embryos are transferred, there is a possibility of confined placental mosaicism, true foetal mosaicism, or UPD/LOH. Confined placental mosaicism may affect the placental function and cause intrauterine foetal growth restriction or preterm birth, even if no abnormalities are detected in the foetus [12]. In true foetal mosaicism, depending on the mosaic ratio and chromosome position, foetal morphological abnormalities and foetal growth may be detected [6]. Indeed, in one case, the same mosaicism observed on PGT-A has been reported in infants after birth [13]. Therefore, anxiety often persists during ongoing pregnancy, even when adequate genetic counselling is provided prior to mosaic embryo transfer. Currently, the number of reports on mosaic embryo transfer is increasing, but there are not enough reported cases to evaluate the effects of each specific mosaic composition and mosaicism rate on the pregnancy outcome and foetus. Therefore, it is important to continue to accumulate detailed clinical and genetic data on mosaic embryo transfers in the future.

In conclusion, we performed postnatal chromosome analysis of the cord blood and chorionic villi of two babies after mosaic embryo transfer. Our results may provide useful information for genetic counselling before embryo transfer and prenatal testing.

Acknowledgments

This research was supported by the Jikei University Research Grant for the Career Development of Female Researchers with Children and the Jikei University Research Fund (Grant Number 2021-006SR).

References

[1] E. Fragouli, S. Alfarawati, K. Spath et al., "Analysis of implantation and ongoing pregnancy rates following the transfer of

mosaic diploid-aneuploid blastocysts," *Human Genetics*, vol. 136, no. 7, pp. 805–819, 2017.

[2] D. S. Cram, D. Leigh, A. Handyside et al., "PGDIS position statement on the transfer of mosaic embryos 2019," *Reproductive Biomedicine Online*, vol. 39, Supplement 1, pp. e1–e4, 2019.

[3] S. Munne, F. Spinella, J. Grifo et al., "Clinical outcomes after the transfer of blastocysts characterized as mosaic by high resolution next generation sequencing- further insights," *European Journal of Medical Genetics*, vol. 63, no. 2, article 103741, 2020.

[4] A. R. Victor, J. C. Tyndall, A. J. Brake et al., "One hundred mosaic embryos transferred prospectively in a single clinic: exploring when and why they result in healthy pregnancies," *Fertility and Sterility*, vol. 111, no. 2, pp. 280–293, 2019.

[5] T. Sato, O. Samura, N. Kato et al., "Novel TFAP2A mutation in a Japanese family with branchio-oculo-facial syndrome," *Human Genome Variation*, vol. 5, no. 1, pp. 1–5, 2018.

[6] L. G. Biesecker and N. B. Spinner, "A genomic view of mosaicism and human disease," *Nature Reviews. Genetics*, vol. 14, no. 5, pp. 307–320, 2013.

[7] L. K. Conlin, B. D. Thiel, C. G. Bonnemann et al., "Mechanisms of mosaicism, chimerism and uniparental disomy identified by single nucleotide polymorphism array analysis," *Human Molecular Genetics*, vol. 19, no. 7, pp. 1263–1275, 2010.

[8] R. L. Kramer, B. Feldman, S. A. Ebrahim, S. B. Kasperski, M. P. Johnson, and M. I. Evans, "Molecular cytogenetic analysis of a de novo 5q31q33 deletion associated multiple congenital anomalies: case report," *American Journal of Medical Genetics*, vol. 82, no. 2, pp. 143–145, 1999.

[9] S. L. Dugan, E. Panza, A. Openshaw, L. D. Botto, J. A. Camacho, and R. M. Toydemir, "Delineation of the 9q31 deletion syndrome: genomic microarray characterization of two patients with overlapping deletions," *American Journal of Medical Genetics. Part A*, vol. 176, no. 12, pp. 2901–2906, 2018.

[10] Y. Segawa, N. Itokazu, A. Hirose, S. Nakagawa, and S. Takashima, "A case of partial 14q- with facial features of holoprosencephaly and hydranencephaly," *Pediatric Neurology*, vol. 37, no. 1, pp. 51–54, 2007.

[11] D. Goodrich, X. Tao, C. Bohrer et al., "A randomized and blinded comparison of qPCR and NGS-based detection of aneuploidy in a cell line mixture model of blastocyst biopsy mosaicism," *Journal of Assisted Reproduction and Genetics*, vol. 33, no. 11, pp. 1473–1480, 2016.

[12] J. Toutain, D. Goutte-Gattat, J. Horovitz, and R. Saura, "Confined placental mosaicism revisited: Impact on pregnancy characteristics and outcome," *PLoS One*, vol. 13, no. 4, article e0195905, 2018.

[13] S. Kahraman, M. Cetinkaya, B. Yuksel, M. Yesil, and C. C. Pirkevi, "The birth of a baby with mosaicism resulting from a known mosaic embryo transfer: a case report," *Human Reproduction*, vol. 35, no. 3, pp. 727–733, 2020.

19

Case Series of Intrauterine Subamniotic Hemorrhage

Momoko Owada, Yoshie Shibata, and Shunji Suzuki

Department of Obstetrics and Gynecology, Japanese Red Cross Katsushika Maternity Hospital, Tokyo, Japan

Correspondence should be addressed to Shunji Suzuki; czg83542@mopera.ne.jp

Academic Editor: Giovanni Monni

We present here 9 cases of intrauterine subamniotic hemorrhage to describe the pathological sequence. The definite diagnosis of subamniotic hemorrhage was mainly made macroscopically with the presence of hemorrhage or hematoma wrapped in the membrane on the fetal surface by postnatal examining of the placenta. In 7 of them (78%), the presence of gradual subamniotic hemorrhage in the second trimester of pregnancy was suspected. In the cases, severe fetal growth restriction and preterm delivery were recognized in 2 (29%) and 4 cases (57%), respectively. In the other 2 cases (22%), acute anemia associated with acute subamniotic hemorrhage was clinically suspected. This may be the first report examining the clinical characteristics of acute or gradual intrauterine subamniotic hemorrhage. Both patterns of subamniotic hemorrhage seemed to be associated with the adverse perinatal outcomes.

1. Introduction

Subamniotic hemorrhage is defined as a hemorrhage between the amniotic membrane and the fetal chorionic plate, following a tear in one of the branches of an umbilical vessel. It is sometimes seen in cases of excessive umbilical cord traction during the third stage of delivery [1, 2] associated with the raised umbilical venous pressure [3]. However, the occurrence of intrauterine subamniotic hemorrhage is relatively rare. Vessel trauma leading to subamniotic hemorrhage in the latter sequence has been supposed to be caused by sudden traction due to fetal movements or to external pressure or spontaneously by the intravascular pressure at a focus of lower vascular wall resistance [3]. To date, some cases concerning various pathological mechanisms associated with subamniotic hemorrhage have been reported [1, 2, 4–8].

We present here our 9 cases of subamniotic hemorrhage to describe the pathological sequence.

2. Case Series

The material reviewed consisted of the total population of women who delivered at 22 weeks' gestation or later at Japanese Red Cross Katsushika Maternity Hospital between 2006 and 2015. All the data are stored in a computer of our hospital. In our institute, all placentae were screened identically by trained staff (plural Japanese obstetrics specialists). Informed consent concerning analysis from a retrospective database was obtained from all subjects. The definite diagnosis of subamniotic hemorrhage was made macroscopically with the presence of hemorrhage or hematoma wrapped in the membrane on the fetal surface postnatally and confirmed by placental pathology with hematoma lying between the chorionic plate and amnion associated with the rupture of chorionic vessels.

During the study period, there were 20,118 deliveries at 22 weeks' gestation or later at our hospital. In 9 of them, subamniotic hemorrhage was confirmed in the placenta postnatally as shown in Table 1. Therefore, the incidence of subamniotic hemorrhage that can be confirmed postnatally is estimated to be about 0.04%.

In 7 of the 9 cases (78%), the subamniotic hemorrhage was shown as oval-shaped mass wrapped in the amniotic membrane at the placental cord insertion site in the fetal surface of the placenta (Figure 1), while it was shown as marginal irregular traces of bleeding under the broken amniotic membrane in 2 cases (22%, Figure 2). In our institute, the screening of placental hemorrhage has been routinely performed using ultrasound in all cases. In the former cases, the subamniotic hemorrhage was shown as cystic lesion

Table 1: Cases of subamniotic hemorrhage managed at our hospital.

Maternal age (y)	Parity	GA at diagnosis (w)	Ultrasonographic findings	GA at delivery (w)	Delivery mode	Birth weight (g)	Macroscopic finding of the placenta	Apgar score (1/5 minutes)	UApH
34	0	19	Cystic lesion protruding from the fetal plate (4x3x2 cm)	38	Vaginal delivery	2,954	Oval-shaped mass wrapped in the membrane	8/9	7.254
40	2	21	Cystic lesion protruding from the fetal plate (4x3x3 cm)	38	Vaginal delivery	2,742	Oval-shaped mass wrapped in the membrane	9/9	7.198
36	1	22	Cystic lesion protruding from the fetal plate (4x4x3 cm)	40	Vaginal delivery	3,128	Oval-shaped mass wrapped in the membrane	8/9	7.289
26	0	24	Cystic lesion protruding from the fetal plate (6x4x3 cm)	33	CS due to nonreassuring fetal status	1,254 (SGA)	Oval-shaped mass wrapped in the membrane	4/7	7.157
24	0	27	Cystic lesion protruding from the fetal plate (5x4x3 cm)	27	CS due to labor	678 (SGA)	Oval-shaped mass wrapped in the membrane	5/8	7.200
27	0	27	Cystic lesion protruding from the fetal plate (6x5x3 cm)	34	Vaginal delivery	2,154	Oval-shaped mass wrapped in the membrane	8/8	7.169
24	0	29	Cystic lesion protruding from the fetal plate (4x4x3 cm)	30	Vaginal delivery	1,426	Oval-shaped mass wrapped in the membrane	6/8	7.118
31	1	37 (after delivery)	No abnormal findings	37	CS due to nonreassuring fetal status	2,618	Extensive subamniotic hemorrhage	2/6	7.012
33	0	38 (after delivery)	No abnormal findings	38	Still birth	2,599	Extensive subamniotic hemorrhage	-	-

GA, gestational age; CS, cesarean section; SGA, small for gestational age; UApH, umbilical artery pH.

protruding from the fetal plate by ultrasonography during the pregnancy (Figure 3), while any abnormal findings were not recognized by ultrasonography in the latter cases. In the former cases, severe fetal growth restriction and preterm delivery were occurred in 2 (29%) and 4 cases (57%), respectively. In Doppler ultrasound examination, the decreased cerebroplacental ratio was observed in the 2 cases of fetal growth restriction; however, the middle cerebral artery-peak systolic velocities were normal. In addition, there were no abnormal findings of placental pathology leading to the development of fetal growth restriction except subamniotic hemorrhage.

On the other hand, there were no events until the onset labor pains at term in the latter cases. In Case 8, the neonatal hemoglobin concentration was 10.9 g/dL (normal: 13-22 g/dL) with reticulocyte counts of 0.9% (normal: < 7%). Although the amniotic fluid was bloody, any findings suggesting abruption or ulceration in the placenta were not recognized. The maternal hemoglobin-F was 0.5% (normal: < 1.0%). In Case 9, intrauterine fetal demise was recognized when the mother visited the hospital due to onset of labor pains at 38 weeks' gestation. The skin of the neonate was pale. Any findings suggesting abruption or ulceration in the placenta were not recognized and the maternal hemoglobin-F was normal (0.6%). Therefore, Cases 8 and 9 were clinically diagnosed as acute anemia associated with acute subamniotic hemorrhage. By placental pathology, there were no abnormal findings except subamniotic hematoma in the 2 cases.

On the other hand, the presence of gradual subamniotic hemorrhage in the second trimester of pregnancy was suspected in the former cases (Cases 1-7). In the 7 cases, there were no neonates complicated by anemia or adverse long-term outcomes.

3. Discussion

This may be the first report examining the clinical characteristics of acute or gradual intrauterine subamniotic hemorrhage.

The gradual subamniotic hematoma appeared as an oval-shaped soft mass wrapped in the membrane, while acute hemorrhage was recognized as marginal irregular traces of bleeding under the broken membrane. In the latter, the acute massive hemorrhage was thought to cause the collapse of the thin amniotic membrane, and then the bloody amniotic fluid

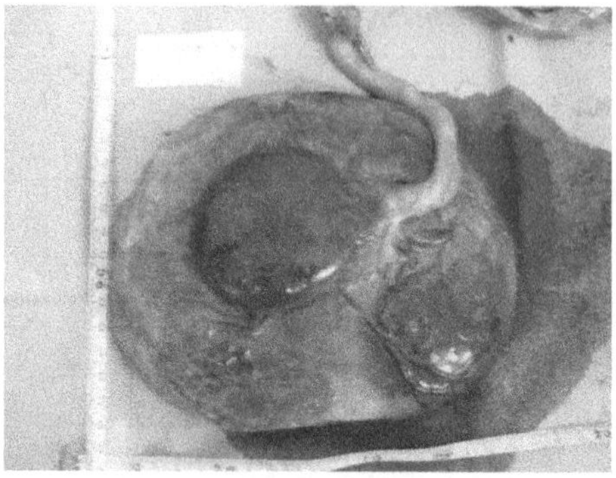

FIGURE 1: Macroscopic view of the placenta in Case 4 at delivery, showing an oval-shaped structure wrapped in the amniotic membrane.

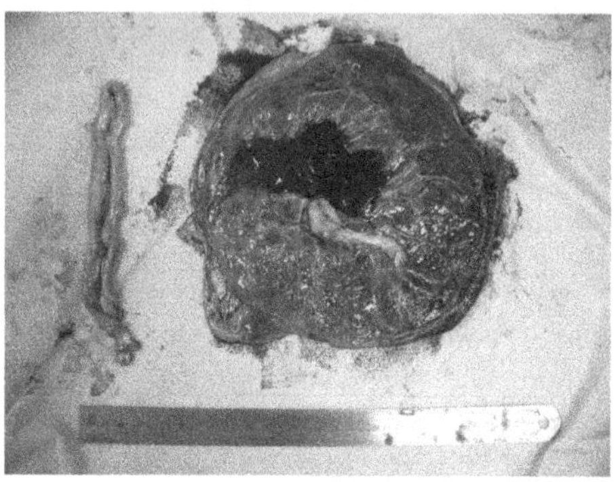

FIGURE 2: Macroscopic view of the placenta in Case 8 at delivery, showing marginal irregular traces of bleeding under the broken amniotic membrane.

was generated in Case 8. On the other hand, the difference in pathogenesis between acute and gradual subamniotic hemorrhages has not been well examined. Based on the difference in clinical courses, we speculate that acute subamniotic hemorrhage is related to the presence of uterine contraction leading to external pressure while gradual subamniotic hemorrhage occurs spontaneously by the intravascular pressure at a focus of lower vascular wall resistance. However, Van Den Bosch et al. [4] reported that the case of gradual subamniotic hematoma was suggested to occur due to the episode of premature contraction. Cases of intrauterine subamniotic hemorrhage are rare; however we expect the elucidation of pathogenesis of acute and gradual subamniotic hemorrhage by accumulation of the same case reports.

In some earlier literatures, subamniotic hemorrhage has not been thought to cause severe intrapartum complications [2, 4] except the cases of acute massive hemorrhage [5, 7]; however severe fetal growth restriction and preterm delivery occurred in 2 (29%) and 4 cases (57%), respectively, in our cases with gradual subchorionic hemorrhage. In this study, the fetal growth restriction might be due to the insufficient blood supply to the fetuses associated with the subamniotic hemorrhage based on the findings of the Doppler ultrasound examination. Classically, it had been thought that large hematoma of average cyst size was larger than 4.5 cm, more

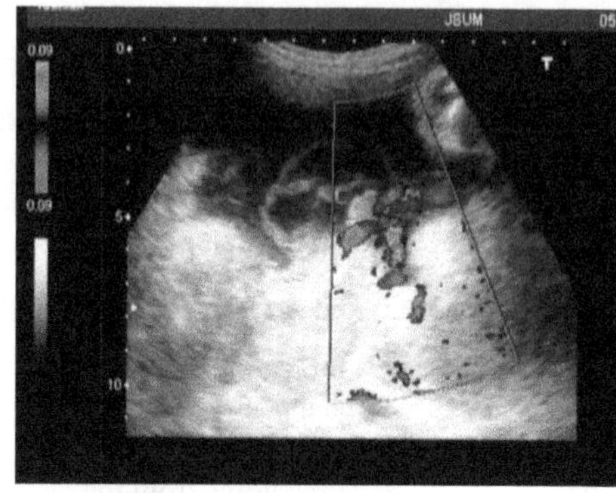

FIGURE 3: Ultrasonographic image showing subamniotic hematoma at 27 weeks in Case 4.

than 3 in number or at the placental cord insertion site leading to fetal growth restriction and nonreassuring fetal status [1, 8–10]. In recent years, however, the conception has tended to be denied [2, 4]. Unfortunately, we could not find any factors affecting the adverse perinatal outcomes associated with the presence of gradual subamniotic hematoma in the clinical courses or placenta findings of our cases. Therefore, a strict fetal surveillance including frequent Doppler ultrasound examination may be needed in all cases complicated by gradual subamniotic hematoma.

We present here the clinical characteristics of acute or gradual intrauterine subamniotic hemorrhage. However, we understand that the sample size of this study is too small to examine the etiology or pathology of intrauterine subamniotic hemorrhage as one of serious limitations because the sequence is very rare. To clarify the etiology and pathology of intrauterine subamniotic hemorrhage, a further study with accumulation of the same case reports is needed.

References

[1] D. J. Desa, "Rupture of fetal vessels on placental surface," *Archives of Disease in Childhood*, vol. 46, no. 248, pp. 495–501, 1971.

[2] E. Jauniaux and S. Campbell, "Ultrasonographic assessment of placental abnormalities," *American Journal of Obstetrics & Gynecology*, vol. 163, no. 5, pp. 1650–1658, 1990.

[3] P. M. Dunn, "The placental venous pressure during and after the third stage of labour following early cord ligation," *BJOG: An International Journal of Obstetrics & Gynaecology*, vol. 73, no. 5, pp. 747–756, 1966.

[4] T. Van Den Bosch, D. Van Schoubroeck, A. Cornelis, and M. Dubin, "Prenatal diagnosis of a subamniotic hematoma," *Fetal Diagnosis and Therapy*, vol. 15, no. 1, pp. 32–35, 2000.

[5] T.-K. Lo, A. Lee, W.-P. Chan et al., "Severe intrapartum asphyxia from subamniotic hemorrhage," *Fetal and Pediatric Pathology*, vol. 35, no. 6, pp. 416–419, 2016.

[6] A. Deans and E. Jauniaux, "Prenatal diagnosis and outcome of subamniotic hematomas," *Ultrasound in Obstetrics & Gynecology*, vol. 11, no. 5, pp. 319–323, 1998.

[7] T. Yoshimura, S. Satoh, S. Yanai, K. Tsukimori, T. Hirakawa,

and H. Nakano, "A case report of intrauterine fetal demise and subamniotic hematoma due to suspected rupture of placental vessels," *Nihon Sanka Fujinka Gakkai Zasshi*, vol. 53, no. 5, pp. 851–854, 2001 (Japanese).

[8] Y. Hiraizumi, M. Satomi, N. Ouchi et al., "Two cases of subamniotic hematoma," *Obstetrics & Gynecology*, vol. 78, no. 9, pp. 1155–1158, 2011 (Japanese).

[9] D. L. Brown, D. N. DiSalvo, M. C. Frates, K. M. Davidson, and D. R. Genest, "Placental surface cysts detected on sonography: Histologic and clinical correlation," *Journal of Ultrasound in Medicine*, vol. 21, no. 6, pp. 641–646, 2002.

[10] P. Kirkinen and P. Jouppila, "Intrauterine membranous cyst: a report of antenatal diagnosis and obstetric aspects in two cases," *Obstetrics & Gynecology*, vol. 67, no. 3, pp. 26S–30S, 1986.

20

Conservative Management of Cesarean Scar Pregnancy: A Case Report and Literature Review

Manuel Sánchez-Prieto, María Jesús Puy, Núria Barbany, Betlem Graupera, Maria Angela Pascual, and Pere Barri-Soldevila

Department of Obstetrics and Gynecology, Instituto Universitario Dexeus, Barcelona, Spain

Correspondence should be addressed to Manuel Sánchez-Prieto; mansan@dexeus.com

Academic Editor: Kyousuke Takeuchi

Cesarean scar pregnancy (CSP) is a rare form of ectopic pregnancy located in the lower uterine segment. The current increase in the percentage of cesarean sections is accompanied by significant growth in the incidence of CSP, while advances in ultrasound diagnostic techniques have led to a greater number of CSP diagnoses. A misdiagnosed CSP, or one that is diagnosed too late, is life-threatening to the pregnant patient and predisposes her to complications such as uterine bleeding or rupture, which often require hysterectomy and thus result in the irreversible loss of fertility. We present the case of a 50-year-old woman with a history of undiagnosed CSP after multiple consultations for intermittent bleeding and hemorrhage. She was diagnosed by ultrasound and the diagnosis was confirmed by hysteroscopy. She underwent conservative medical treatment that was successful.

1. Introduction

Cesarean scar pregnancy (CSP) is a type of ectopic pregnancy in which the gestational sac (GS) implants into the anterior wall of the lower uterine segment in an anterior cesarean scar [1]. It is the rarest form of ectopic pregnancy, representing 6% of all ectopic pregnancies in patients with a history of a previous cesarean section [1]. The incidence of CSP has increased, in parallel with the increase in the rate of cesarean sections and the widespread use of ultrasound in early pregnancy [2].

Abnormal implantation of the embryo within the myometrium and fibrous tissues of a previous scar can lead to uterine rupture, placental accreta, and uncontrolled bleeding, which can lead to hysterectomy and the permanent loss of fertility or even maternal death [3].

Early and accurate diagnosis and prompt management are very important to reduce life-threatening complications and preserve fertility [4]. Despite the large number of clinical reports and different therapeutic approaches, there is no consensus on the treatment of CSP [5].

Methotrexate (MTX) is an antimetabolite drug that has been used in the treatment of molar and ectopic pregnancies, including CSP [6, 7]. Although MTX is considered a safe and effective therapy, the optimal dose, route, and protocol for its use have yet to be determined for CSP [6].

We present a case of CSP detected in a symptomatic woman at the beginning of her pregnancy, and we review the management of the pathology.

2. Case report

A 50-year-old woman (Gravida 4, Para 1), with a history of 1 cesarean section and 3 rectovaginal fistula repairs -due to a complication of debridement of a Bartholin's gland abscess-, presented a menstrual delay. A urine pregnancy test was performed and was positive. Two days later, she started heavy bleeding. She went to the emergency department of an outer center, was diagnosed with an abortion in progress and underwent emergency dilation and curettage (D&C).

One month later, she consulted to another Center due to persistent bleeding and was diagnosed by ultrasound with chorionic remains in the left horn. A diagnostic hysteroscopy was recommended, but it was not performed since she expelled spontaneously. In the next 20 days, she had intermittent spotting.

On the day of her visit to our service, she came in due to vaginal bleeding with abundant clots. In the admission examination, abundant bleeding with clots at the level of the cervix was found, which were extracted with Foerster forceps. A transvaginal ultrasound was performed, which showed an endometrial thickness of 7 mm, with the cervical canal occupied by abundant blood content and clots with a size of 34 mm (Figures 1 and 2).

While waiting for ultrasound, she developed vasovagal syncope. Hypotension was evidenced, moderate bleeding continued with abundant clots, and the cervix was dilated to 1 cm.

Urgent analysis was performed, resulting in a hemoglobin level of 11.1 g/dL, correct coagulation, and a β-human chorionic gonadotropin (β-hCG) level of 2,000 mUI/mL.

D&C was performed by aspiration guided with transabdominal ultrasound, and 0.25 mg/ml of carboprost was administered intramuscularly. Correct hemostasis and no active bleeding were observed at the end of curettage.

Ultrasound and analytical control were recommended after one week.

The histological result of the curettage showed hematic material with fragments of decidua. Regarding analytical control, her β-hCG level had increased to 2188 mIU/mL.

Control transvaginal ultrasound revealed the following: At the level of the cesarean section scar, a 29 x 16 mm nodular image with a heterogeneous pattern was observed (Figure 3), and a color Doppler study showed vascularization (Figure 4). The image was compatible with organized and vascularized hematic material and compatible with probable placental remains, although it could not be conclusively ruled out that it had been an ectopic pregnancy.

Diagnostic hysteroscopy was recommended to confirm the suspected diagnosis; ectopic pregnancy was evidenced on the cesarean section scar (Figure 5).

The diagnosis of ovular remains in the previous cesarean section scar was confirmed, without being able to specify the gestation time. Given the diagnostic confirmation of ectopic pregnancy on the cesarean section scar, both surgical and medical treatment with methotrexate (MTX) was proposed so the patient could make an informed decision. She opted for conservative treatment. A single dose of MTX was administered. At 7 days, there was a >15% decrease in the β-hCG levels compared to the control on the 4th day, so no further doses were administered. On the 10th day, there was a >15% decrease compared to the 7th day, for which weekly clinical and analytical control was decided until β-hCG became negative. There was a gradual decrease in the β-hCG levels until negativization, 38 days after the administration of MTX (Figure 6).

Clinical and imaging controls were requested 2 months after MTX treatment. Ultrasound control was carried out, resulting in normality (Figure 7). A 12 x 4 mm niche was observed (Figure 8).

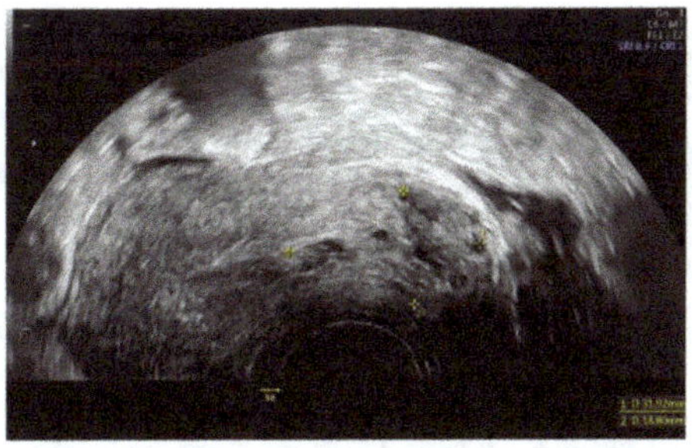

FIGURE 1: Transvaginal ultrasonographic study of the pelvic-abdomen region shows a retroverted uterus with a biometry of 70 mm x 40 mm. The uterine morphology was regular, and the myometrial ultrasound pattern was homogeneous. The endometrial thickness was 7 mm. The cervical canal was occupied by abundant blood content and clots with a size of 34 mm.

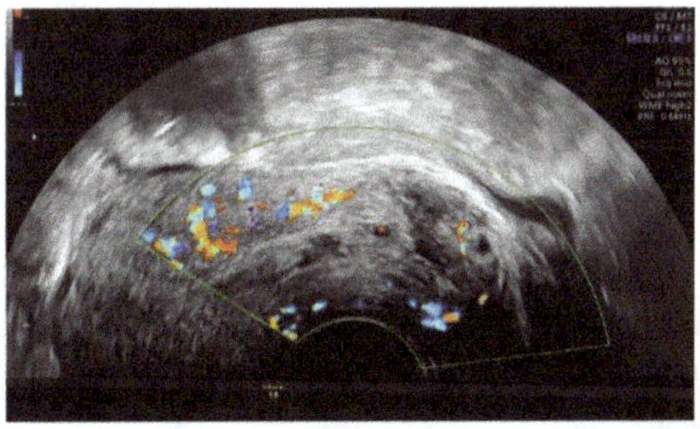

FIGURE 2: Color Doppler study did not provide new data for diagnosis.

3. Discussion

Ectopic pregnancies in cesarean section scars (CSPs) are extremely rare, representing 0.4% of all pregnancies and constituting 6% of all ectopic pregnancies in patients with a history of a previous cesarean section [1]. They constitute a continuous pathology that ranges from gestation with implantation on a properly healed scar (superficial CSP) to those implanted in a dehiscent scar ("niche") (deep CSP) which have a worse prognosis than those that are inserted on the scar [8].

The niche was defined as a cleft at the site of the cesarean section scar with a depth of at least 2 mm [9]. Basic measurements, including the niche length and depth, residual and adjacent myometrial thickness in the sagittal plane, and niche width in the transverse plane, were considered essential.

The ultrasound diagnostic criteria for CSP were defined as follows [4, 10, 11]:

(1) Empty uterus with clearly visualized endometrium

(2) Empty cervical canal

(3) Gestational sac implanted in the lower anterior uterine segment at the presumed site of the cesarean section incision scar

(4) Thin or absent myometrium between the gestational sac and the bladder (the majority of cases have a myometrium thickness<5 mm). "Sliding organ sign"

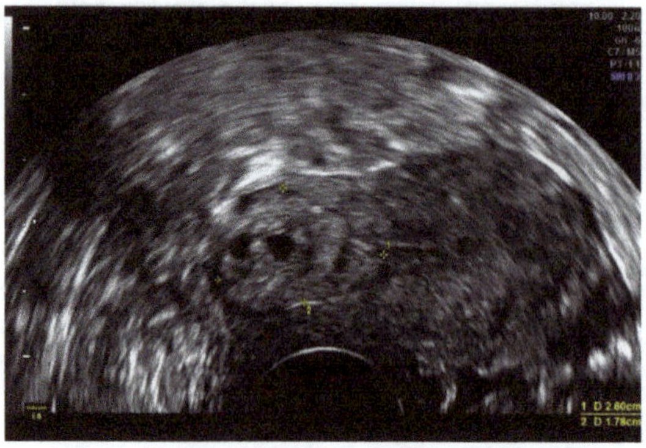

FIGURE 3: Transvaginal ultrasonographic study of the pelvic-abdominal region showing a retroverted uterus, with a biometry of 64 mm x 38 mm. The uterine morphology was regular, and the myometrial ultrasound pattern was homogeneous. Ultrasound signs of cavitary pathology were not observed. The endometrial thickness was 2 mm. At the level of the cesarean section scar, a 29x16 mm nodular image was observed, with a heterogeneous pattern.

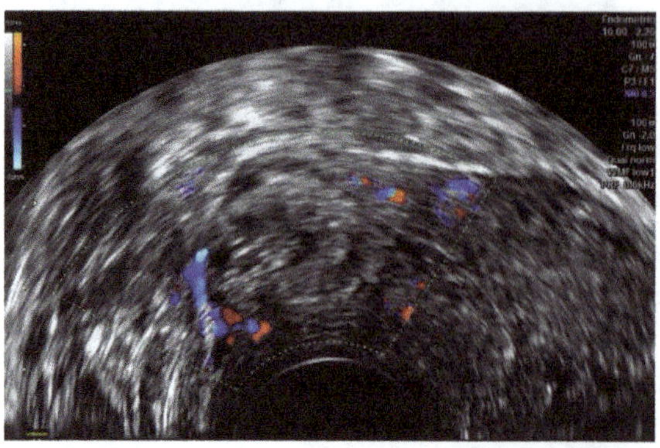

FIGURE 4: The color Doppler study showed vascularization.

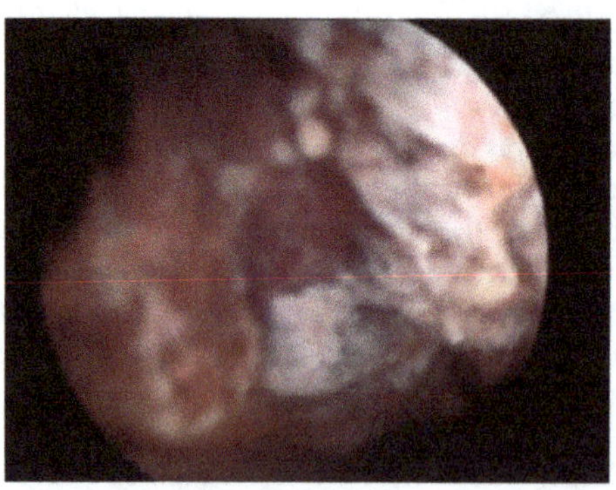

FIGURE 5: Hysteroscopic image showing an ectopic pregnancy at the level of the cesarean section scar.

(5) Doppler Flow at the previous cesarean scar

Although hysteroscopy and laparoscopy are not recommended diagnostic modalities, surgical findings at the time of surgical treatment are valuable in confirming the diagnosis of CSP [12].

3.1. Risk Factors. In a multivariate analysis, smoking in the first trimester (adjusted odds ratio (OR) 3.03, 95% CI 1.01-9.07), higher parity (adjusted OR 1.30, 95% CI 1.03-1.64) and more than 1 previous cesarean section (adjusted OR 3.43, 95% CI 1.35–8.66) were independently predictive of CSP [13]. An elective cesarean section in the index pregnancy was associated with an increased risk of CSP, but it did not remain significant in the multivariate analysis.

It is unknown whether the surgical technique of cesarean section affects the risk of a subsequent CSP [13].

3.2. Clinical Findings. In the early stages of pregnancy, most patients are asymptomatic. As the pregnancy progresses, vaginal bleeding can occur with or without pain [13]. The uterus can rupture and cause hemoperitoneum and hypovolemic shock.

In a review of 112 published cases and case series, the mean gestational age at presentation was 7.5 ± 2.5 weeks [13]. Among the 57 patients with presentation information, 37 percent were asymptomatic and diagnosed by ultrasound after remission for evaluation to rule out ectopic pregnancy, 39 percent had painless vaginal bleeding, 16 percent had abdominal pain and bleeding and 9 percent had only abdominal pain.

3.3. Risk Factors for Massive Bleeding. Multiple pregnancy, a big gestation sac, large gestation days, a high serum β-hCG level, an abundant blood supply to the pregnancy sac, and a thin myometrium may be risk factors for massive bleeding during CSP treatment [3].

3.4. Expectant Management. The meta-analysis by Calì et al. [14] showed that expectantly managed CSP with positive embryonic/fetal cardiac activity is associated with a high catastrophic maternal disease burden, including early uterine rupture, severe hemorrhage, abnormally invasive severe placenta, and hysterectomy.

Although the relative risk of maternal morbidity from the expectant management of CSP without cardiac activity is low, the risk of uterine rupture is as high as 13.4% [14]. The 2020 *Society for Maternal-Fetal Medicine* guideline also recommends against the expectant management of CSP (Grade 1B) [15].

3.5. Medical Treatment. Conservative treatment with systemic MTX is considered the treatment of choice in clinically stable patients with a desire to preserve fertility [1, 6, 7, 16].

In cases of positive embryocardium, as an alternative to the injection of 2 ml of KCl, the combined medical treatment with intrasaccular MTX + intramuscular MTX can be considered, since it is associated with an earlier negativization of β-HCG, the disappearance of the image of earlier ectopic gestation and a shorter hospitalization time [7].

3.6. Surgical Treatment. In some selected cases of CSP, the surgical option may be considered [1, 7, 16, 17]:

(i) Uterine curettage: Some authors [18] proposed performing aspiration curettage as the first therapeutic option in patients with superficial implantation who meet all the following diagnostic criteria: <8 weeks'

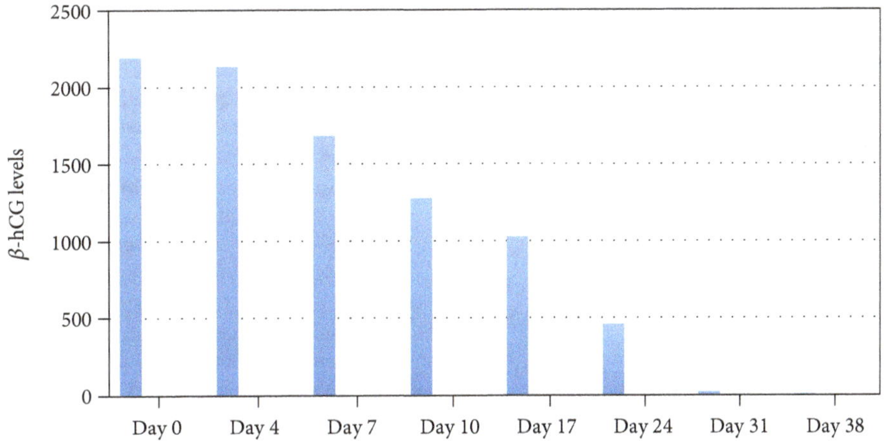

FIGURE 6: Chronogram of the serum β-hCG values.

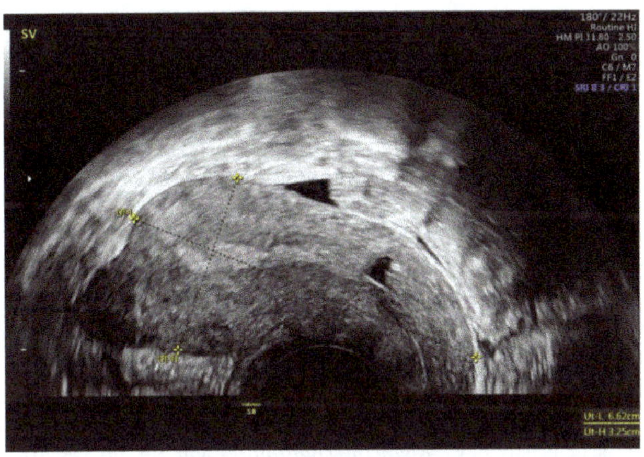

FIGURE 7: Transvaginal ultrasonographic study of the pelvic-abdominal region showed a retroverted uterus, with a biometry of 66 mm x 33 mm. Images of cavitary pathology were not observed. The endometrial thickness was 4 mm.

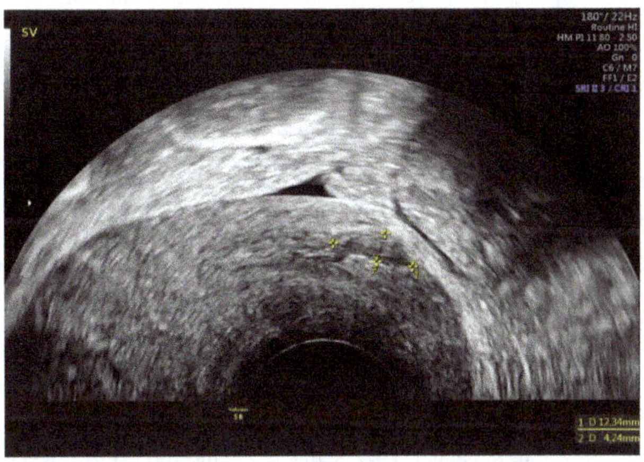

FIGURE 8: .12 mm x 4 mm niche.

gestation; a myometrial thickness between the bladder and gestational sac of >2 mm; and hemodynamic stability. In the case of suction curettage, it should be performed guided by transabdominal ultrasound, with a small cannula (4 or 6) and with a maximum suction pressure of 300 mmHg. It can be performed simultaneously with the help of a Foley balloon [18].

(ii) Hysteroscopy: It is a therapeutic option with a low complication rate [19, 20] that can be considered as an alternative to curettage in patients with the same criteria described for uterine curettage

(iii) Surgical resection by laparoscopy or laparotomy [17]: It is an option in cases in which there is bladder infiltration [20], as well as in cases of suspected uterine rupture

(iv) Hysterectomy may be indicated in cases of uncontrollable bleeding or the impossibility of conservative treatment [7].

In cases of acute bleeding, selective embolization of the uterine arteries can be considered prior to any of the previously proposed therapeutic options [21, 22].

3.7. Outcomes of Reproduction after CSP. Women with a history of CSP still have a high pregnancy rate, but the risk of recurrence and miscarriage is also increased [23, 24]. The effect of different treatments on subsequent pregnancy is unclear [24].

There is a need to further evaluate whether cesarean section scar resection and repair can improve reproductive outcomes [24, 25].

4. Conclusion

Cesarean scar pregnancy (CSP) is a type of ectopic pregnancy in which the gestational sac (GS) implants into the anterior wall of the lower uterine segment in an anterior cesarean scar. Before a diagnosis of abortion in a woman with a history of uterine scarring, we must rule out the possibility of implantation in the scar. Knowledge of the specific ultrasound characteristics of the rare locations of ectopic pregnancies, such as CSP, is crucial to making a correct diagnosis and initiating prompt treatment to prevent complications and preserve a patient's fertility. Early pregnancy termination should be considered, and treatment options should be individualized.

Authors' Contributions

All authors were involved in patient care. MAP and BG contributed to the image acquisition and interpretation. MSP researched the literature and wrote the first draft of the manuscript. MSP and MJP wrote the final version of the manuscript. NB and PBS critically reviewed the content of the manuscript. All authors reviewed and approved the final version of the manuscript.

References

[1] F. A. Gulino, C. Ettore, and G. Ettore, "A review on management of caesarean scar pregnancy," *Current Opinion in Obstetrics & Gynecology*, vol. 33, no. 5, pp. 400–404, 2021.

[2] M. A. Begam, H. Mirghani, W. Al Omari et al., "Caesarean scar pregnancy: time to explore indications of the caesarean sections?," *Journal of Obstetrics and Gynaecology*, vol. 39, no. 3, pp. 365–371, 2019.

[3] Y. Zhang, Z. Zhang, X. Liu, L. Zhang, F. Hong, and M. Lu, "Risk factors for massive hemorrhage during the treatment of cesarean scar pregnancy: a systematic review and meta-analysis," *Archives of Gynecology and Obstetrics*, vol. 303, no. 2, pp. 321–328, 2021.

[4] I. E. Timor-Tritsch, A. Monteagudo, G. Calì, F. D'Antonio, and A. A. Kaelin, "Cesarean scar pregnancy: diagnosis and pathogenesis," *Obstetrics and Gynecology Clinics of North America*, vol. 46, no. 4, pp. 797–811, 2019.

[5] W. Zhou, X. Feng, J. Yu, Z. Chai, L. Zheng, and F. Qi, "The efficacy of different treatments for type 2 cesarean scar pregnancy," *Fertility and Sterility*, vol. 32, no. 4, pp. 255–262, 2022.

[6] N. Salari, M. Kazeminia, S. Shohaimi, A. A. Nankali, and M. Mohammadi, "Evaluation of treatment of previous cesarean scar pregnancy with methotrexate: a systematic review and meta-analysis," *Reproductive Biology and Endocrinology*, vol. 18, no. 1, p. 108, 2020.

[7] L. S. Morente, A. I. G. León, M. P. E. Reina, J. R. A. Herrero, E. G. Mesa, and J. S. J. López, "Cesarean scar ectopic pregnancy-case series: treatment decision algorithm and success with medical treatment," *Medicina (Kaunas, Lithuania)*, vol. 57, no. 4, p. 362, 2021.

[8] N. Gonzalez and T. Tulandi, "Cesarean scar pregnancy: a systematic review," *Journal of Minimally Invasive Gynecology*, vol. 24, no. 5, pp. 731–738, 2017.

[9] I. P. M. Jordans, R. A. de Leeuw, S. I. Stegwee et al., "Sonographic examination of uterine niche in non-pregnant women: a modified Delphi procedure," *Ultrasound in Obstetrics & Gynecology*, vol. 53, no. 1, pp. 107–115, 2019.

[10] I. P. M. Jordans, C. Verberkt, R. A. de Leeuw et al., "Definition and sonographic reporting system for cesarean scar pregnancy in early pregnancy: modified Delphi method," *Ultrasound in Obstetrics & Gynecology*, vol. 59, no. 4, pp. 437–449, 2021.

[11] L. Shi, L. Huang, L. Liu et al., "Diagnostic value of transvaginal three-dimensional ultrasound combined with color Doppler ultrasound for early cesarean scar pregnancy," *Ann Palliat Med.*, vol. 10, no. 10, pp. 10486–10494, 2021.

[12] L. Liu, W. T. Ross, A. L. Chu, and T. A. Deimling, "An updated guide to the diagnosis and management of cesarean scar pregnancies," *Current Opinion in Obstetrics & Gynecology*, vol. 32, no. 4, pp. 255–262, 2020.

[13] B. Gull, V. Klerelid, A. Jormeus, and A. Strandell, "Potential risk factors for caesarean scar pregnancy: a retrospective case-control study," *Human Reproduction Open*, vol. 2021, no. 2, 2021.

[14] G. Calì, I. E. Timor-Tritsch, J. Palacios-Jaraquemada et al., "Outcome of cesarean scar pregnancy managed expectantly: systematic review and meta-analysis," *Ultrasound in Obstetrics & Gynecology*, vol. 51, no. 2, pp. 169–175, 2018.

[15] Z. OuYang, J. Wu, and B. Zhong, "Society for Maternal-Fetal Medicine Consult Series for cesarean scar pregnancy: each treatment option has its indications," *American Journal of Obstetrics and Gynecology*, vol. 224, no. 1, pp. 134-135, 2021.

[16] K. Birch Petersen, E. Hoffmann, C. Rifbjerg Larsen, and N. H. Svarre, "Cesarean scar pregnancy: a systematic review of treatment studies," *Fertility and Sterility*, vol. 105, no. 4, pp. 958–967, 2016.

[17] C. M. Pickett, N. Minalt, O. M. Higgins, C. Bernard, and K. M. Kasper, "A laparoscopic approach to cesarean scar ectopic pregnancy," *American Journal of Obstetrics and Gynecology*, vol. 10, no. 21, pp. S0002–S9378, 2021.

[18] M. Aslan and Ş. Yavuzkir, "Suction curettage and Foley balloon as a first-line treatment option for caesarean scar pregnancy and reproductive outcomes," *International Journal of Women's Health*, vol. 13, no. 13, pp. 239–245, 2021.

[19] X. Zhang, Y. Pang, Y. Ma et al., "A comparison between laparoscopy and hysteroscopy approach in treatment of cesarean scar pregnancy," *Medicine (Baltimore)*, vol. 99, no. 43, article e22845, 2020.

[20] Y. Lin, C. Xiong, C. Dong, and J. Yu, "Approaches in the treatment of cesarean scar pregnancy and risk factors for intraoperative hemorrhage: a retrospective study," *Frontiers in Medicine*, vol. 8, no. 8, article 682368, 2021.

[21] H. K. Ko, J. H. Shin, G. Y. Ko et al., "Efficacy of prophylactic uterine artery embolization before obstetrical procedures with high risk for massive bleeding," *Korean Journal of Radiology*, vol. 18, no. 2, pp. 355–360, 2017.

[22] J. Ou, P. Peng, C. Li, L. Teng, and X. Liu, "Assessment of the necessity of uterine artery embolization during suction and curettage for caesarean scar pregnancy: a prospective cohort study," *BMC Pregnancy and Childbirth*, vol. 20, no. 1, p. 378, 2020.

[23] M. Morlando, D. Buca, I. Timor-Tritsch et al., "Reproductive outcome after cesarean scar pregnancy: a systematic review and meta-analysis," *Acta Obstetricia et Gynecologica Scandinavica*, vol. 99, no. 10, pp. 1278–1289, 2020.

[24] J. Wu, J. Ye, Z. OuYang et al., "Outcomes of reproduction following cesarean scar pregnancy treatment: a systematic review and meta-analysis," *European Journal of Obstetrics, Gynecology, and Reproductive Biology*, vol. 262, pp. 80–92, 2021.

[25] M. Shapira, R. Mashiach, N. Meller et al., "Clinical success rate of extensive Hysteroscopic cesarean scar defect excision and correlation to histologic findings," *Journal of Minimally Invasive Gynecology*, vol. 27, no. 1, pp. 129–134, 2020.

21

Significant Clinical Manifestations in Ballantyne Syndrome, after a Case Report and Literature Review: Recognizing Preeclampsia as a Differential Diagnosis

Silvia F. Navarro-Perez,[1] Karen Corona-Fernandez,[2] José L. Rodriguez-Chavez,[3] A. Bañuelos-Franco,[3] and María G. Zavala-Cerna[2]

[1] *Unidad de Investigación en Ginecología y Alto Riesgo Obstétrico, División de Ginecología y Obstetricia del Hospital General de Occidente, Av. Zoquipan #1050, Col. Seattle, 45170, Mexico*
[2] *Immunology Research Laboratory, International Program of Medicine, Universidad Autonoma de Guadalajara, 44100, Mexico*
[3] *Unidad de Investigación en Ginecología y Alto Riesgo Obstétrico, División de Ginecología y Obstetricia del Hospital General de Occidente, Mexico*

Correspondence should be addressed to María G. Zavala-Cerna; g_zavala_78@hotmail.com

Academic Editor: Maria Grazia Porpora

Ballantyne syndrome (BS) also called mirror syndrome is defined by the presence of a clinical triad that includes fetal hydrops and placental and maternal edema. Here we present a clinical case of a 34-year-old woman with a 29 weeks' pregnancy, who developed BS and fetal loss probably due to failure in prompt recognition of a rapidly growing sacrococcygeal teratoma (SCT). Due to similarities in clinical presentation with preeclampsia and the importance in early identification of the source for BS, we underwent a literature review in order to identify significant signs and symptoms, as well as sonographic changes, in order to help clinicians to make this prompt recognition, identification of the cause, and early management of BS, which will have an important impact in maternal and fetal survival.

1. Introduction

Ballantyne syndrome (BS) also called mirror syndrome or triple edema is defined by the presence of a clinical triad that includes fetal hydrops and placental and maternal edema [1]. The term mirror as the name implies is due to an edema that is mirrored in both, the fetus and the mother [2]. John William Ballantyne in 1892 was the first to acknowledge the syndrome, originally thought to be the consequence of rhesus isoimmunization; however currently more than 80 different causes have been described and not all of them have an immunological origin [3], with only a few reported cases [4]. The syndrome appears in one out of 3,000 pregnancies; however the incidence can be underestimated, due to similarities in clinical presentation with preeclampsia (PE) [1, 3], which include maternal edema (80-100%), hypertension (60%), proteinuria (20-56%), anemia (46%), rapid weight gain, progressive dyspnea, and albuminuria [5]. Unlike preeclampsia in BS patients are hemodiluted according to blood indices with a typical low hematocrit [6]. In addition to similarities in their clinical presentation, preeclampsia and BS can coexist and compromise to a greater extent pregnancy resolution, as well as the maternal and fetal prognosis. In preeclampsia the recognition of abnormal placentation with defective spiral artery remodeling, favoring progressive placental ischemic reperfusion and excessive oxidative stress has been clearly established [7]. These changes result in a pathological imbalance among angiogenic (VEFG) and anti-angiogenic circulating factors (sFlt, activin) [8]. On the contrary, the etiology and pathogenic mechanisms in BS are still partially described and remain unclear, probably due to a limited number of papers [9]. Some factors that have been previously associated with the development of BS include diverse conditions, such as nonstructural causes:

rhesus isoimmunization, fetal supraventricular tachycardia, vertical cytomegalovirus, parvovirus B19 and Coxsackie virus infection, and laser photocoagulation for twin-to-twin transfusion syndrome, as well as structural alterations: aneurysm of Galen's vein, sacrococcygeal teratoma (SCT), or placental chorioangioma [10, 11].

It is extremely important for clinicians to identify similarities and differences between BS and preeclampsia, since diagnosis and management of BS might be possible when the source is readily identified [3]. Here, we present a case report of BS probably secondary to SCT that was not promptly identified. Additionally, we underwent a literature review to identify clinical similarities and differences between preeclampsia and BS, in order to provide hallmarks for prompt recognition and treatment of the base pathology that is responsible for BS, which will decrease maternal and newborn fatalities.

2. Case Report

A 34-year-old woman gravida 5, para 3, abortion 1 presented to the ER of our hospital, at 29 weeks' gestation, due to uterine contractions that increased in frequency and intensity in the last 5 hours, with no other symptomatologies added (Figure 1). Her past medical history was unremarkable with O + hemotype; she had an abortion due to an anembryonic pregnancy that required curettage, which was performed without complications. The patient had 3 healthy previous pregnancies which resulted in 3 healthy living children. Currently in her fifth pregnancy, she denies pregnancy care; only one obstetric ultrasound performed at 24 weeks' gestation in another clinic reported the following: harmonic fetal growth and no fetal malformations; however polyhydramnios was present. During her observation in the ER, a new ultrasound examination was ordered, which revealed an apparently large placenta with approximate weight of 1,800 gr, suggestive of placental edema; the fetus appeared with polyhydramnios, and no heartbeats nor fetal movements were registered; she was then referred to the high risk obstetric department, where she was found to have normal vital signs, mild edema of the ankles without fovea, and a gravid uterus occupied by a single longitudinal cephalic fetus with lateralized back to the left; fetal heart rate was not detected with doptone; she had regular uterine dynamics palpable at a rate of 3 contractions lasting 60 seconds each, within a time frame of 10 minutes; at vaginal examination the cervix was softened with 4 cm of dilation and 70% thinned, intact amniotic membranes, without bleeding or leucorrhoea. Laboratory tests reported the following: hemoglobin 11.5 g/dl, hematocrit 34.8%, and no other abnormal results including normal renal and hepatic function. Due to increased frequency of contractions, she was immediately sent to the expulsive room, where a single female sex without vitality was spontaneously delivered, with data of hydrops and macerated skin, weight: 1,730 gr, with a grayish and hemorrhagic sacral mass (Figure 2). After resection of the tumor and pathologic examination the following report was made: An 820 gr Type I sacrococcygeal teratoma (SCT) with mature and immature elements as well as blood sequestration areas, partially encapsulated with extensive areas of coagulation and necrosis. Placenta was grossly edematous and weighed 1,280 gr with a marked hydropic change of the villi, with an area of intervillous fibrinoid infarct was noticed. Amnion and chorion had no alterations. The umbilical cord had three blood vessels with marked edema of Wharton's jelly. The patient received counseling and was discharged 3 days after delivery without edema or any other physical alteration.

3. Discussion

In the present case, the diagnosis of BS was established after the findings of fetal hydrops, placental edema, and mild maternal edema. Presumably in this case, BS developed secondary to SCT. The SCT was not evident in the first ultrasound at 24 weeks' gestation, neither were fetal hydrops; however polyhydramnios was present at that time. SCT is a rare congenital disease of the newborn that happens in 1 out of 20,000-40,000 pregnancies, predominantly in female newborns with a ratio of 3:1 [12]. The perinatal mortality of SCT has been estimated from 40 to 50% [13]. Death occurs in fetuses with fast growing, solid, and highly vascularized teratomas which can originate high-output cardiac failure, which is a consequence of the tumor acting as a large arteriovenous malformation that steals vascular supply from the fetus [14]. Goto et al. published the report of two cases of SCT in which only one was associated with BS and a fetal outcome for the fetus [15].

The etiopathogenic mechanisms of BS remain partially understood; it has been suggested that the placenta is the source of the problem, since resolution of the pregnancy with the removal of the placenta resolves the mirroring edema [16]. Some previous reports have stated that compensatory mechanisms originate as a consequence of placental ischemia and are responsible for an increased placental blood flow with a rise in placental renin up to 10-fold, which will aid in increased maternal aldosterone a fluid retention [17]. Furthermore, some molecules have been identified in association with endothelial dysfunction in BS, such as Activin A and follistatin; other molecules are involved in inflammation and increased vascular permeability including ICAM-1 and vWF; the potent vasoconstrictor ET-1 [10]; and the anti-angiogenic factor sVGEFR-1 [18]. Nevertheless, it would be of interest to determine the abnormalities in the fetus that will later give rise to these alterations in the placenta that finally manifest in BS, which is a life threatening condition for the mother and the fetus [19].

In the fetus, the development of hydrops secondary to SCT can be explained by a high output failure caused by either anemia due to tumor hemorrhage and/or an arteriovenous shunt in a low resistance, rapidly growing tumor [20, 21]. Cardiac failure can give rise to an alteration in the regulation of the fluid dynamics between vascular and interstitial spaces, with an imbalance of interstitial fluid production and lymphatic return, which will eventually lead to fetal hydrops [19]. The fetus is particularly susceptible to interstitial fluid accumulation because of its greater capillary permeability compliant interstitial compartments

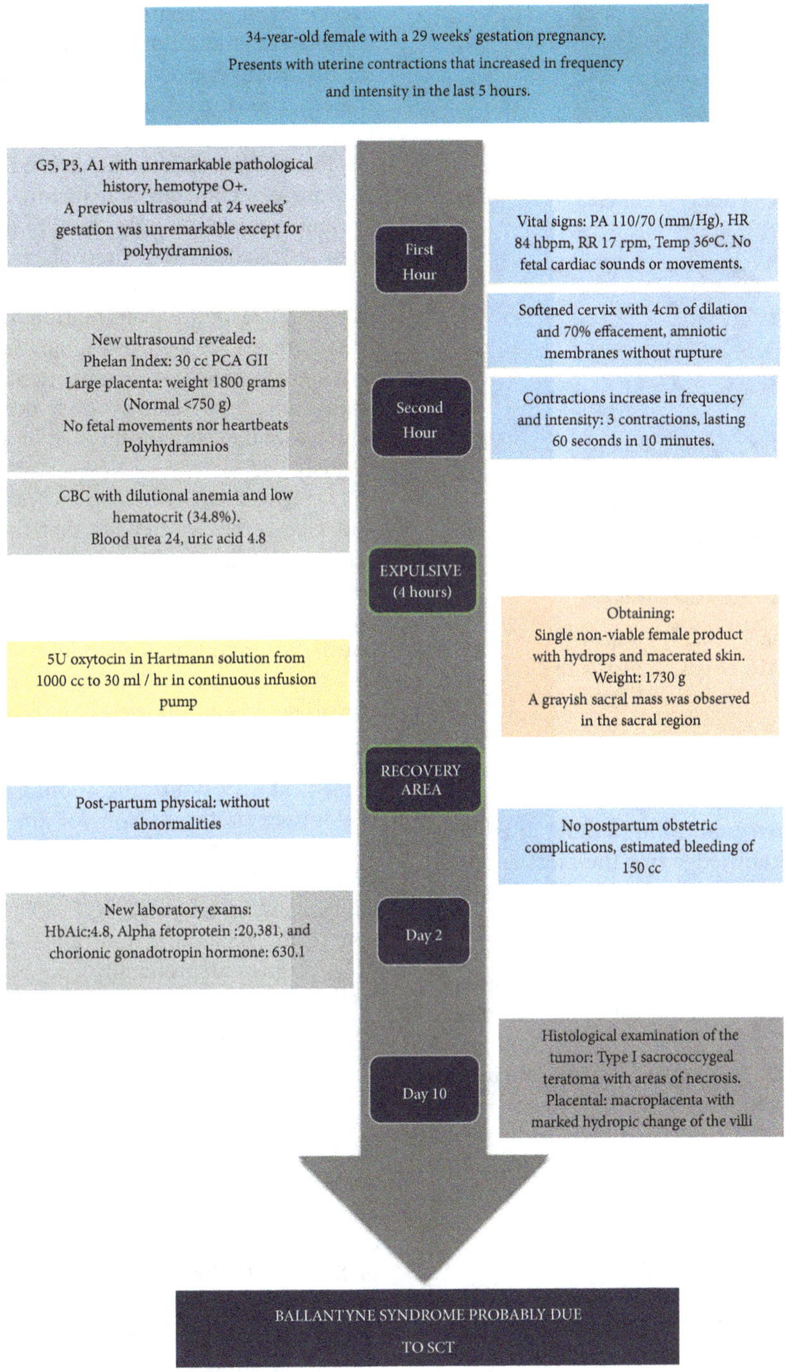

FIGURE 1: Timeline of patient's clinical evolution with diagnostic tests and treatments. SCT: sacrococcygeal teratoma.

and vulnerability to venous pressure on lymphatic return. Compensatory mechanism to maintain homeostasis during hypoxia results in increased venous pressure and interstitial fluid accumulation, developing the characteristic hydropic changes [22]. In our case the histologic examination of the tumor demonstrated signs of bleeding; nevertheless the presence of an arteriovenous shunt was not examined. The presence of fetal hydrops in our case was evident at delivery, established by accumulation of fluid in the skin and abdomen (Figure 2), in accordance with fetal hydrops definition [23].

Furthermore, rapid growth of SCT (>150 cm^3 per week) and hypervascularity are associated with increased risk in perinatal mortality [12]. A previous study stated that SCT bigger than 5 cm can be involved in the formation of high volume arteriovenous shunts that can lead to cardiac failure, placentomegaly, hydrops, and preeclampsia or BS [14]. This seems to be in accordance with our case; although the growth of the tumor was not registered by week, it was evident that most of the growth happened after 24 weeks' gestation and before 29 weeks' gestation.

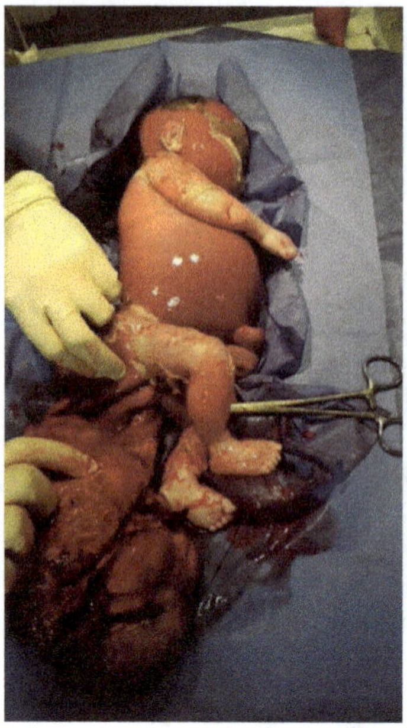

FIGURE 2: Single female sex without vitality spontaneously delivered, with hydrops and macerated skin, weight: 1730 g, with a grayish and hemorrhagic sacral mass, later described as a Type I sacrococcygeal teratoma (SCT).

Differential Diagnosis. When establishing a differential diagnosis, it is important to acknowledge that the most common complications in pregnancy are hypertensive disorders such as preeclampsia with an estimated prevalence of 10-12% worldwide; nevertheless it may coexist with other pathologies including BS. It is yet to be determined whether the treatment of the underlying cause of BS could improve preeclampsia as well.

In order to distinguish BS from preeclampsia, one important variable is time for presentation since BS can present earlier, with the first becoming evident as soon as 16 weeks' gestation and the latter presenting after 20 weeks' gestation [1]. Please refer to Table 1 in order to compare this and other considerations for each pathology.

Maternal rapid weight gain, marked skin edema, and uterine distention can also be distinguishable features in BS, whereas elevated blood pressure and proteinuria can be present in both [11]. Although maternal edema is an important clinical consideration, our case presented with only mild maternal edema; we found only few cases where maternal edema could be absent or mild in BS secondary to SCT [11].

Renal failure can appear in both; however, it has been described in a higher frequency for BS; postpartum hemorrhage and pulmonary edema have also been described in BS [24]. Other unspecific findings common to both include headache, nausea, vomiting, dyspnea, oliguria, pulmonary edema, anemia, elevated uric acid/creatinine, and elevated liver enzymes [25]. Laboratory findings of special interest for differential diagnosis are a dilutional anemia with low hematocrit, thrombocytopenia, and low serum albumin which are characteristic of BS, whereas in preeclampsia patients typically present with hemoconcentration [1, 26]. Dilutional anemia and thrombocytopenia in BS might be explained through the finding of high maternal serum vasopressin and atrial natriuretic factor [11].

First-trimester uterine artery Doppler ultrasound examination, placental growth factor, and pregnancy-associated plasma protein-A help to predict pregnancy complications associated with uteroplacental insufficiency such as preeclampsia before the onset of clinical features [27]. Also, during ultrasound examination in BS the most common fetal findings are hydrops fetalis (involving peritoneal compartment, cutaneous compartment, pleural space, pericardial space, and fetal scalp), polyhydramnios, placental edema, fetal anomalies, organomegaly, or a tumor, alone or simultaneously [1].

Development of BS can increase the risk of preeclampsia and vice versa; we believe that there is a common ground for the development of both pathologies, a ground that favors an angiogenic-antiangiogenic imbalance that might contribute to an even worse prognosis when both entities coexist; therefore it is mandatory to alert physicians about this possibility in order to remain vigilant and prescribe early treatment when indicated.

Treatment. BS syndrome should be treated accordingly to the source or the reason for the endothelial dysfunction. Placental or fetal malignancies are rare complications during pregnancy, but when they occur, they may present significant challenges. In our case SCT was identified as the possible source for BS. The importance in this association is that SCT diagnosed prenatally can be managed to avoid fetal fatalities [14]. Fetal surgery of SCT is a viable option for treatment in selected patients that demonstrate signs of cardiovascular decline during gestation, or when the mother is at risk [28]. Beyond 27 weeks' gestation, however, the risk for the development of complications related to the surgery increases significantly; therefore early delivery (27 to 32 weeks' gestation) with immediate SCT resection has been shown to be a better option than "watchful waiting" documented by Baumgartner et al. with a survival rate of 81.8% [13]. Important considerations for the success of earlier delivery include a low compromised hydropic fetus, absence of high-output cardiovascular failure, absence of tumor bleeding or fetal anemia, and having appropriate facilities for neonatal intervention and immediate surfactant administration [13].

Maternal complications of BS, such as hypertension and pulmonary edema, should be immediately treated if there is a decision to wait with continuous observation and the administration of diuretics, calcium channel blockers, and beta-blockers [29].

4. Conclusions

We presented a case report with BS probably following to the development of SCT after 24 weeks' gestation, with polyhydramnios, hydrops fetalis, placental edema, and mild

Table 1: Clinical considerations in establishing a differential diagnosis for BS.

Variable	PE	BS	Case Report
	Maternal		
Gestational age	< 20	16-34	24-29
Edema	++	++	+
Hypertension (> 130/80)	+++	+	-
Proteinuria (> 300mg/day)	+++	+	+
Hyperreflexia (OTR)	+	-	-
Liver function test abnormalities	+++	+	+
Creatinine	++	+	+
Urea	++	+	+
Creatinine:urea ratio	++	+	+
Thrombocytopenia	+++	+	-
Uterine bleeding	++	+	-
Renal failure	++	+++	-
Pulmonary edema	+	+++	-
Anemia	Hemoconcentration	Hemodilution	Hemodilution
Placental edema	-	+++	+++
	Fetal		
Hydrops	+	+++	+++
Polyhydramnios	+	+++	+++
Cardiac affection	+	++	Unknown
Intrauterine growth restriction	+	-	-
Associated tumor	-	+	+
Fetal death	+	++	++

maternal edema. Since the most common cause for the development of hydrops fetalis is preeclampsia, we thought it could be important to identify clinical differences that could help in a prompt diagnosis since management of both entities is different, especially in BS where the source for endothelial dysfunction can be recognized prenatally. Preeclampsia and BS share some similarities in clinical presentation; even more, they can occur simultaneously, increasing the risk of maternal and fetal death. Some clinical considerations that point towards BS in the mother are time of onset (<20 weeks), edema, renal affection, and hemodilution; in the fetus ultrasound examination: polyhydramnios, cardiac affection, and fetal anomalies, including tumors. Finally, we would like to emphasize that in our case the initial manifestation was polyhydramnios; therefore, it is mandatory that patients with this abnormality are adequately observed during the following weeks' gestation with a Doppler ultrasound or fetal MRI for the evaluation of hydrops fetalis, and, in the case of a tumor, growth rate and vascularity. Then, each case should be evaluated for either early termination of pregnancy or fetal surgical intervention, in order to decrease the risk of fetal mortality, as well as maternal morbidity and mortality associated to BS.

Additional Points

Highlights. (i) Ballantyne syndrome and preeclampsia have different etiologies but similar clinical presentations; (ii) identification of significant clinical differences between both will contribute to accurate prompt diagnosis; (iii) prompt treatment of BS will have a beneficial impact in maternal and fetal survival.

Consent

Informed consent was obtained from the patient; her personal data was protected always, during the elaboration and publication of the manuscript.

Disclosure

This article does not contain studies with human participants or animal subjects of experimentation.

Authors' Contributions

Silvia F. Navarro-Perez, Karen Corona-Fernandez, and María

G. Zavala-Cerna were responsible for gathering information; Silvia F. Navarro-Perez, Karen Corona-Fernandez, María G. Zavala-Cerna, José L. Rodriguez-Chavez, and A. Bañuelos-Franco carried out the analysis of the information and medical literature; Silvia F. Navarro-Perez, Karen Corona-Fernandez, José L. Rodriguez-Chavez, A. Bañuelos-Franco, and María G. Zavala-Cerna were responsible for draft writing and approval of the final version; María G. Zavala-Cerna was responsible for draft submission.

References

[1] S. Allarakia, H. A. Khayat, M. M. Karami et al., "Characteristics and management of mirror syndrome: a systematic review (1956–2016)," *Journal of Perinatal Medicine*, vol. 45, no. 9, pp. 1013–1021, 2017.

[2] D. Y. Midgley and K. Harding, "The mirror syndrome," *European Journal of Obstetrics & Gynecology and Reproductive Biology*, vol. 88, no. 2, pp. 201-202, 2000.

[3] D. V. Valsky, H. Daum, and S. Yagel, "Reversal of mirror syndrome after prenatal treatment of Diamond-Blackfan anemia," *Prenatal Diagnosis*, vol. 27, no. 12, pp. 1161–1164, 2007.

[4] S. Ren, T. Bhavsar, and J. Wurzel, "CHAOS in the mirror: Ballantyne (mirror) syndrome related to congenital high upper airway obstruction syndrome," *Fetal and Pediatric Pathology*, vol. 31, no. 6, pp. 360–364, 2012.

[5] A. Brandão, A. Domingues, E. Fonseca, T. Miranda, and J. Moura, "Mirror syndrome after fetoscopic laser treatment - a case report," *Revista Brasileira de Ginecologia e Obstetrícia*, vol. 38, no. 11, pp. 576–579, 2016.

[6] R. B. Gherman, M. H. Incerpi, D. A. Wing, and T. M. Goodwin, "Ballantyne syndrome: Is placental ischemia the etiology?" *The Journal of Maternal-Fetal and Neonatal Medicine*, vol. 7, no. 5, pp. 227–229, 1998.

[7] J. W. Meekins, R. Pijnenborg, M. Hanssens, I. R. McFadyen, and A. van Asshe, "A study of placental bed spiral arteries and trophoblast invasion in normal and severe pre-eclamptic pregnancies," *British Journal of Obstetrics and Gynaecology*, vol. 101, no. 8, pp. 669–674, 1994.

[8] R. J. Levine, S. E. Maynard, C. Qian et al., "Circulating angiogenic factors and the risk of preeclampsia," *The New England Journal of Medicine*, vol. 350, no. 7, pp. 672-83, 2004.

[9] J. Y. Lee and J. Y. Hwang, "Mirror syndrome associated with fetal leukemia," *Journal of Obstetrics and Gynaecology Research*, vol. 41, no. 6, pp. 971–974, 2015.

[10] S. R. Hobson, E. M. Wallace, Y. F. Chan, A. G. Edwards, M. W. Teoh, and A. P. Khaw, "Mirroring preeclampsia: the molecular basis of Ballantyne syndrome," *The Journal of Maternal-Fetal & Neonatal Medicine*, pp. 1–6, 2019.

[11] T. Braun, M. Brauer, I. Fuchs et al., "Mirror syndrome: a systematic review of fetal associated conditions, maternal presentation and perinatal outcome," *Fetal Diagnosis and Therapy*, vol. 27, no. 4, pp. 191–203, 2010.

[12] R. D. Wilson, H. Hedrick, A. W. Flake et al., "Sacrococcygeal teratomas: prenatal surveillance, growth and pregnancy outcome," *Fetal Diagnosis and Therapy*, vol. 25, no. 1, pp. 15–20, 2009.

[13] H. D. Baumgarten, J. S. Gebb, N. Khalek et al., "Preemptive delivery and immediate resection for fetuses with high-risk sacrococcygeal teratomas," *Fetal Diagnosis and Therapy*, pp. 1–8, 2018.

[14] J. C. Langer, M. R. Harrison, K. G. Schmidt et al., "Fetal hydrops and death from sacrococcygeal teratoma: Rationale for fetal surgery," *American Journal of Obstetrics & Gynecology*, vol. 160, no. 5, pp. 1145–1150, 1989.

[15] S. Goto, N. Suzumori, S. Obayashi, Y. Ozaki, and M. Sugiura-Ogasawara, "Two cases of prenatally diagnosed sacrococcygeal teratoma type I with different clinical features," *Congenital Anomalies*, vol. 53, no. 2, pp. 92–94, 2013.

[16] S. Hayashi, H. Sago, R. Hayashi et al., "Manifestation of mirror syndrome after fetoscopic laser photocoagulation in severe twin-twin transfusion syndrome," *Fetal Diagnosis and Therapy*, vol. 21, no. 1, pp. 51–54, 2005.

[17] D. M. Paternoster, F. Manganelli, D. Minucci et al., "Ballantyne syndrome: a case report," *Fetal Diagnosis and Therapy*, vol. 21, no. 1, pp. 92–95, 2005.

[18] J. Espinoza, R. Romero, and J. K. Nien, "A role of the anti-angiogenic factors VEGFR-1 in the 'mirror syndrome' (Ballantyne's syndrome)," *The Journal of Maternal-Fetal and Neonatal Medicine*, vol. 19, no. 10, pp. 607–613, 2006.

[19] T. Van Mieghem, A. Al-Ibrahim, J. Deprest et al., "Minimally invasive therapy for fetal sacrococcygeal teratoma: case series and systematic review of the literature," *Ultrasound in Obstetrics & Gynecology*, vol. 43, no. 6, pp. 611–619, 2014.

[20] A.-X. Holterman, D. Filiatrault, M. Lallier, and S. Youssef, "The natural history of sacrococcygeal teratomas diagnosed through routine obstetric sonogram: a single institution experience," *Journal of Pediatric Surgery*, vol. 33, no. 6, pp. 899–903, 1998.

[21] S. J. Bond, M. R. Harrison, K. G. Schmidt et al., "Death due to high-output cardiac failure in fetal sacrococcygeal teratoma," *Journal of Pediatric Surgery*, vol. 25, no. 12, pp. 1287–1291, 1990.

[22] C. Bellini and R. C. Hennekam, "Non-immune hydrops fetalis: a short review of etiology and pathophysiology," *American Journal of Medical Genetics Part A*, vol. 158A, no. 3, pp. 597–605, 2012.

[23] X. González-De Chirivella, D. Silva-García, M. Rivas-Gómez, and C. Medina-Gómez, "Diagnóstico prenatal de hidrops fetal no inmune: Serie de nueve casos. Revisión de la literatura," *Revista Colombiana de Obstetricia y Ginecología*, vol. 63, pp. 148–154, 2012.

[24] R. M. Burwick, R. A. Pilliod, S. E. Dukhovny, and A. B. Caughey, "Fetal hydrops and the risk of severe preeclampsia," *The Journal of Maternal-Fetal and Neonatal Medicine*, pp. 1–5, 2017.

[25] G. Hirata, S. Aoki, K. Sakamaki, T. Takahashi, F. Hirahara, and H. Ishikawa, "Clinical characteristics of mirror syndrome: a comparison of 10 cases of mirror syndrome with non-mirror syndrome fetal hydrops cases," *The Journal of Maternal-Fetal and Neonatal Medicine*, vol. 29, no. 16, pp. 2630–2634, 2016.

[26] R. Iciek, M. Brązert, A. Klejewski, M. Pietryga, and J. Brązert, "Ballantyne syndrome (the Mirror syndrome) associated with severe non-immune fetal hydrops – a case report," *Polish Gynaecology*, vol. 86, no. 9, pp. 706–711, 2015.

[27] S. L. Khong, S. C. Kane, S. Brennecke, and F. da Silva Costa, "First-trimester uterine artery Doppler analysis in the prediction of later pregnancy complications," *Disease Markers*, vol. 2015, Article ID 679730, 10 pages, 2015.

[28] N. S. Adzick, T. M. Crombleholme, M. A. Morgan, and T. M. Quinn, "A rapidly growing fetal teratoma," *The Lancet*, vol. 349, no. 9051, p. 538, 1997.

[29] C. Brochot, P. Collinet, N. Provost, and D. Subtil, "Mirror syndrome due to parvovirus B19 hydrops complicated by severe maternal pulmonary effusion," *Prenatal Diagnosis*, vol. 26, no. 2, pp. 179-180, 2006.

22

Hemorrhage from Umbilical Cord Ulceration Identified on Real-Time Ultrasound in a Fetus with Duodenal Atresia

William M. Curtin,[1,2] Jaimie L. Maines,[1] Christina T. DeAngelis,[3] Niamh A. Condon,[1] Serdar H. Ural,[1,4] and Karmaine A. Millington[2,5]

[1]*Division of Maternal-Fetal Medicine, Penn State University Milton S. Hershey Medical Center, Penn State College of Medicine, Hershey, Pennsylvania, USA*
[2]*Department of Pathology & Laboratory Medicine, Penn State University Milton S. Hershey Medical Center, Penn State College of Medicine, Hershey, Pennsylvania, USA*
[3]*Department of Obstetrics & Gynecology, Penn State University Milton S. Hershey Medical Center, Penn State College of Medicine, Hershey, Pennsylvania, USA*
[4]*Department of Radiology, Penn State University Milton S. Hershey Medical Center, Penn State College of Medicine, Hershey, Pennsylvania, USA*
[5]*Department of Pathology, Perinatal Pathology, North well Health/Cohen Children's Medical Center/Long Island Jewish Medical Center, New Hyde Park, New York, USA*

Correspondence should be addressed to William M. Curtin; wcurtin@pennstatehealth.psu.edu

Academic Editor: Kyousuke Takeuchi

Umbilical cord ulceration has been associated with congenital upper intestinal (duodenal or jejunal) atresia and can lead to fatal fetal intrauterine hemorrhage. We report a case of spontaneous hemorrhage from the umbilical cord, incidentally noted at the time of ultrasound in a 33-week fetus with suspected duodenal atresia, in which immediate delivery resulted in a good outcome. Despite many reports in the literature of congenital upper intestinal atresia and its association with umbilical cord ulceration, the propensity for this lesion for fetal hemorrhage, and the resulting perinatal morbidity and mortality, there appears to be a gap in the dissemination of this knowledge. In fetuses with suspected congenital upper intestinal atresia, recognition of the entity of umbilical cord ulceration may be improved by ultrasound with special attention to the amount of Wharton's jelly within the cord. Routine antepartum fetal surveillance may reduce perinatal morbidity and mortality from this condition. A high index of suspicion is needed to make the diagnosis of umbilical cord ulceration in association with congenital upper intestinal atresia. The role of amniotic fluid bile acids in the genesis of this disorder needs further study.

1. Introduction

Umbilical cord ulceration is an unusual lesion characterized by degenerative changes in Wharton's jelly and overlying amnion, thinning of vessel walls, and superficially located, friable vessels prone to hemorrhage. This lesion, its association with congenital upper intestinal (duodenal or jejunal) atresia, and its association with increased perinatal morbidity and mortality have been well documented in the literature; despite this, awareness of this condition and the potential associated lethality remains limited [1]. Because of spontaneous and catastrophic intramniotic bleeding, fetal exsanguination and stillbirth can occur in a high frequency of cases. We describe a case of umbilical cord ulceration in a 33-week fetus with suspected duodenal atresia where active intramniotic hemorrhage from the umbilical cord was identified during real-time ultrasound imaging that led to a prompt delivery and a good outcome.

2. Case

A 27-year-old nullipara presented to her local hospital at 33 weeks' gestation with decreased fetal movement, uterine contractions, and possible leakage of fluid from the vagina.

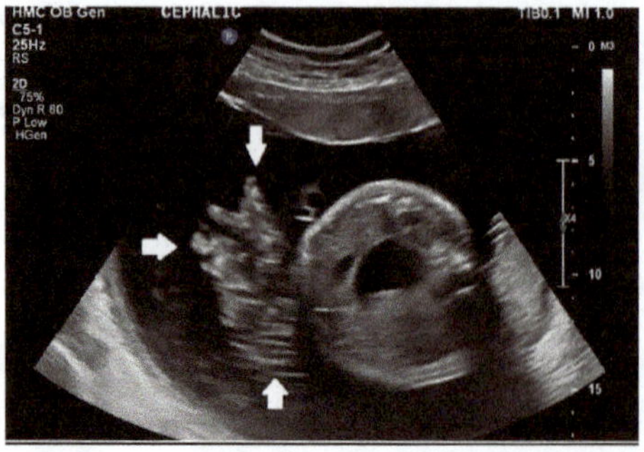

FIGURE 1: Ultrasound image of fetal blood swirling (arrows) into the amniotic fluid from the umbilical cord adjacent to a transverse view of the fetal abdomen/pelvis.

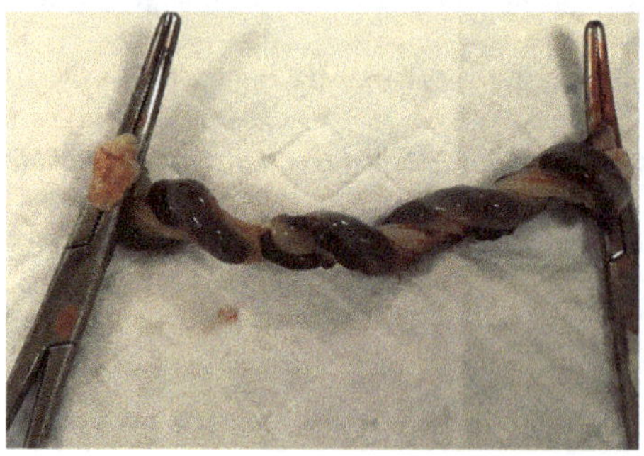

FIGURE 2: Gross photograph of clamped segment of umbilical cord demonstrating segments of exposed spiraling umbilical arteries.

Testing confirmed rupture of membranes; therefore, the patient was started on antibiotics to increase latency and was given betamethasone to hasten fetal lung maturity. An ultrasound at the community hospital showed polyhydramnios and a fetal double bubble sign consistent with duodenal atresia. The mother was transferred to Penn State Milton S Hershey Medical Center for anticipation of preterm delivery in a fetus that would require postnatal surgery.

After transfer, fetal monitoring showed normal fetal heart rate variability with accelerations and occasional decelerations related to contractions. An ultrasound confirmed the double bubble sign and polyhydramnios. Blood was observed in real-time swirling into the amniotic fluid from the umbilical cord (Figure 1). The patient was taken to the operating room and an emergent cesarean section was performed. The amniotic fluid was grossly bloody. A viable male infant weighing 2295 grams was delivered with Apgar scores of 7 and 8 at one and five minutes, respectively.

The umbilical cord overall length was 29.5 cm and there were 13, 0.5- 1 cm exposed segments of the umbilical arteries spiraling along the length of the cord (Figure 2). A discrete area from which the hemorrhage emanated was not identified. The placental disk was of normal weight and appeared grossly normal. Histopathologic examination of the cord showed absence of Wharton's jelly covering the umbilical artery, extreme attenuation of the media in the portion of the vessel exposed to the amniotic fluid, and degeneration of the overlying amnion (Figures 3(a) and 3(b)).

The infant had no stigmata of Down syndrome. He appeared pale at birth and an initial hematocrit was 29.4% that was treated by a blood transfusion upon admission to the neonatal intensive care unit. Postnatally the abdominal X-ray revealed air in the stomach and first portion of the duodenum with the remainder of the abdomen appearing gasless, consistent with duodenal atresia. A nasogastric tube was placed and 37 ml of bloody secretions were suctioned. The infant underwent laparotomy on the second day of life where an atresia was noted in the third portion of the duodenum and duodenojejunostomy was performed. He did well postoperatively and was discharged on day 30 of life.

3. Comment

The association between fetal hemorrhage from umbilical cord ulceration and congenital intestinal atresia was first noted in 1991 by Bendon et al. [2] when they reported three cases of intestinal atresia associated with linear ulcerations of the umbilical cord. Two of the cases occurred in fetuses that were delivered by cesarean section for fetal distress and the infants were found to be anemic; the third was a stillbirth with hydrops, in the latter the authors presumed secondary to fetal anemia. Since that time, numerous cases of umbilical cord ulceration have been reported in association with upper intestinal atresia. Globally, a large number of cases have been documented in Japan [3]. Only one prior case reported capturing the hemorrhage as it occurred during real-time ultrasound [4]. As in our case, nonreassuring fetal heart rate patterns were noted prior to the ultrasound and prompt cesarean delivery of an anemic infant resulted in a good outcome.

The frequency of umbilical cord ulceration and fetal hemorrhage in fetuses with congenital upper intestinal atresia is estimated to be 15-20% [1, 5, 6]. The typical clinical presentation is preterm labor, nonreassuring fetal heart rate monitoring, and delivery of an anemic infant. In one literature review of 38 cases there was a 32% incidence of fetal demise, 32% incidence of postnatal death, and an overall survival rate of 37% [1]. Macroscopic features of cord lesions in umbilical cord ulceration are variable and may include ulcers that are single or multiple, linear, helical, or punctate. As in our case, other features include visibly exposed umbilical arteries that upon histologic examination show absent Wharton's jelly, thinned or necrotic vessel walls, and overlying necrotic amniotic epithelium. The area of rupture and hemorrhage from the vessels may not be apparent.

The etiology of umbilical cord ulceration in conjunction with congenital upper intestinal atresia is not precisely known. Bendon et al. [2] addressed this association with three hypotheses: (1) vascular reactivity and ischemia leading to the intestinal atresia and the cord ulcer, (2) a primary epithelial cell abnormality in both cord and intestine, and (3) regurgitation of gastric or duodenal contents into amniotic fluid that cause the cord ulceration. Ichinose et al. [6] performed histological examination of the umbilical cord in 20 cases of duodenal or jejunal atresia, only 3 of which were clinically diagnosed, i.e., presented with fetal hemorrhage secondary to umbilical cord ulceration, and compared them

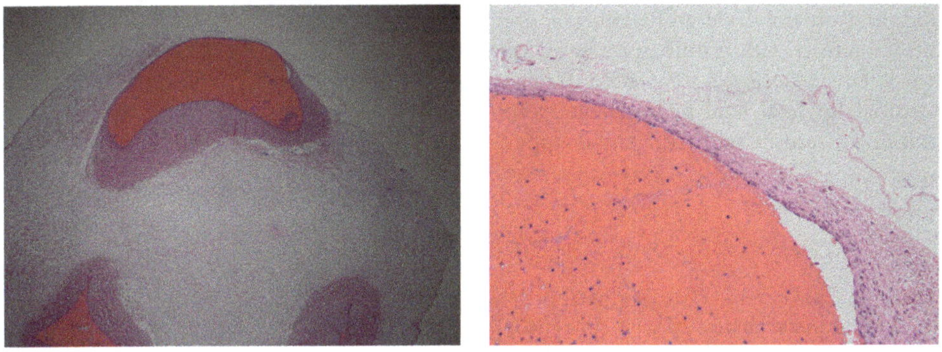

(a) (b)

FIGURE 3: (a). Low power photomicrograph of section of umbilical cord showing superficial location of the umbilical artery (top) with absence of overlying Wharton's jelly, attenuated vascular media, and degeneration of the amnion. This is in contrast to the umbilical vein (lower left) and other umbilical artery (lower right) both of which were completely surrounded by Wharton's jelly and amnion (complete views not in the field). H &E, X 20. (b). High power photomicrograph of ulcerated umbilical artery demonstrating markedly thinned media, absent Wharton's jelly, and degeneration of the overlying amnion. H &E, X 200.

to 28 controls. They devised a grading scheme to characterize the degree of ulceration: grade 0, no ulceration; grade 1, loss of amniotic epithelium; grade 2, detachment of basal lamina of amniotic epithelium; grade 3, loss of Wharton's jelly with widespread grade 2 change; and grade 4, exposed umbilical artery or vein. They found that 28/28 controls had no or grade 1 ulceration as compared to 16/20 duodenal or jejunal atresia cases that had grade 2 or greater ulceration. They concluded that these findings suggested gradual pathologic changes in the umbilical cords of fetuses affected by upper intestinal atresia that precede clinical presentation.

Substances that could cause the umbilical cord ulceration in upper intestinal atresia might include gastric acid, digestive enzymes and bile. It is estimated that 85% of duodenal atresia cases are located distal to the ampulla of Vater and the other 15% proximal [7]. In the atresia noted distal to the ampulla of Vater, gastric acid, digestive enzymes, and bile would be anticipated to reflux into the amniotic fluid, while in the atresia located proximally only gastric acid would reflux. Ichinose et al. [6] reported eight cases of duodenal atresia with obstruction proximal to the ampulla of Vater; four of the eight had grade 3 ulcerations of the umbilical cord, suggesting that gastric contents alone may be sufficient to cause ulceration. Their study also reported three fetuses with upper intestinal atresia that presented with nonreassuring fetal status during routine fetal heart rate monitoring and were delivered by emergency cesarean section; however, all three died in the neonatal period and all had intestinal obstruction distal to the ampulla of Vater. These findings suggest that clinically apparent ulceration of the umbilical cord may be more likely in the fetus with duodenal atresia distal to the ampulla of Vater and provides further support that substances from the hepatobiliary tree may have the corrosive effect upon the umbilical cord. Trypsin and bile acids, assayed from amniotic fluid from a 33-week fetus with duodenal atresia, were found to be elevated when compared to fetuses without duodenal atresia, and could be useful markers for diagnosis of the condition [8]. Ohyama et al. [5] suggested that measurement of total bile acids in amniotic fluid may identify fetuses at high risk for umbilical cord ulceration.

The potential role of bile acids in the causation of umbilical cord ulceration is further supported by the potentially corrosive effect that meconium can have on umbilical cord vessels. Meconium contains bile acids similar in composition to those from the fetal gallbladder [9]. Meconium has been associated with vascular myonecrosis of the umbilical cord and umbilical cord ulceration [10]. Segmental hemorrhage from the umbilical cord has been documented in a term pregnancy with suspected prolonged meconium stained amniotic fluid [11]. Complete dissolution of Wharton's jelly associated with exposure of coiled vessels from a 34-week fetus with meconium staining has been documented [12]. Cases such as these lend support to the theory that bile acids may have a toxic effect upon the structural integrity of the umbilical cord.

The lesson learned from our case report was that, despite previous reporting of the association between fetuses with suspected upper intestinal atresia and umbilical cord ulceration, we were unaware of this association and its attendant fetal morbidity and mortality. It is likely that others are also unaware of this association and there is a need to disseminate this information. Pregnancies complicated by suspected congenital upper intestinal atresia may need to have management altered to address the increased risk of fetal hemorrhage. Ultrasound assessment of cross-sectional areas of the umbilical cord with calculation of the area occupied by the Wharton's jelly [13] could be useful to detect asymptomatic umbilical cord ulceration in fetuses with congenital upper intestinal atresia. Routine antepartum surveillance with fetal nonstress testing may be important for all fetuses with suspected upper intestinal atresia. Many of the cases of hemorrhage from umbilical cord ulceration have come to clinical attention when the mother presents with preterm labor and is found to have nonreassuring fetal testing. The clinician will need to have a high index of suspicion for the diagnosis of umbilical cord ulceration and fetal hemorrhage when a patient presents with this clinical scenario. Further studies on whether measurement of total bile acids in amniotic fluid obtained via amniocentesis are needed to determine if there is a discriminatory level for umbilical ulceration risk. For now, efforts are needed to raise awareness of the potential for fatal fetal hemorrhage from umbilical cord ulceration in fetuses with congenital upper intestinal atresia.

References

[1] D. Aronowitz, S. Dolgin, E. Bornstein et al., "Perinatal hemorrhage from ulceration of the umbilical cord: A potentially catastrophic association with duodenal and jejunal obstruction," *Journal of Pediatric Surgery*, vol. 53, no. 9, pp. 1669–1674, 2018.

[2] R. W. Bendon, R. W. Tyson, V. J. Baldwin, K. A. Cashner, F. Mimouni, and M. Miodovnik, "Umbilical cord ulceration and intestinal atresia: A new association?" *American Journal of Obstetrics & Gynecology*, vol. 164, no. 2, pp. 582–586, 1991.

[3] M. Ohyama, Y. Itani, H. Ishikawa, and Y. Tanaka, "Is umbilical cord ulcer associated with congenital upper intestinal atresia so rare? Japanese case series and review of the literature," *Fetal Diagnosis and Therapy*, vol. 28, no. 4, pp. 236-237, 2010.

[4] A. Nijagal, L. Rand, R. Goldstein, L. Poder, and D. Miniati, "Intrauterine umbilical cord hemorrhage with associated jejunal atresia captured by real-time ultrasound," *American Journal of Obstetrics & Gynecology*, vol. 200, no. 3, pp. e5–e6, 2009.

[5] M. Ohyama, Y. Itani, M. Yamanaka et al., "Umbilical cord ulcer: A serious in utero complication of intestinal atresia," *Placenta*, vol. 21, no. 4, pp. 432–435, 2000.

[6] M. Ichinose, T. Takemura, K. Andoh, and M. Sugimoto, "Pathological analysis of umbilical cord ulceration associated with fetal duodenal and jejunal atresia," *Placenta*, vol. 31, no. 11, pp. 1015–1018, 2010.

[7] E. A. Boyden, J. G. Cope, and A. H. Bill, "Anatomy and embryology of congenital intrinsic obstruction of the duodenum," *The American Journal of Surgery*, vol. 114, no. 2, pp. 190–202, 1967.

[8] M. Legge and H. C. Potter, "Prenatal diagnosis of duodenal atresia using third trimester amniotic fluid immunoreactive trypsin," *Australian and New Zealand Journal of Obstetrics and Gynaecology*, vol. 24, no. 61, 1984.

[9] N. Naritaka, M. Suzuki, H. Sato et al., "Profile of bile acids in fetal gallbladder and meconium using liquid chromatography-tandem mass spectrometry," *Clinica Chimica Acta*, vol. 446, pp. 76–81, 2015.

[10] G. Altshuler, M. Arizawa, and G. Molnar-Nadasdy, "Meconium-Induced umbilical cord vascular necrosis and ulceration: A potential link between the placenta and poor pregnancy outcome," *Obstetrics & Gynecology*, vol. 79, no. 5, pp. 760–766, 1992.

[11] G. Larciprete, ME. Romanini, D. Arduini et al., "Umbilical cord segmental hemorrhage and fetal distress," *International Journal of Biomedical Science*, vol. 2, pp. 185-186, 2006.

[12] K. Benirschke, G. J. Burton, and R. N. Baergen, "Anatomy and pathology of the placental membranes," in *Pathology of the Human Placenta*, K. Benirschke, G. J. Burton, and R. N. Baergen, Eds., vol. 6th, p. 276, Springer, Heidelberg, Germany, 2012.

[13] L. Raio, F. Ghezzi, E. Di Naro, M. Franchi, H. Brühwiler, and K. P. Lüscher, "Prenatal assessment of Wharton's jelly in umbilical cords with single artery," *Ultrasound in Obstetrics & Gynecology*, vol. 14, no. 1, pp. 42–46, 1999.

23

Expectant Management of Monochorionic-Triamniotic Triplets Complicated by Selective *In Utero* Growth Restriction: Report of 2 Cases

Laurence Carmant, Sandrine Wavrant, and Elisabeth Codsi

Department of Obstetrics and Gynecology, Division of Maternal Fetal Medicine, Sainte-Justine Mother and Child University Hospital, 3175 Chemin de la Côte Sainte Catherine, Montreal, QC, Canada H3T 1C5

Correspondence should be addressed to Laurence Carmant; lcarmant@gmail.com

Academic Editor: Cem Ficicioglu

The optimal management of monochorionic-triamniotic (MCTA) triplet pregnancies is not clearly established, and there is no literature to guide management of MCTA complicated with selective intrauterine growth restriction (sIUGR). This gap in knowledge and the concern for higher risk of severe complications have led some medical societies to recommend selective termination of nontrichorionic triplet pregnancies. We sought to report the favourable outcomes of two MCTA complicated by sIUGR expectantly managed at Sainte-Justine Hospital, Montreal, Canada. The first case is of a 42-year-old woman with spontaneous MCTA triplets diagnosed at 18 weeks with type II sIUGR who opted for expectant management. The second patient was a 22-year-old woman with a spontaneous MCTA triplet pregnancy diagnosed at 18 weeks with type III sIUGR. Our experience shows that close serial ultrasounds could potentially allow physicians to foresee fetal deterioration. In our opinion, expectant management should be considered as a management option for MCTA complicated by sIUGR.

1. Introduction

In North America, triplets and higher-order multifetal gestations account for approximately 153.4 per 100 000 live births. The increasing incidence of multifetal gestations reflects older maternal age at conception and the growing use of assisted reproductive technologies. These pregnancies are associated with increased fetal and neonatal morbidity and mortality mainly due to prematurity [1]. Literature has also shown that perinatal morbidity and mortality in multifetal gestations are strongly linked to chorionicity [2, 3]. Indeed, dichorionic-triamniotic (DCTA) and monochorionic-triamniotic (MCTA) triplet pregnancies are at higher risk of complications compared to trichorionic-triamniotic (TCTA) pregnancies [4, 5]. This has led the North American Fetal Therapy Network (NAFTNet) to state that because of the higher complication rates, parents of nontrichorionic triplets should be counseled about the option of selective fetal reduction of the monochorionic pair [6]. However, when faced with MCTA triplets, the optimal management is less clear. Moreover, there is no literature to guide management of MCTA complicated with selective intrauterine growth restriction (sIUGR). Therefore, we sought to report the outcomes of two MCTA complicated by sIUGR that were expectantly managed at the Sainte-Justine Mother and Child University Hospital.

2. Case Presentation #1

A 42-year-old woman, gravida 3 para 1 avorta 1, was diagnosed with spontaneous MCTA triplets during nuchal translucency (NT) ultrasound. All fetuses had a normal NT. Selective fetal reduction was discussed, but the patient opted for expectant management. Low-dose aspirin was initiated. All her first trimester laboratory tests were normal. She proceeded with amniocentesis at 15 weeks. All 3 karyotypes were normal. At 18 weeks, morphology ultrasound was normal but showed sIUGR of fetus B, for which she was referred to our center. A detailed level II ultrasound confirmed the diagnosis of type II sIUGR in triplet B. Indeed, triplet B estimated fetal weight was less than the fifth percentile, there was intertriplet discordance of more than twenty-five percent and its umbilical artery (UA) Doppler showed absent diastolic flow. However, its middle cerebral artery (MCA) and ductus venosus (DV) Dopplers were both normal. Twin B had a velamentous cord insertion. There was no sign of twin-twin transfusion syndrome (TTTS) or twin anemia polycythemia sequence (TAPS). Selective fetal reduction using radiofrequency ablation was again discussed with the new findings; however, the patient opted for expectant management. She underwent weekly ultrasound. At 22 weeks, she underwent fetal echocardiography, which only showed a mild pulmonary valve dysplasia on fetus A. Triplet B followed its <5th percentile growth curve and Dopplers remained stable from week to week, and the patient underwent caesarean section at 32 weeks after a course of betamethasone. All three babies had a normal pH and APGAR at birth and now have normal development at 1 year of age. The patient was discharged from the hospital postpartum day 5 because she suffered a nonsevere postpartum preeclampsia. Her blood pressure and laboratory testing were back to normal at her 6 weeks' postpartum follow-up visit.

3. Case Presentation #2

A 22-year-old woman primigravida with a spontaneous MCTA triplet pregnancy was referred to our center for a suspicion of sIUGR of triplet B at 18 weeks. A detailed level II ultrasound confirmed the diagnosis of type III sIUGR in triplet B. Indeed, triplet B estimated fetal weight was less than the fifth percentile, there was intertriplet discordance of more than twenty-five percent, and it showed intermittently absent/reverse diastolic flow in the umbilical artery of twin B. Middle cerebral artery and ductus venosus Dopplers were both normal. Twin B had a velamentous cord insertion. Selective fetal reduction was discussed, but the patient opted for expectant management. She underwent weekly ultrasound. Triplet B followed its <3rd percentile growth curve. At 27 weeks, the DV Doppler of triplet B showed a pulsatility index above the 95th percentile. Occasional spontaneous heart rate decelerations were also noted. The patient was immediately hospitalised and underwent a C-section after a course of betamethasone and four hours of magnesium sulfate. All three babies had normal pH and APGAR at birth and have normal development at 1 year of age.

4. Discussion

Monochorionic-triamniotic triplets are inherently at higher risk of adverse pregnancy outcomes than higher chorionic multiple gestation pregnancy. With added complications such as TTTS, TAPS, or sIUGR, it seems reasonable to opt for selective fetal reduction as it can correct both the complication and the burden of having a higher order multiple fetal gestation. However, fetal therapy is not without significant risk for the pregnancy and the neurological prognosis of the remaining cotriplet. Van Schoubroeck and colleagues published a case series in which 3 MCTA triplets underwent cord occlusion for TRAP, 1 for fetal anomaly and 1 laser photocoagulation for TTTS. They reported outcomes similar to those described in larger series of twin pregnancies. They therefore concluded that laser photocoagulation was preferable to expectant management in MCTA complicated with TTTS. Moreover, they deemed second-trimester cord occlusion a reasonable option for TRAP or major discordant anomaly [7]. However, they did not have cases of MCTA complicated by sIUGR. NAFTNet states in their 2015 consensus that for type II or III sIUGR, selective feticide can be considered but laser photocoagulation should remain experimental [3]. Gratacos and colleagues also prefer cord occlusion to laser photocoagulation for type II and III sIUGR when fetal therapy is the chosen option [8].

Our experience with these MCTA triplets shows that we can achieve good outcomes with expectant management. Close serial ultrasounds allow the physician to foresee fetal deterioration even in more unpredictable sIUGR such as type III. As shown in the literature, abnormal DV Doppler is associated with adverse outcomes in monochorionic-diamniotic twins, which may be extrapolated to MCTA [9]. In our 2 cases, DV Dopplers were normal, suggesting that the findings in MCDA could potentially be extrapolated to MCTA pregnancies. It is important to emphasize that these patients were managed in a quaternary care hospital with optimal resources. The outpatient follow-up protocol in our institution consisted of weekly ultrasound for UA/MCA/DV Doppler and fluid assessment with biweekly assessment of fetal growth. Management of MCTA complicated with sIUGR should be tailored to institutional resources and parents' wishes, and in our opinion, expectant management should be at least considered as a management option. An international registry of complicated MCTA triplets should be considered to help determine the best treatment option because of the paucity of cases.

Disclosure

The abstract of this manuscript was presented as an electronic poster at the 29th World Congress on Obstetrics and Gynecology in Berlin.

References

[1] Committee on Practice B-O, Society for Maternal-Fetal M, "Practice Bulletin No. 169: multifetal gestations: twin, triplet, and higher-order multifetal pregnancies," *Obstetrics and Gynecology*, vol. 128, no. 4, pp. e131–e146, 2016.

[2] A. Geipel, C. Berg, A. Katalinic et al., "Prenatal diagnosis and obstetric outcomes in triplet pregnancies in relation to chorionicity," *BJOG : An International Journal of Obstetrics and Gynaecology*, vol. 112, no. 5, pp. 554–558, 2005.

[3] S. P. Emery, M. O. Bahtiyar, K. J. Moise, and North American Fetal Therapy N, "The North American Fetal Therapy Network consensus statement," *Obstetrics and Gynecology*, vol. 126, no. 3, pp. 575–584, 2015.

[4] H. Kawaguchi, K. Ishii, R. Yamamoto, S. Hayashi, N. Mitsuda, and Perinatal Research Network Group in Japan, "Perinatal

death of triplet pregnancies by chorionicity," *American journal of obstetrics and gynecology*, vol. 209, no. 1, pp. 36.e1–36.e7, 2013.

[5] J. Curado, F. D'Antonio, A. T. Papageorghiou, A. Bhide, B. Thilaganathan, and A. Khalil, "Perinatal mortality and morbidity in triplet pregnancy according to chorionicity: systematic review and meta-analysis," *Ultrasound in Obstetrics & Gynecology*, vol. 54, no. 5, pp. 589–595, 2019.

[6] M. O. Bahtiyar, S. P. Emery, J. S. Dashe et al., "The North American Fetal Therapy Network consensus statement: prenatal surveillance of uncomplicated monochorionic gestations," *Obstetrics and Gynecology*, vol. 125, no. 1, pp. 118–123, 2015.

[7] D. Van Schoubroeck, L. Lewi, G. Ryan et al., "Fetoscopic surgery in triplet pregnancies: a multicenter case series," *American Journal of Obstetrics and Gynecology*, vol. 191, no. 5, pp. 1529–1532, 2004.

[8] E. Gratacos, L. Lewi, B. Munoz et al., "A classification system for selective intrauterine growth restriction in monochorionic pregnancies according to umbilical artery Doppler flow in the smaller twin," *Ultrasound in Obstetrics & Gynecology*, vol. 30, no. 1, pp. 28–34, 2007.

[9] C. Monaghan, E. Kalafat, J. Binder, B. Thilaganathan, and A. Khalil, "Prediction of adverse pregnancy outcome in monochorionic diamniotic twin pregnancy complicated by selective fetal growth restriction," *Ultrasound in Obstetrics & Gynecology*, vol. 53, no. 2, pp. 200–207, 2019.

Placenta Accreta Spectrum Disorder in a Patient with Six Previous Caesarean Deliveries: Step by Step Management

Gloria Calagna,[1] Salvatore Polito,[1] Francesco Labate,[1] Rosa Anna Guiglia,[2] Francesca De Maria,[2] Chiara Bisso,[2] Gaspare Cucinella,[3] and Giuseppe Calì[1]

[1]*Obstetrics and Gynecology, "Villa Sofia-Cervello" Hospital, Palermo, Italy*
[2]*University of Palermo, Palermo, Italy*
[3]*Obstetrics and Gynecology, "Villa Sofia-Cervello" Hospital, University of Palermo, Palermo, Italy*

Correspondence should be addressed to Gloria Calagna; gloria.calagna83@gmail.com

Academic Editor: Daniel Martin

The definition *placenta accreta spectrum disorders* (PAS) introduced by FIGO (International Federation of Gynaecology and Obstetrics) indicates an abnormal, pathological adherence or invasion of the placenta. The growing worldwide incidence of this pathological entity, and the possible serious correlated surgical risks, has caused a significant increase in attention among the scientific community. Previous caesarean delivery and presence of placenta previa are the main risk factors for the onset of PAS. Here, we present the intriguing case of a 39-year-old woman, at the 33rd week of gestation, with six previous caesarean sections and with a diagnosis of placenta previa accreta. At our referral center for PAS disorders, we successfully managed this difficult case with the help of a multidisciplinary skilled team.

1. Introduction

Placenta accreta spectrum disorders (PAS) is a heterogeneous group of abnormalities of placental adherence or invasion, for which previous caesarean sections and placenta previa represent main risk factors [1]. The American College of Obstetricians and Gynaecologists (ACOG) reported a PAS incidence ten times during the last fifty years, probably with an increase of the incidence of caesarean deliveries (CDs) [2, 3]. The occurrence of PAS is 1-3% in patients without a history of CD and increases to 24% in the case of one CD, to 40-50% in the case of three CDs, and finally to 67% in patients with six CDs [3, 4].

PAS are traditionally classified according to the "invasion depth" criterion, identifying three different conditions of increasing severity: placenta accreta, increta, and percreta [5]. However, this is a histopathological classification and thus only retrospective: it does not provide information on treatment plans or in vivo anatomical and vascular features.

More recently, "ultrasound (US) prenatal PAS staging" has been suggested and introduced in our clinical evaluation of patients, based on the presence of so-called *US invasion signs*, in order to stratify the prenatal risk and postsurgery outcome [6]. It should be mandatory to perform an in vivo analysis of PAS cases by prenatal imaging to establish the correct management and define particular surgical management.

Here, we describe the challenging management at our referral center of a unique PAS disorder in a patient with a history of six caesarean sections, focusing on focusing on the importance on the collaboration of a skilled multidisciplinary group.

2. Case Presentation

A 39-year-old woman, G7 P6, with 6 living children by caesarean delivery, was referred to our center at 33.1 weeks of gestation with a suspected PAS. She was Caucasian, 19 BMI, with normal vital signs, a personal history of appendectomy, and a more recent surgical treatment of pelvic endometriosis. Blood tests were normal, there was no clinical evidence of vaginal bleeding, and there were no US signs of urinary tract obstructions nor of hydronephrosis. Fetal growth was adequate.

At presentation, ultrasound (US) examination showed an anterior placenta previa and a careful evaluation of prenatal PAS signs was performed by an expert sonographer (GC). Surprisingly, most of the PAS signs were absent: abnormal placental lacunae, bladder-line interruption, and myometrial thinning which was identified (Figure 1). The only ultrasound findings were the partial absence of the "clear zone," that is, the loss of the hypoechoic plane in the myometrium underneath the placental bed and a moderate uterovesical hypervascularity (Figure 2). Diagnosis of PAS 1/2 was given [6].

After an in-depth study, implemented by a multidisciplinary team including gynaecologists, radiologists, neonatologist, and anaesthesiologists, it was decided to perform a CD at gestational age of 34 weeks, with a possibility of a hysterectomy, under support of highly qualified and experienced interventional radiology with temporary occlusion of hypogastric artery. After adequate counselling, the patient signed the informed consent form.

The patient underwent epidural anaesthesia. First, the interventional radiology procedure was performed, with a balloon catheter positioned in the hypogastric arteries, bilaterally. Subsequently, the caesarean section was performed according to the *Kustner technique*, on the previous scar [7]. Once the abdomen was opened, a large area dilated vessels were visible in the lower uterine segment; for this reason, we performed a vertical incision of the uterus in the upper part, away from the placental insertion, and a male foetus was extracted, alive and vital in breech presentation (Apgar score 9-10).

After clamping the umbilical cord and before carrying out the hysterectomy, inflation of the catheters previously inserted in the hypogastric arteries was performed. In the meantime, an inspection of the placental site was carried out: after developing a bladder flap clearing the lower uterine segment, the bulging of the invasion of the placenta in a very thin myometrium with intense vascularization was evident on the anterior surface of the external anterior uterus (Figure 3); no parameters and bladder infiltration were present. The uterine incision was closed leaving the placenta and umbilical cord stump in situ.

As a third surgical step, a total hysterectomy was performed, with ovary preservation, considering the patient's wish and her age. The uterus was submitted for histological examination, which confirmed the US diagnosis of placenta increta with focal percreta (PAS 1/2-US partial absence of the "clear zone" and a moderate uterovesical hypervascularity) [6].

During surgery, all vital signs were normal and stable. Intraoperative transfusion of one homologous blood transfusion was given considering an estimated blood loss of about 600 ml. On the 3rd postoperative day. she was discharged and the one-week follow-up revealed normal course.

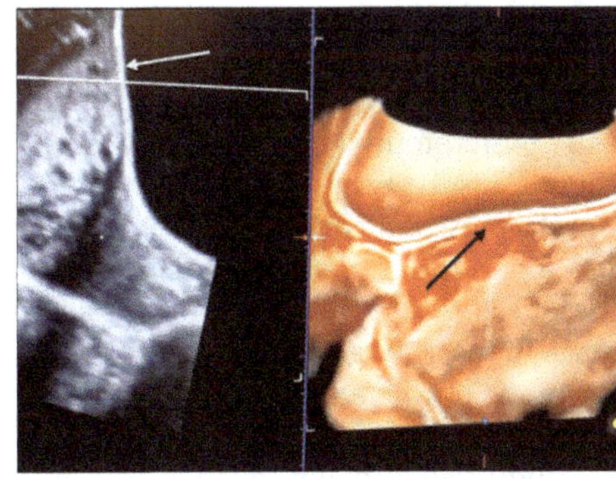

Figure 1: 3D ultrasound image. White arrow indicates normal bladder line; black arrow indicates the perimetrial interruption.

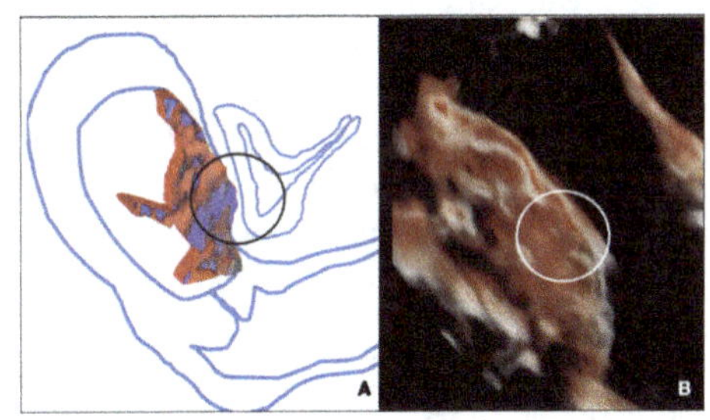

Figure 2: (a, b) Images of utero-bladder relationship. Graphic reconstruction (a) and 3D-ultrasound image (b) of the focal myometrial invasion without involvement of the bladder and integrity of the posterior bladder wall.

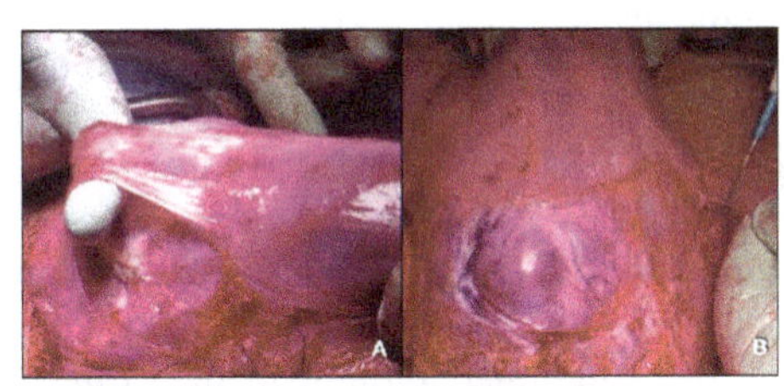

Figure 3: (a, b) Intraoperative images of vesicouterine peritoneum detachment (a) and evidence of placental "bulging" (b).

3. Discussion

In the last decade, there has been a notable increase in incidence of CDs, with relative short- and long-term complications, such as slower recovery, rise in blood loss, infections, thrombosis, possible bladder, intestinal injury, and even hysterectomy [8]. The occurrence of PAS in successive pregnancies is a relevant risk, mainly due to the related maternal and fetal mortality and morbidity [8]. Despite the relevant clinical impact of the disease, PAS disorders remain undiagnosed before delivery in half to two-thirds of cases still today [9–11]. Given the difficulty and subjectivity in the interpretation of "typical" findings or signs by two-dimensional US and colour Doppler imaging; the recent literature reported variable sensitivity and specificity regarding markers of PAS [12]. However, there are no clear guidelines worldwide to define how and when to screen and evaluate women with previous CDs.

Recent studies have ascertained the histopathological correlation between caesarean scar pregnancy (CSP) and PAS disorders [13]. CSP is defined as the gestational sac located on the hysterotomy scar created by a previous caesarean section. This type of pregnancy is a pathological one, and if undiagnosed, it could have serious consequences and complications such as uncontrollable haemorrhage and need for hysterectomy [14]. Furthermore, an associated placenta previa in the setting of CSP suggests placental invasion. The diagnosis of CSP at the early first trimester is possible, and in this sense, CSP can be considered a surrogate marker for a future abnormally invasive placenta [15–18]. In particular, the study of the gestational-sac implantation site using COS ("cross-over" sign) criteria is a simple and reproducible tool for ascertaining the relationship between the ectopic sac, cesarean scar, and anterior uterine wall [19, 20].

Based on the possible severe consequences of a misdiagnosed PAS, patients may have the best possible outcome if referred to the closest "reference center" with multidisciplinary team for diagnosis, staging, and adequate management [21].

Our case demonstrates the importance of correct diagnosis and related surgical planning. The careful organization of the cesarean section at the 34th week, the execution by highly skilled operators in election regimen (avoiding the urgency), and the support of intensive care unit and interventional radiology have allowed a desired and favorable result. In particular, reduced intraoperative bleeding was possible mainly thanks to the help of interventional radiology, achieving the reduction of the uterine vascularization during this delicate surgery and then ensuring a better maternal outcome.

In 2015, early first trimester US examination of pregnant women was incorporated into obstetrics and gynecology practice guidelines; it is a notable step forward in this field, because the identification of specific markers is a fundamental check point in order to carry out effective screening and therefore adequate diagnosis of a PAS disorder [22]. At the same time, the additional training in detecting the ultrasound signs of PAS using a standardized protocol has emerged as an essential tool significantly improving the diagnostic sensitivity of operators with only a basic obstetric ultrasound training [23]. In fact, high reproducibility and low interobserver variability of ultrasound imaging of PAS are essential to implement a screening program for women at a high risk of PAS [23].

Our experience highlights that a management by an experienced team reduces the risk of both maternal and fetal mortality and morbidity. In regional health facilities or smaller hospitals, which may lack the experience and the necessary support, PAS disorder (particularly the invasive forms) can result in numerous intra- and postoperative complications, such as massive haemorrhage secondary to attempts to separate the placenta from the uterus, in cases of pathology underdiagnosed. Based on the surgical risks and the perioperative challenges presented by PAS disorders, the transfer to a center of excellence relies on the recognition of the risk of PAS disorders, on accurate prenatal diagnosis, and on delivery with the help of a multidisciplinary experienced care team.

References

[1] G. Calì, *Le anomalie dell'invasione placentare*, EDITEAM, 2015.

[2] Committee on Obstetric Practice, "ACOG committee opinion. Placenta accreta. Number 266, January 2002," *International Journal of Gynaecology and Obstetrics: The Official Organ of the International Federation of Gynaecology and Obstetrics*, vol. 77, no. 1, pp. 77-78, 2002.

[3] R. M. Silver, M. B. Landon, D. J. Rouse et al., "Maternal morbidity associated with multiple repeat cesarean deliveries," *Obstetrics and Gynecology*, vol. 107, no. 6, pp. 1226–1232, 2006.

[4] S. L. Clark, P. P. Koonings, and J. P. Phelan, "Placenta previa/accreta and prior cesarean section," *Obstetrics and Gynecology*, vol. 66, no. 1, pp. 89–92, 1985.

[5] R. Resnik and R. M. Silver, *Clinical features and diagnosis of placenta accreta spectrum (placenta accreta, increta, and percreta)*, UpToDate, 2018.

[6] G. Cali, F. Forlani, C. Lees et al., "Prenatal ultrasound staging system for placenta accreta spectrum disorders," *Ultrasound in Obstetrics & Gynecology*, vol. 53, no. 6, pp. 752–760, 2019.

[7] P. Vercellini, G. Bolis, and P. G. Crosignani, "The Kustner technique: a neglected transverse lower abdominal incision," *American Journal of Obstetrics & Gynecology*, vol. 174, no. 4, pp. 1394-1395, 1996.

[8] E. Jauniaux, D. Ayres-de-Campos, and for the FIGO Placenta Accreta Diagnosis and Management Expert Consensus Panel, "FIGO consensus guidelines on placenta accreta spectrum disorders: Introduction,," *International Journal of Gynecology & Obstetrics*, vol. 140, no. 3, pp. 261–264, 2018.

[9] J. L. Bailit, W. A. Grobman, M. M. Rice et al., "Morbidly adherent placenta treatments and outcomes," *Obstetrics and Gynecology*, vol. 125, no. 3, pp. 683–689, 2015.

[10] K. E. Fitzpatrick, S. Sellers, P. Spark, J. J. Kurinczuk, P. Brocklehurst, and M. Knight, "The management and outcomes of placenta accreta, increta, and percreta in the UK: a population-based descriptive study," *BJOG*, vol. 121, no. 1, pp. 62–71, 2014.

[11] L. Thurn, P. G. Lindqvist, M. Jakobsson et al., "Abnormally invasive placenta – prevalence, risk factors and antenatal suspicion: results from a large population-based pregnancy cohort study in the Nordic countries," *BJOG*, vol. 123, no. 8, pp. 1348–1355, 2016.

[12] F. D'Antonio, C. Iacovella, and A. Bhide, "Prenatal identification of invasive placentation using ultrasound: systematic review and meta-analysis," *Ultrasound in Obstetrics & Gynecology*, vol. 42, no. 5, pp. 509–517, 2013.

[13] I. E. Timor-Tritsch, A. Monteagudo, G. Cali et al., "Cesarean scar pregnancy and early placenta accreta share common histology," *Ultrasound in Obstetrics & Gynecology*, vol. 43, no. 4, pp. 383–395, 2014.

[14] I. E. Timor-Tritsch and A. Monteagudo, "Unforeseen consequences of the increasing rate of cesarean deliveries: early placenta accreta and cesarean scar pregnancy. A review," *American Journal of Obstetrics and Gynecology*, vol. 207, no. 1, pp. 14–29, 2012.

[15] I. E. Timor-Tritsch, F. D'Antonio, G. Calí, J. M. Palacios-Jaraquemada, J. Meyer, and A. Monteagudo, "Early first-trimester transvaginal ultrasound is indicated in pregnancy after previous cesarean delivery: should it be mandatory?,"

Ultrasound in Obstetrics & Gynecology, vol. 54, no. 2, pp. 156–163, 2019.

[16] J. Panaiotova, M. Tokunaka, K. Krajewska, N. Zosmer, and K. H. Nicolaides, "Screening for morbidly adherent placenta in early pregnancy," *Ultrasound in Obstetrics & Gynecology*, vol. 53, no. 1, pp. 101–106, 2019.

[17] F. D'Antonio, I. E. Timor-Tritsch, J. Palacios-Jaraquemada et al., "First-trimester detection of abnormally invasive placenta in high-risk women: systematic review and meta-analysis," *Ultrasound in Obstetrics & Gynecology*, vol. 51, no. 2, pp. 176–183, 2018.

[18] R. Granese, E. Gitto, G. D'Angelo et al., "Preterm birth: seven-year retrospective study in a single centre population," *Italian Journal of Pediatrics*, vol. 45, no. 1, pp. 1–6, 2019.

[19] G. Cali, F. Forlani, I. E. Timor-Tritsch, J. Palacios-Jaraquemada, G. Minneci, and F. D'Antonio, "Natural history of cesarean scar pregnancy on prenatal ultrasound: the crossover sign," *Ultrasound in Obstetrics & Gynecology*, vol. 50, no. 1, pp. 100–104, 2017.

[20] Y. Wang, G. Tan, X. Cheng, Y. Xu, F. Xu, and P. Qu, "Association of hemorrhage at termination in caesarean scar pregnancy using the crossover sign of ultrasound image," *Journal of Obstetrics and Gynaecology Research*, vol. 46, no. 8, pp. 1378–1383, 2020.

[21] G. Cali, F. Forlani, L. Giambanco et al., "Prophylactic use of intravascular balloon catheters in women with placenta accreta, increta and percreta," *European Journal of Obstetrics, Gynecology and Reproductive Biology*, vol. 179, pp. 36–41, 2014.

[22] SIEOG, *Linee guida società italiana di Ecografia Ostetrica e Ginecologica e metodologie biofisiche*, 2015.

[23] I. Dimitrova, E. Jauniaux, N. Zosmer et al., "Development of a training program for the ultrasound screening of placenta accreta spectrum disorders," *International Journal of Gynecology & Obstetrics*, vol. 147, no. 1, pp. 73–77, 2019.

Undiagnosed Abdominal Term Pregnancy with Good Neonatal Outcome

Phoy Cheng Chun , Ka-Hee Chua, Mohamed Siraj Shahul Hameed, Manisha Mathur, and Wai Kheong Ryan Lee

Department of Obstetrics and Gynecology, Kandang Kerbau Women's and Children's Hospital, 229899, Singapore

Correspondence should be addressed to Phoy Cheng Chun; phoycheng.chun@mohh.com.sg

Academic Editor: Giovanni Monni

Abdominal pregnancy is a rare occurrence and it represents only 1% of ectopic pregnancy. We report a case of an abdominal pregnancy that resulted in a term live baby. Diagnosis is unsurprisingly difficult in advanced gestation. A high index of suspicion detailed clinical and imaging examinations are needed to make the diagnosis. Multidisciplinary team involvement is crucial in the management of abdominal pregnancy.

1. Introduction

Ectopic pregnancy is a rare occurrence and represents 1–2% of overall pregnancy [1]. 95% of ectopic pregnancy involves the fallopian tube. Abdominal pregnancy represents only 1% of ectopic pregnancy [1], in which the implantation occurs within the peritoneal cavity, outside the fallopian tube and ovary. The incidence rate of abdominal pregnancy is estimated to be 1 : 10000 [1]. It is important to identify such pregnancies as they carry higher mortality and morbidity for both the mother and baby. We report a case of an abdominal pregnancy that resulted in a term live baby.

2. Case Report

The patient, a 31-year-old Malay lady, Gravida 2 Para 0 + 1 presented at 38 + 6 weeks of pregnancy with constant lower abdominal pain for 1 day duration associated with back pain.

She had a history of right ectopic pregnancy 7 years ago and was treated with single dose methotrexate. For her current pregnancy, she presented at 35 weeks of gestation for her first antenatal visit. A trans-abdominal (TA) ultrasonography was performed and confirmed a single viable foetus in breech presentation with head circumference (HC) of 309 mm and femur length (FL) of 61 mm, corresponding to 35 weeks and 33 weeks of gestation, respectively. Clinically, her symphysio-fundal height (SFH) was 35 cm. She defaulted her subsequent antenatal appointments.

On arrival, her vitals were stable. Her abdomen was soft with palpable contractions. SFH was 38 cm, longitudinal lie with breech presentation. Speculum examination revealed a closed cervix.

A bedside TA ultrasonography showed a live foetus in breech presentation, HC and FL corresponding to 37 weeks of gestation and AC corresponding to 38 weeks of gestation with estimated foetal weight of 3.3 kg, placenta low covering internal orifice of uterus, and a cervical fibroid measuring 7.6 cm. A repeat TA ultrasonography performed by a dedicated obstetrics sonographer revealed similar findings. Patient was then consented for caesarean section, keeping in view hysterectomy. Preoperative haemoglobin (Hb) was 10.6 g/dL. Four pints of packed red cell (PCT) were arranged.

Patient was placed on regional anaesthesia (combined spinal epidural). A Pfannenstiel skin incision was made and her uterus was found to be intact and small upon entering her abdomen. The foetus was found in her abdomen surrounded by a large amniotic membrane filled with clear liquor. The amniotic membrane was incised, and the foetus was delivered cephalic. The foetal Apgar scores were 9 and 9 at one and five minutes, respectively, with birth weight of 2821 gram. The

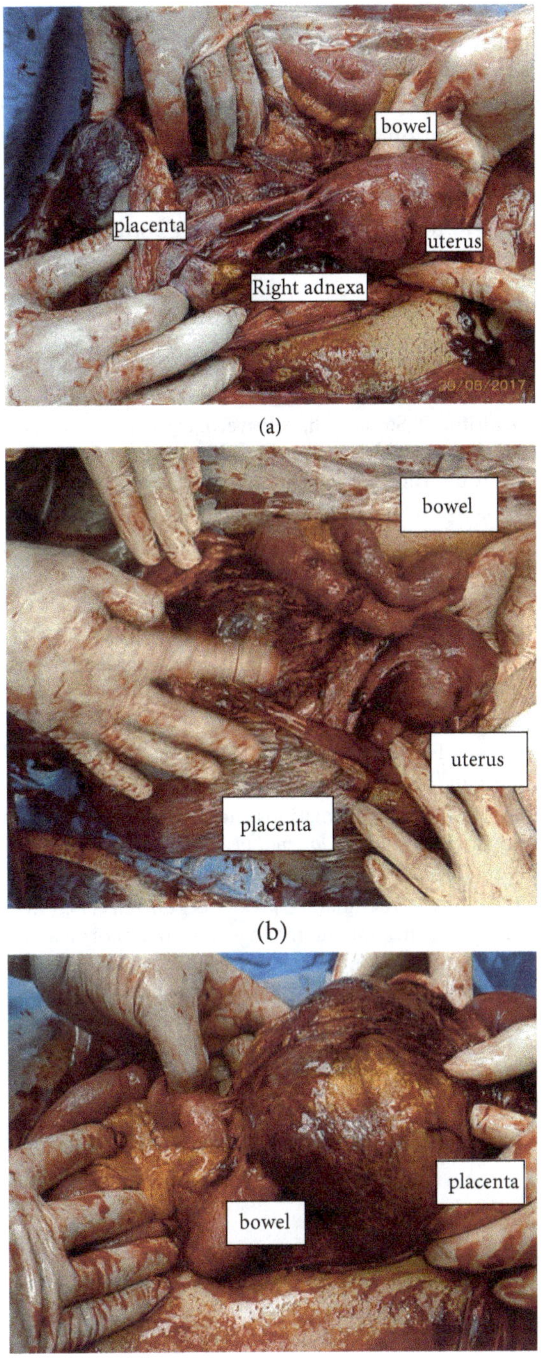

FIGURE 1: The placenta is located outside of the uterus, attached to the right adnexa, terminal ileum, proximal caecum, and appendix.

placenta was attached to the right adnexa, terminal ileum, proximal caecum, and appendix (Figure 1(a)–1(c)). Placenta attachments were dissected and ligated, starting from the adnexa and lastly the bowel. Parts of placenta membrane were left in-situ to avoid bowel injury (Figure 2). The left fallopian tube and ovary were seen with the left tube fimbriae end attached to placenta. This was dissected and the left fallopian tube was preserved (Figure 3). The right fallopian tube and ovary were not seen despite a thorough search. There was bleeding from the right uterine vessels, and they were ligated.

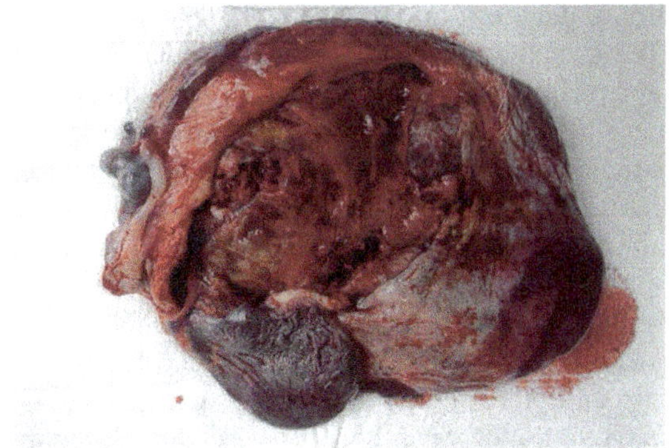

FIGURE 2: Incomplete placenta. Parts of placenta membrane were left in-situ to avoid bowel injury.

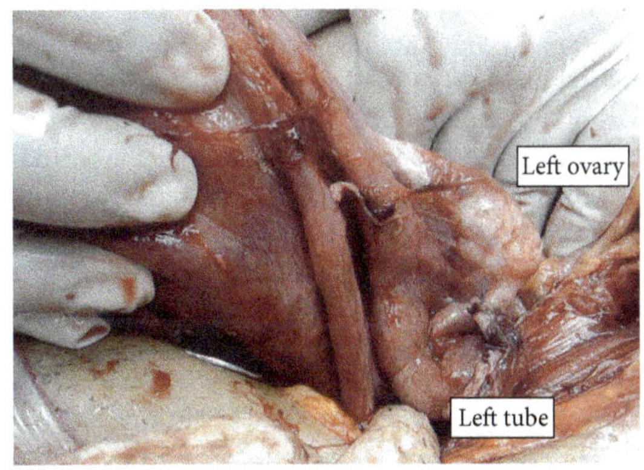

FIGURE 3: Left fallopian tube and left ovary were identified.

Intravenous therapy tranexamic acid 1 g was given. Estimated blood loss was 2 litres with Hb of 6.6 g/dL. Two pints of PCT was transfused intraoperatively. Her vitals remained stable. Abdominal redivac drain size #12 was inserted. The duration of operation was 100 min. She was transferred to Intensive Care Unit (ICU) after operation. Posttransfusion Hb was 11.2 g/dL and coagulation profile was normal. Her urine output and vitals remained stable throughout her stay in hospital. Drain output was minimal. Beta HCG 2 days postdelivery was 3617.4 IU/L. She was discharged home on postoperative day 3. Her baby did not require ICU or high dependency unit admission after birth. Placenta histology revealed an intra-abdominal implantation with villous ischemic change and infarction; fimbriae of fallopian tube was seen in specimen; however, ovary was not seen. Patient defaulted follow up after discharge from hospital.

3. Discussion

Advanced abdominal pregnancy is extremely rare. Most of the abdominal pregnancy cases are secondary, where a tubal pregnancy ruptures and implants in the peritoneal cavity [2]. In this case, the pregnancy was likely secondary to an undiagnosed ruptured right fallopian tube as placenta histology showed fimbriae end of fallopian tube. Of note, patient had a previous right ectopic pregnancy which was treated conservatively with methotrexate.

Clinical diagnosis and ultrasonography can be difficult at advanced gestation. A diagnosis of extrauterine abdominal pregnancy is frequently missed, with only 45% diagnosed during antenatal period and the rest are diagnosed during surgery [3]. Patients typically have persistent abdominal and/or gastrointestinal symptoms, which were not present in our patient other than the abdominal pain at 38 weeks of gestation.

Sonography is the most effective method in diagnosing abdominal pregnancy. There is report by Radhakrishnan that MRI is a useful adjunct tool to locate the placenta and delineate its origin and attachments as well as confirm the diagnosis. Perioperative angiogram might be useful in mapping the vascular supply of the placenta preoperatively, also, embolization or balloon obturation of vessels to control haemorrhage [4].

Major criteria for diagnosis of intra-abdominal pregnancy listed by Allibone et al. include: (1) demonstration of a foetus in gestational sac outside the uterus, or the depiction of an abdominal or pelvic mass identifiable as the uterus separate from the foetus, (2) failure to see a uterine wall between the foetus and the urinary bladder, (3) recognition of a close approximation of the foetus to the maternal abdominal wall, and (4) localization of placenta outside the confines of the uterine cavity [5]. Other additional criteria include oligohydramnios, abnormal foetal lie, placenta praevia appearance, and maternal bowel gas impending foetal visualization. On retrospective review of the ultrasound images, there was indeed no uterine wall between the foetus and urinary bladder, and the placenta appeared to be praevia. However, these signs were not picked up prior to Caesarean section.

Stevens (1993) reported a 21% birth defect risk associated with extra-uterine pregnancies, which include, central nervous system malformations, facial and cranial asymmetry, joint abnormalities and limb defects [6]. The lack of amniotic fluid buffer leading to foetal compression may be the cause of these defects. The patient's baby was examined by neonatology team and no malformation was found on the baby upon delivery.

One of the major concerns intraoperatively was the management of placenta. Bleeding from placenta implantation site can be life-threatening especially if the blood supply cannot be identified or ligated completely. Expectant management can be considered in such situation. By leaving the placenta in situ, blood loss and blood transfusion requirement are less compared to removal of placenta [7]. However, this approach can be associated with postoperative morbidity and mortality such as peritonitis, abscess formation, and prolonged hospital stay [8]. Till date, discussion on this issue is still ongoing. Careful assessment should be carried out when deciding the suitable approach for each patient. In this case, the blood supply to the placenta was identified and almost all of the placenta was removed with minimal placenta tissues attached to the bowel. Human chorionic gonadotropin (HCG) level was measured postsurgery, with a plan of repeat HCG level during postnatal follow up in outpatient clinic.

4. Conclusion

Abdominal pregnancy with resultant healthy live newborn is a rare occasion. Diagnosis is unsurprisingly difficult in advanced gestation. A high index of suspicion, detailed clinical and imaging examinations are needed to make the diagnosis.

In addition, the surgeon's experience and clinical judgment, co-operation with the anaesthetists and neonatologist teams, availability of blood products for potential massive blood transfusions, immediate detection, and rapid surgical repair help to minimise life-threatening complications.

References

[1] E. I. Nwobodo, "Abdominal pregnancy. a case report," *Annals of African Medicine*, vol. 3, no. 4, pp. 195–196, 2004.

[2] B. Amritha, T. Sumangali, B. Priya, S. Deepak, and S. Rai, "A rare case of term viable secondary abdominal pregnancy following rupture of a rudimentary horn. a case report," *Journal of Medical Case Reports*, vol. 3, no. 1, 2009.

[3] D. Nkusu Nunyalulendho and E. M. Einterz, "Advanced abdominal pregnancy: case report and review of 163 cases reported since 1946," *Rural Remote Health*, vol. 8, no. 4, p. 1087, 2008.

[4] K. Radhakrishnan, "Intra-abdominal pregnancy," *Applied Radiology*, vol. 44, no. 5, 44 pages, 2015.

[5] G. W. Allibone, C. J. Fagan, and S. C. Porter, "The sonographic features of intra-abdominal pregnancy," *Journal of Clinical Ultrasound*, vol. 9, no. 7, pp. 383–387, 1981.

[6] C. A. Stevens, "Malformations and deformations in abdominal pregnancy," *American Journal of Medical Genetics*, vol. 47, no. 8, pp. 1189–1195, 1993.

[7] S. L. Collins, B. Alemdar, H. J. Van Beekhuizen et al., "Evidence-based guidelines for the management of abnormally invasive placenta: recommendations from the international society for abnormally invasive placenta," *American Journal of Obstetrics and Gynecology*, vol. 220, pp. 511–526, 2019.

[8] Z. Jianping, L. Fen, and S. Qiu, "Full-term abdominal pregnancy. a case report and review of the literature," *Gynecologic and Obstetric Investigation*, vol. 65, no. 2, pp. 139–141, 2008.

26

Diagnosis of an Umbilical Vein Aneurysm at 30 Weeks Gestation

Meredith S. Campbell,[1] Amanda M. Craig,[2] Jeff Reese,[1] Alicia K. Crum,[2,3] and Soha S. Patel[2,3]

[1]*Division of Neonatology, Department of Pediatrics, Monroe Carell Jr. Children's Hospital at Vanderbilt, Nashville, TN, USA*
[2]*Department of Obstetrics and Gynecology, Vanderbilt University Medical Center, Nashville, TN, USA*
[3]*Division of Maternal-Fetal Medicine, Department of Obstetrics and Gynecology, Vanderbilt University Medical Center, Nashville, TN, USA*

Correspondence should be addressed to Meredith S. Campbell; meredith.campbell@vumc.org

Academic Editor: Maria Grazia Porpora

Background. Fetal umbilical vein aneurysm is an uncommon anomaly without clear guidelines regarding the management of these pregnancies. *Case Presentation.* We describe an ultrasound diagnosis of this condition involving a 38-year-old multigravid woman who presented at 30 weeks and 3 days gestation with severe fetal growth restriction, reverse end-diastolic flow on umbilical artery dopplers, elevated ductus venosus doppler, and an umbilical vein aneurysm. Due to nonreassuring fetal assessment in the setting of an umbilical vein aneurysm, she underwent a cesarean delivery with a favorable neonatal outcome. *Conclusions.* There are currently no guidelines for the management of an umbilical vein aneurysm. This case demonstrates a successful multidisciplinary approach for creating a plan of care focused on achieving a favorable outcome for a fetus with a large umbilical vein aneurysm. The approach took into account timing of delivery given the potential for fetal morbidity and mortality, while factoring in the risk of prematurity.

1. Introduction

An umbilical vein aneurysm is a rare prenatal diagnosis with limited literature available regarding management. Fetal umbilical vein aneurysm was first described in 1978 [1] and accounts for less than 4% of umbilical cord malformations [2, 3]. Possible complications include aneurysm rupture, thrombosis, and compression of the umbilical cord leading to poor fetal outcome [4]. Published studies have been small, with contradictory results regarding increased risk of fetal anomalies or poor perinatal outcomes associated with this ultrasonographic finding. Some authors have reported normal fetal outcomes [4, 5] while other authors have cited fetal mortality rates over 40% [6, 7]. A review of 23 cases identified no fetal or neonatal deaths; however, these authors did find a high rate of fetal malformations with 34.8% of infants having major congenital anomalies including multiple-anomaly syndromes and severe cardiac defects [8].

Our case highlights a multidisciplinary approach to the care of a woman at 30 weeks gestation whose pregnancy was complicated by this abnormality. We recommend that obstetrical providers consider earlier timing of delivery in the setting of umbilical vein aneurysm due to the potential for severe fetal morbidity and mortality.

2. Case Presentation

2.1. Maternal History. A 38-year old gravida 2, para 1001 mother presented at 30 weeks and 3 days gestation as a transfer of care from an outside hospital for reverse end-diastolic flow on umbilical artery Doppler assessment, elevated ductus venosus doppler, and umbilical vein aneurysm in the setting of severe fetal growth restriction, less than the 3rd percentile for gestational age. Her pregnancy was also complicated by type 2 diabetes mellitus, a prior history of cesarean delivery, and an increased risk for trisomy 21

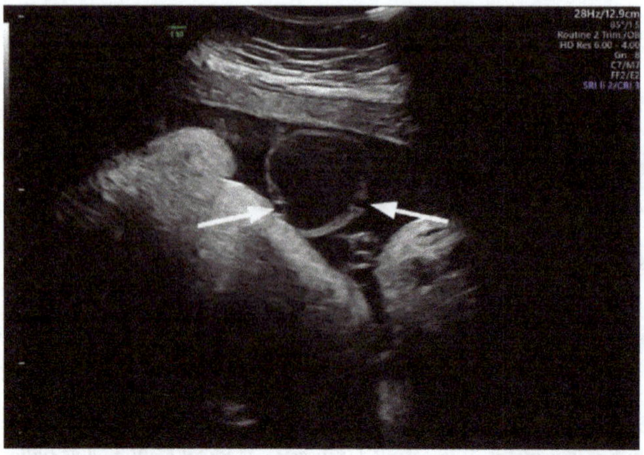

Figure 1: Cross-sectional view of the umbilical vein aneurysm with arrows pointing towards the umbilical arteries on either side.

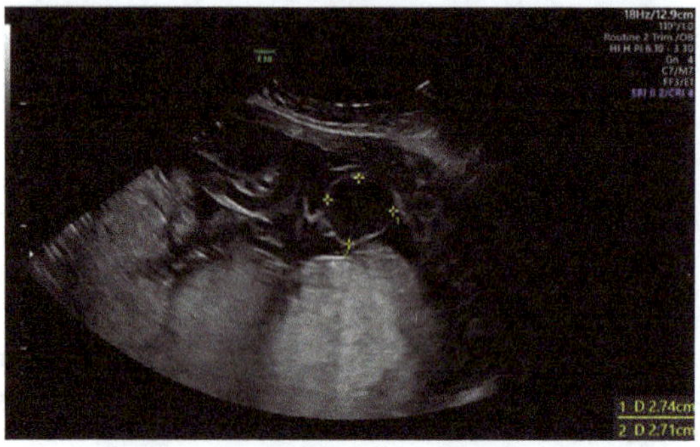

(a)

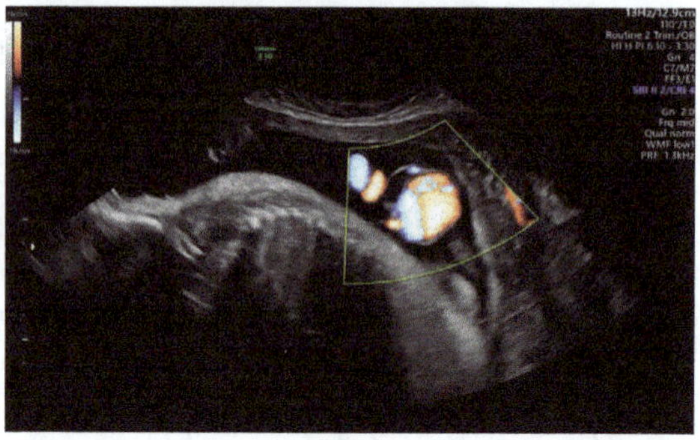

(b)

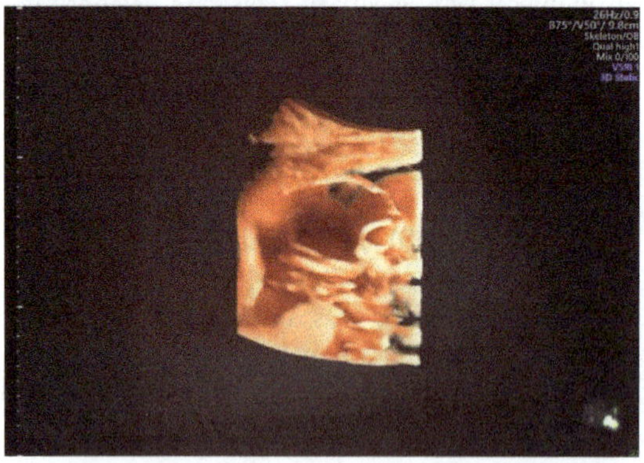

(c)

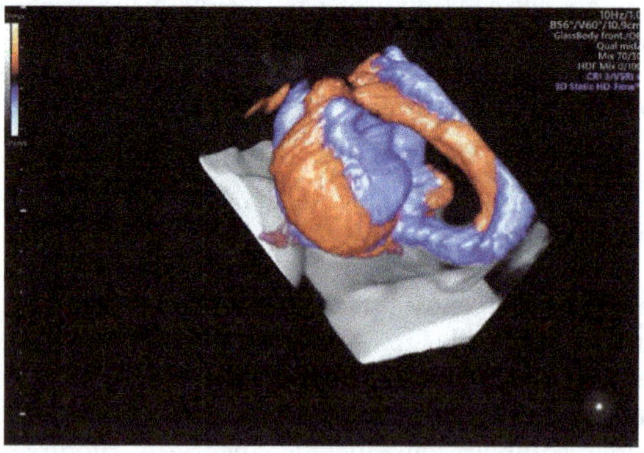

(d)

Figure 2: (a) Top left—2.7 cm umbilical vein aneurysm free-floating cord. (b) Top right—color doppler demonstrating bidirectional flow within umbilical vein aneurysm. (c) Bottom left—high definition live 3D rendering of umbilical vein aneurysm. (d) Bottom right—color 3D rendering of umbilical vein aneurysm.

(1 : 80) on first trimester screen. Prior to transfer to our hospital, she received two doses of betamethasone and a magnesium sulfate infusion for fetal neuroprotection.

She was admitted to the hospital for observation and continuous electronic fetal monitoring. Repeat ultrasound on arrival confirmed the abnormal Doppler findings. Elevated flow through the ductus venosus with intermittent reversal of end-diastolic flow. More concerning, there was a 3-4 cm thin-walled umbilical vein aneurysm in the free-floating cord with nonpulsatile, turbulent flow (Figure 1). The following day, given her ultrasound findings, and increased risk for fetal compromise, the decision was made to schedule a repeat cesarean section. The surgery was tolerated well with no complications. Postoperatively, she was diagnosed with HELLP syndrome (hemolysis, elevated liver enzymes, low platelet count) and started on magnesium sulfate for seizure prophylaxis. She was subsequently discharged on postoperative day 3.

2.2. Birth History and Neonatal Evaluation. A 1320 gram male infant, born at less than the 1st percentile for weight, was delivered with APGAR scores of 6 and 7 at 1 and 5 minutes, respectively. Resuscitation included stimulation and continuous positive airway pressure (CPAP). The infant

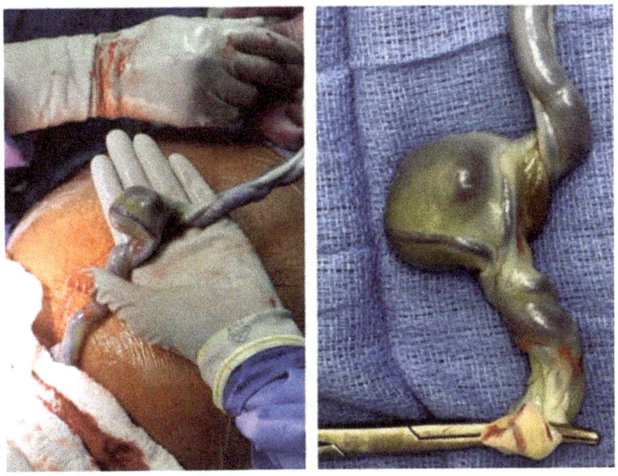

FIGURE 3: Gross specimen of the umbilical cord and umbilical cord aneurysm.

was admitted to the neonatal intensive care unit for management of prematurity and respiratory distress.

Laboratory tests revealed a hemoglobin of 15.9 gm/dL, platelet count 23 × 103/mcL, requiring platelet transfusion. Neonatal thrombocytopenia was considered secondary to maternal HELLP syndrome and prematurity, although a relationship to the umbilical cord anomaly such as thrombus formation within the umbilical aneurysm was also considered. Abdominal ultrasound was performed to evaluate secondary causes of thrombocytopenia including sequestration at the umbilical cord site, arteriovenous malformation, or vascular lesions, which was negative. There were no signs of intracranial or intraventricular bleeding on ultrasound. Further studies including urine cytomegalovirus, karyotype, and chromosomal microarray analysis were negative.

The extra-abdominal umbilical vein aneurysm measured approximately 3.5 × 3 cm (Figures 2 and 3). Placental pathology showed uneven villous maturation, fetal thrombotic vasculopathy with endothelial cushion lesions, hemorrhagic endovasculitis, and focal acute deciduitis. The placenta was grossly normal with a normal placental cord insertion.

Initial chest X-ray showed decreased lung volumes, diffuse granularity, and air bronchograms most consistent with respiratory distress syndrome. The infant required intubation, a single dose of surfactant, and mechanical ventilation for 1 day. After extubation, he remained on nasal CPAP until 34 weeks gestation followed by low flow nasal cannula until 37 weeks gestation, consistent with mild bronchopulmonary dysplasia. The infant was discharged on day of life 67.

3. Discussion and Conclusion

Recommendations regarding evaluation and antenatal surveillance are not well established but are aimed at recognizing early evidence of fetal distress to potentially prevent poor fetal outcomes. Authors from a case report of an intrauterine fetal demise at 41 weeks gestation have suggested that the increased umbilical cord blood flow in pregnancy may increase fetal compromise with advancing gestational age, which might explain why cases of intrauterine death have been presented later in pregnancy [9]. These authors hypothesized that there is a significantly increased risk of vessel rupture with uterine contractions in labor and rupture of membranes [9]. Due to the uncertainties regarding the relationship of this hemodynamically significant lesion with poor neonatal outcomes, obstetric providers should consider earlier timing of delivery after administration of betamethasone given the potential for severe fetal morbidity and mortality [10–13].

Abbreviations

CPAP:	Continuous positive airway pressure
HELLP syndrome:	Hemolysis, elevated liver enzymes, low platelet count.

Consent

Written informed consent was obtained from the patient for publication of this case report and any accompanying images. A copy of the written consent is available for review by the Editor-in-Chief of this journal.

Authors' Contributions

MSC and AMC wrote the first draft and final manuscript. JR and SSP reviewed and edited the manuscript. All authors were involved in the case of the patients described in the report. All authors read and approved the final manuscript.

Acknowledgments

We would like to thank Alicia Crum for capturing the fetal ultrasound images of the umbilical vein aneurysm.

References

[1] D. W. Fortune and A. G. Ostör, "Umbilical artery aneurysm," *American Journal of Obstetrics and Gynecology*, vol. 131, no. 3, pp. 339-340, 1978.

[2] S. R. Giannubilo, A. Pasculli, A. Cecchi, A. Biagini, and A. Ciavattini, "Fetal intra-abdominal umbilical vein aneurysm," *Obstetrical & Gynecological Survey*, vol. 72, no. 9, pp. 547–552, 2017.

[3] B. Kostantinova, "Malformations of the umbilical cord," *Acta Geneticae Medicae et Gemellologiae*, vol. 26, pp. 259–266, 1977.

[4] S. P. White and A. Kofinas, "Prenatal diagnosis and management of umbilical vein varix of the intra-amniotic protion of the umbilical vein," *Journal of Ultrasound in Medicine*, vol. 13, pp. 992–994, 1994.

[5] J. A. Estroff and B. R. Benecerraf, "Fetal umbilical vein varix: sonographic appearance and postnatal outcome," *Journal of Ultrasound in Medicine*, vol. 11, pp. 69–73, 1992.

[6] W. Sepulveda, A. Mackenna, J. Sanchez, E. Corral, and A. Cartens, "Fetal prognosis in varix of the intrafetal umbilical vein," *Journal of Ultrasound in Medicine*, vol. 17, pp. 171–175, 1998.

[7] B. S. Mahoney, J. P. McGahan, D. A. Nyberg, and D. P. Reisner, "Varix of the fetal intra-abdominal umbilical vein: com-

parison with normal," *Journal of Ultrasound in Medicine*, vol. 11, pp. 73–76, 1992.

[8] A. Rahemtullah, E. Leiberman, C. Benson, and M. Norton, "Outcome of pregnancy after prenatal diagnosis of umbilical vein varix," *Journal of Ultrasound in Medicine*, vol. 20, pp. 135–139, 2001.

[9] N. M. Vandevijver, R. H. Hermans, C. C. Schrander-Stumpel, J. W. Arends, L. L. Peeters, and P. L. Moerman, "Aneurysm of the umbilical vein: case report and review of literature," *European Journal of Obstetrics & Gynecology and Reproductive Biology*, vol. 89, pp. 85–87, 2000.

[10] E. Beuraud, C. Rozel, J. Milon, and P. Darnault, "Umbilical vein varix: importance of ante- and post-natal monitoring by ultrasound," *Diagnostic and Interventional Imaging*, vol. 96, pp. 21–26, 2014.

[11] J. H. Lee, J. H. Cho, H. Y. Kwon, Y. W. Park, and Y. H. Kim, "A huge umbilical vein aneurysm: case report and a brief review of literatures describing umbilical vessel aneurysm," *Korean Journal of Perinatology*, vol. 25, no. 3, pp. 178–183, 2014.

[12] E. Leinsinger, "Varix thrombose der Nabelschnur," *Zeitschrift für Geburtshilfe und Gynäkologie*, vol. 171, pp. 82–87, 1969.

[13] M. Akar, D. Dilli, G. Sandal, M. Y. Öncel, Ö. Erdeve, and U. Dilmen, "Prenatally diagnosed umbilical vein aneurysm with good prognosis," *Journal of Clinical Ultrasound*, vol. 40, no. 6, pp. 368-369, 2012.

27

Case Report of a Triplet Pregnancy with Complete Hydatidiform Mole and Coexisting Twins

Marjorie H. Thompson,[1] Nathaniel R. Miller,[2] Shelby L. Haugan,[3] and Michael C. Gordon[4]

[1]*University of Washington School of Medicine, USA*
[2]*Providence Sacred Heart Maternal and Fetal Medicine, USA*
[3]*Billings Clinic Bozeman, USA*
[4]*Billings Clinic Maternal Fetal Medicine, USA*

Correspondence should be addressed to Michael C. Gordon; packergord@aol.com

Academic Editor: Seung-Yup Ku

Background. Triplet pregnancy with complete hydatidiform mole and coexisting twin fetuses is extremely rare with an unknown incidence. *Case.* Here, we present a case report of a pregnancy with twin fetuses and concurrent hydatidiform mole that resulted in the preterm delivery of one viable baby, the unfortunate intrauterine demise of the other twin, and successful treatment of gestational trophoblastic neoplasia in the postpartum period. *Conclusion.* This case highlights several important questions that arise for women who choose to carry a multiple gestation pregnancy with complete hydatidiform mole and describes complications that can occur. It is imperative to accurately assess risks and counsel individuals who elect to carry these pregnancies to provide the best possible outcomes.

1. Introduction

Twin pregnancy with complete hydatidiform mole and concurrent fetus is rare with an estimated occurrence of 1 in every 22,000 to 100,000 pregnancies [1–5]. The incidence of triplet pregnancies with twin fetuses and concurrent hydatidiform mole is unknown due to rarity of case reports.

Multiple gestation with a complete mole and coexisting fetus (CHMCF) is complicated by increased risk in spontaneous abortion, intrauterine fetal demise, preeclampsia, preterm labor, and hyperthyroidism. The chance of delivering a viable baby appears to be less than 50% according to current data [1, 6, 7]. Risk of progression of the mole to gestational trophoblastic neoplasia (GTN) does not appear to be increased for individuals who choose to carry CHMCF pregnancies to birth; however, it is considered somewhat controversial in the limited literature on this subject [5, 6]. Additionally, gestational age at molar evacuation or early termination of pregnancy does not appear to influence rate of progression to GTN [1, 8].

Here, we present a case report of a pregnancy with twin fetuses and concurrent hydatidiform mole that resulted in the delivery of one viable baby, the unfortunate intrauterine demise of the other twin, and successful treatment of gestational trophoblastic neoplasia in the postpartum period.

2. Case Presentation

A 32-year-old healthy nulliparous woman achieved a diamniotic-dichorionic twin pregnancy with one cycle of clomiphene and timed intrauterine insemination. Her initial ultrasound was done at 7 weeks, and this exam noted 2 fetuses with an irregular third sac with no yolk sac or fetal pole and was thought to be a triplet pregnancy that was triamniotic-trichorionic. An ultrasound at 14 weeks noted a diamniotic-dichorionic twin with a posterior mass that was thought to be a degenerating fibroid. An 18-week ultrasound showed normal twin growth and anatomy, but a posterior uterine vascular mass was seen with a differential diagnosis of a fibroid versus a chorioangioma versus other multicystic uterine lesions. She presented for a comprehensive anatomic ultrasound at 21 weeks gestation with maternal fetal medicine to better evaluate this mass. This ultrasound revealed an abnormal third placenta along the posterior uterine wall with large multicystic structures, consistent with diamniotic-dichorionic twin pregnancy with coexisting complete hydatidiform mole (Figures 1 and 2). The abnormal third placenta was separated from the two normal twin placentas. The fetal anatomy was normal on both twins, and they were both appropriately grown. The diagnosis was confirmed by a second maternal-fetal medicine physician and a gynecologic-oncologist was also consulted. The B-human chorionic gonadotropin (B-hCG) was measured to be 276,568 mIU/mL. The chest X-ray was unremarkable. She was experiencing some nausea and fatigue but was otherwise healthy. Risks and benefits were discussed with her. Additionally, the option of pregnancy termination was offered given her increased risk for pregnancy complications and risk of developing persistent GTN. She elected to proceed with the pregnancy.

She was seen weekly by maternal-fetal medicine and had fetal growth ultrasounds obtained every 3-4 weeks. She took a daily 81 mg aspirin and performed home blood pressure readings to monitor for signs of early pre-eclampsia. The pregnancy proceeded without complication until 25 weeks.

At 25 weeks and 4 days gestation, she presented to the hospital for vaginal bleeding and was diagnosed with preterm premature rupture of membranes (PPROM) of twin A. She was given betamethasone, magnesium sulfate, and latency antibiotics. Her blood pressure readings were within normal limits, and a 24-hour urine protein was less than 300 mg. She had a low thyroid stimulating hormone (TSH); however, free thyroxine was within the upper limits of normal. A fetal growth scan was performed and was normal for both twins. The hydatidiform mole once again appeared to be separate and measured 19 cm in its largest diameter.

At 27 weeks and 3 days gestation, she had a transient increase in contractions in the early morning, and twin B was found to have a nonreactive nonstress test (NST). A biophysical profile (BPP) for both babies was 6/8 (−2 due to decreased amniotic fluid in twin A and −2 due to diminished breathing for twin B). Due to the overall BPP of 6/10 for twin B later that day, a repeat BPP was performed and revealed a demise of twin B. Over the next two days, the tocometer showed continued contractions and the NSTs were reactive for twin A.

At 27 weeks and 6 days gestation, due to vaginal bleeding, increased contractions, and cervical change, a placental abruption was suspected. Twin A was subsequently delivered by Cesarean delivery and weighed 2 lb 6 oz (1080 gm) with APGAR scores of 7/8, and there was meconium-stained amniotic fluid, but no obvious placental abruption was found. The suspected molar tissue was extracted completely without difficulty. Pathology confirmed the diagnosis that the third placenta was a complete mole. At autopsy, twin B weighed 2 lb 7 oz (1100 gm), and no gross developmental abnormalities or signs of infection were noted, and the placentas of the twins were unremarkable and confirmed diamniotic placentation.

One day after delivery, serum B-hCG measured 52,243.6 mIU/mL. The B-hCG initially decreased to 8,088.1 mIU/mL two weeks after delivery, but then increased to a peak of 17,562.8 mIU/mL three weeks after delivery. Due to this increase, she was diagnosed with GTN and was treated with intramuscular methotrexate: 30 mg for five consecutive days each week for one month. She desired to preserve fertility and thus hysterectomy was not recommended.

Her GTN responded to methotrexate. B-hCG lowered to 5mIU/mL, and she was treated with one more month of methotrexate and followed with weekly B-hCG. B-hCG was then followed every month for 12 months. She has remained on oral progesterone contraception during this time. One year after delivery, her B-hCG is still negative, and the surviving twin is doing well without any severe complications of prematurity.

3. Discussion

The initial diagnosis of a triplet pregnancy with complete hydatidiform mole and coexisting twin fetuses was challenging because of the rarity of the diagnosis. First trimester diagnosis is possible but appears to be more challenging, and the molar placenta can be incorrectly diagnosed as a subchorionic hematoma or an early miscarriage [9]. When the abnormal mole placenta is seen, the differential diagnosis typically includes a subchorionic hematoma, placental mesenchymal dysplasia, placental chorioangioma, an incomplete molar pregnancy, or triploidy. The important sonographic diagnostic features needed to make the correct diagnosis include seeing a separate atypical placenta with a Swiss cheese or cluster of grape appearance with otherwise normal fetal anatomy of the two intrauterine fetuses [9–11]. In addition, unlike a subchorionic hematoma, the molar placenta enlarges and has blood flow. The diagnosis is made easier with the finding of high B-hCG levels as was found in the case described.

Carrying a complete mole with coexisting fetus (CHMCF) pregnancy appears to have a significant increased risk of adverse perinatal outcomes, particularly a decreased chance of a viable pregnancy and increased risk for prematurity, particularly when compared with twin and triplet pregnancies without coexisting mole. In non-terminated singleton pregnancies with coexisting mole, the chances of a live birth are estimated to be 21-45% [1, 5, 6, 9, 10, 12]. This case study is the fourteenth (of which the authors are aware) to present a triplet pregnancy with twin fetuses and concurrent mole, for which 4 live fetuses have survived the neonatal period (29% live birth rate) [13].

There is also a high rate of preterm delivery in CHMCF. The mean gestational age at delivery for pregnancies that advance beyond 24 weeks gestation is 33.5 weeks gestation [5, 10, 11, 14]. The individual in this case study delivered at 27.9 weeks. Conversely, the average gestation for twin and triplet gestations without concurrent mole are 36 weeks and 32 weeks, respectively.

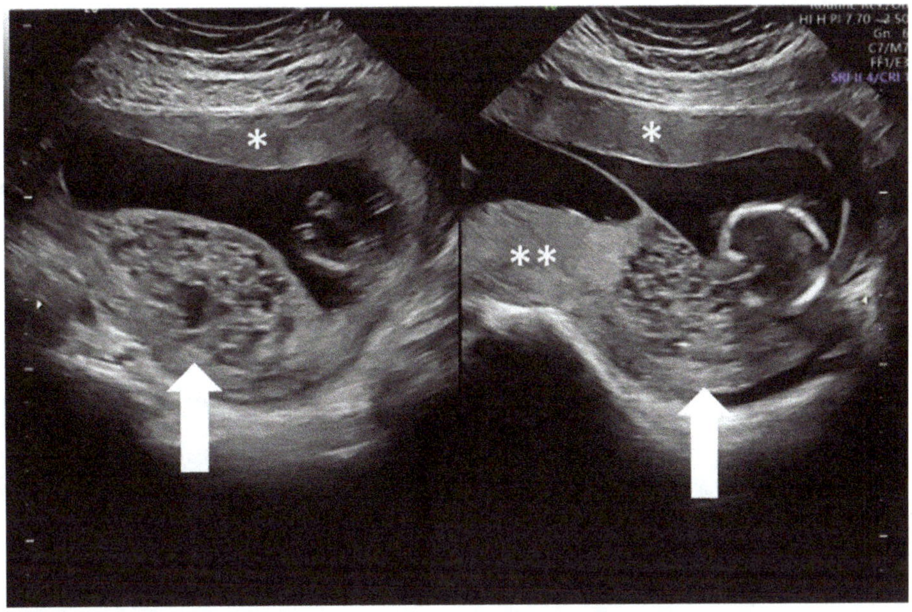

FIGURE 1: Ultrasound at 21 weeks showing three separate placentas and a dividing membrane *Twin A placenta. **Twin B placenta. Up arrow: molar placenta.

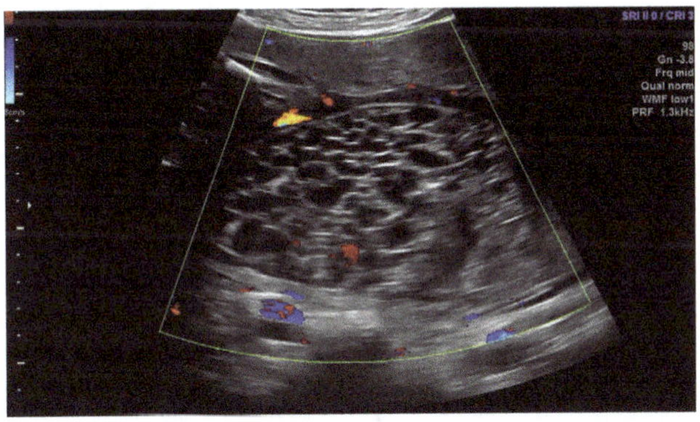

FIGURE 2: Close of color Doppler of molar placenta.

Much of the latest research on CHMCF has focused on risk of molar progression to GTN. However, these studies have also reported the incidence of obstetric complications in CHMCF. Vaginal bleeding is common, with an incidence as high as 76% in one literature review [14]. Risk of hyperthyroidism appears to be much lower, at about 15% estimated incidence [12]. In this case study, vaginal bleeding occurred later in her pregnancy, when she presented to the hospital at 25 weeks gestation and ultimately was diagnosed with a placental abruption. She did not have hyperthyroidism. Although the exact etiology of the cause of the stillbirth on twin B is uncertain, we speculate that it was due to a placental abruption.

The risk of preeclampsia is somewhat controversial. According to one cohort study of 77 CHMCF pregnancies performed by Sebire et al., the incidence of severe preeclampsia was 6%, which is reportedly higher than severe preeclampsia risk in normal twin pregnancies, but similar to rates of singleton complete hydatidiform molar pregnancies [6]. However, according to two literature reviews of cohort studies performed by Sukasi et al. and Wee et al., the estimate of preeclampsia in CHMCF ranges from 20 to 27% [12, 14]. A separate retrospective survey estimated the rate of preeclampsia and/or massive bleeding events at 14% [3]. This discrepancy might be explained by differences in the definitions of preeclampsia used. For example, Sebire et al. only reported the incidence of severe preeclampsia.

Premature rupture of membranes (PROM) was reported in one CHMCF pregnancy out of the reviewed literature [1]. In the literature review of CHMCF with two or more viable fetuses conducted by Takagi et al., they reported on a total of 13 pregnancies, and there were no incidences of PROM [13]. In our case study, it is unclear why this pregnancy was complicated by PPROM, and it is possible that this complication may not be associated with CHMCF or CHMCF with two viable fetuses and may simply have been a complication due to the multifetal pregnancy. In addition, whether the possible abruption was due to the molar placenta or simply a consequence of a multifetal pregnancy with PPROM is unknown. Abruptions are more common with multifetal pregnancies and with PPROM.

CHMCF pregnancies that are carried to birth do not appear to have a significantly increased rate of progression to gestational trophoblastic neoplasia (GTN) or more severe GTN in comparison to pregnancies that are aborted or have early elective terminations [5, 6]. However, this is still thought to be somewhat controversial, with multiple authors recommending that women need to be counseled about the potential benefits of pregnancy termination. The estimated progression to GTN appears to be 20-36% [5, 6, 9, 12]. However, one retrospective review of 14 CHMCF pregnancies reported a 50% rate of progression to GTN [1]. This discrepancy may be due to differences in study size, selection bias, differences in disease classification, or indications for chemotherapy.

4. Conclusion

This case highlights several important questions that arise for women who choose to carry a multiple gestation pregnancy with complete hydatidiform mole. Unfortunately, this pregnancy was complicated by intrauterine fetal demise, vaginal bleeding, and preterm delivery. There was also progression of the complete mole to gestational trophoblastic neoplasia after delivery. It is imperative to accurately assess risks and counsel individuals who elect to carry these pregnancies to provide the best possible outcomes for these women and their children.

References

[1] J. Massardier, F. Golfier, D. Journet et al., "Twin pregnancy with complete hydatidiform mole and coexistent fetus," *European Journal of Obstetrics, Gynecology, and Reproductive Biology*, vol. 143, no. 2, article S0301211509000153, pp. 84–87, 2009, Epub 2009 Feb 3.

[2] W. B. Jones and N. H. Lauersen, "Hydatidiform mole with coexistent fetus," *American Journal of Obstetrics and Gynecology*, vol. 122, no. 3, article 0002937875901659, pp. 267–272, 1975.

[3] H. Matsui, S. Sekiya, T. Hando, N. Wake, and Y. Tomoda, "Hydatidiform mole coexistent with a twin live fetus: a national collaborative study in Japan," *Human Reproduction*, vol. 15, no. 3, pp. 608–611, 2000.

[4] P. Petignat, P. Vassilakos, and A. Campana, "Are fertility drugs a risk factor for persistent trophoblastic tumour?," *Human Reproduction*, vol. 17, no. 6, pp. 1610–1615, 2002.

[5] I. Niemann, L. Sunde, and L. K. Petersen, "Evaluation of the risk of persistent trophoblastic disease after twin pregnancy with diploid hydatidiform mole and coexisting normal fetus," *American Journal of Obstetrics and Gynecology*, vol. 197, no. 1, 2007.

[6] N. J. Sebire, M. Foskett, F. J. Paradinas et al., "Outcome of twin pregnancies with complete hydatidiform mole and healthy co-twin," *The Lancet*, vol. 359, no. 9324, pp. 2165-2166, 2002.

[7] L. H. Lin, I. Maestá, A. Braga et al., "Multiple pregnancies with complete mole and coexisting normal fetus in North and South America: a retrospective multicenter cohort and literature review," *Gynecologic Oncology*, vol. 145, no. 1, pp. 88–95, 2017.

[8] S. Y. Sun, A. Melamed, D. P. Goldstein et al., "Changing presentation of complete hydatidiform mole at the New England Trophoblastic Disease Center over the past three decades: does early diagnosis alter risk for gestational trophoblastic neoplasia?," *Gynecologic Oncology*, vol. 138, no. 1, article S0090825815008719, pp. 46–49, 2015, Epub 2015 May 10.

[9] V. Giorgione, P. Cavoretto, G. Cormio et al., "Prenatal diagnosis of twin pregnancies with complete hydatidiform mole and coexistent normal fetus: a series of 13 cases," *Gynecologic and Obstetric Investigation*, vol. 82, no. 4, pp. 404–409, 2017.

[10] D. A. Fishman, L. A. Padilla, P. Keh, L. Cohen, M. Frederiksen, and J. R. Lurain, "Management of twin pregnancies consisting of a complete hydatidiform mole and normal fetus," *Obstetrics and Gynecology*, vol. 91, no. 4, pp. 546–550, 1998.

[11] M. A. Steller, D. R. Genest, M. R. Bernstein, J. M. Lage, D. P. Goldstein, and R. S. Berkowitz, "Clinical features of multiple conception with partial or complete molar pregnancy and coexisting fetuses," *The Journal of Reproductive Medicine*, vol. 39, no. 3, pp. 147–154, 1994.

[12] M. Suksai, C. Suwanrath, O. Kor-Anantakul et al., "Complete hydatidiform mole with co-existing fetus: predictors of live birth," *European Journal of Obstetrics, Gynecology, and Reproductive Biology*, vol. 212, article S0301211517301161, pp. 1–8, 2017, Epub 2017 Mar 7.

[13] K. Takagi, N. Unno, H. E. Hyodo et al., "Complete hydatidiform mole in a triplet pregnancy coexisting two viable fetuses: case report and review of the literature," *The Journal of Obstetrics and Gynaecology Research*, vol. 29, no. 5, pp. 330–338, 2003.

[14] L. Wee and E. Jauniaux, "Prenatal diagnosis and management of twin pregnancies complicated by a co-existing molar pregnancy," *Prenatal Diagnosis*, vol. 25, no. 9, pp. 772–776, 2005.

28

Meckel's Diverticulum: The "Great Mimic" but Often a Forgotten Cause of Acute Abdomen during Pregnancy

Beatriz Féria,[1] **Madalena Trindade**,[2] **Maria João Palma**,[1] **Joana Figueiredo**,[2] **and Filipa Passos**[1]

[1]*Obstetrics and Gynecology, Hospital Garcia de Orta, Almada, Portugal*
[2]*General Surgery, Hospital Garcia de Orta, Almada, Portugal*

Correspondence should be addressed to Beatriz Féria; beatrizdcferia@gmail.com

Academic Editor: Giuseppe Gullo

Meckel's diverticulitis is an extremely rare event during pregnancy. Its diagnosis is often difficult and can result in higher maternal and fetal morbimortality. We describe a case of a 40-year-old healthy pregnant woman at 33 weeks of gestation who presented with abdominal pain and tender abdomen, leukocytosis, and elevated PCR. The imagiological exams were not conclusive. After an urgent caesarean section due to worsening of clinical status and nonreassuring fetal well-being, a laparotomy revealed a distended, necrotic, and perforated Meckel's diverticulum.

1. Introduction

Acute abdomen during pregnancy is a rare condition, with a reported incidence of one in 500-635 patients [1, 2]. Perforation of Meckel's diverticulum is an exceptional but potentially life-threatening condition during pregnancy. When assessing a pregnant patient with an acute abdomen, its diagnosis must be considered and early management is imperative to avoid complications. We report a rare case of an acute abdomen caused by infection and perforation of Meckel's diverticulum in the third trimester of pregnancy.

2. Case Presentation

A 40-year-old woman, primigravid, presented at our emergency department at 33 weeks of gestation with a diffuse abdominal pain for two days, more intense at the left iliac fossa, sharp and not responsive to analgesia. The pain was associated with nausea, vomiting, and constipation for a day. She had no previous medical, gynecological, or surgical history, and her antenatal course had been uneventful.

On physical examination, the patient had a blood pressure of 117/67 mmHg and pulse rate of 93 bpm and was apyretic. The abdomen was distended and tender. There was no evidence of uterine contractions or fetal distress. The blood work revealed elevated white blood cell count (21,300/mL with 88% neutrophils) and elevated CRP (19,1 mg/dL). Abdominal ultrasound was normal so it was decided to perform an abdominal-pelvic computerized tomography scan (CT scan) that showed densification of pericolic fat tissue suggesting an inflammatory process of indeterminate nature and no other alterations.

Corticosteroids for fetal lung maturation and empirical broad-spectrum antibiotics were initiated with temporarily clinical improvement. Despite that, on the following day, the patient presented intense pain, abdominal guarding, and rebound as well as an increase in inflammatory parameters. A second abdominal ultrasound was performed but was nonconclusive.

Differential diagnosis included appendicitis, bowel obstruction, perforated ulcer, inflammatory bowel disease, and diverticulitis. Obstetrical and gynecological causes were not excluded but were less plausible.

Facing an acute abdomen and also a pathological fetal cardiotocography, an urgent caesarean section was performed followed by a laparotomy. A male infant was born weighing 1966 grams with Apgar score of 9 and 10 at one and five minutes. It was identified purulent discharge on the abdominal cavity as well as a distended and necrotic Meckel's diverticulum with 9 cm in length and 3 cm in diameter, with a perforation site (Figures 1, 2, and 3). Segmental small bowel resection with mechanical anastomosis was performed.

The histological report confirmed the diagnosis and reported no ectopic mucosa nor malignancy. The patient had an eventful recovery and was discharged after four days.

3. Discussion

Meckel's diverticulum (MD) is a true diverticulum containing all layers of the intestinal wall. It is the most common congenital anomaly of the gastrointestinal track and results from the failure of the omphalomesenteric duct to involute during the 5th to 7th weeks of gestation. The reported prevalence in general population is approximately 2%. Symptomatic Meckel's diverticulum during pregnancy is an extremely rare event. There are only 38 cases reported so far since 1949 [3–6] and 21 cases describing perforation of Meckel's diverticulum [5, 6].

This condition has been classically described as the "rule of twos": prevalence of 2% in population, twice as common in men than women, located 2 feet from the ileocecal valve, and can be 2 inches wide and long [7]. Typically, MD is clinically silent and only 2-4% of people become symptomatic, usually in children [7, 8], with the risk decreasing with age.

The most common complications are obstruction, intussusception, inflammation or diverticulitis, hemorrhage, and perforation. Obstruction is more frequent amongst adults, whereas bleeding is most commonly observed in children due to ulceration caused by acid secretion by ectopic gastric mucosa [9]. Rarely, fistulae and malignancy can occur with carcinoid tumor being the most frequent [6, 7]. MD can be discovered incidentally during abdominal exploration or diagnostic imaging.

The diagnosis of MD during pregnancy can be challenging as it often presents with unspecific symptoms such as abdominal pain, nausea, vomiting, and obstipation which overlap with other conditions and can also occur physiologically in pregnancy.

Additionally, anatomical and physiologic changes like gravid uterus changes, mild to moderate leukocytosis, and tachycardia are considered normal, making the evaluation even more difficult. The main differential diagnosis is with appendicitis as it is the first nonobstetric cause of acute abdomen in pregnancy with an incidence of 0.04%-0.2% [10] and both can cause pain on the right iliac fossa. MD complication should be suspected specially if imaging studies reveal a healthy appendix. Other causes of acute abdomen include cholecystitis (1/500 to 1/3000 [11]), pancreatitis (1/10 000 [12]), bowel obstruction, and urolithiasis, amongst others. In pregnancy, symptomatic MD may mimic obstetric conditions like preterm labor, chorioamnionitis, or placental abruption [5]. Ectopic pregnancy is a diagnosis that should be considered at the beginning of the pregnancy as it is an important cause of acute abdomen and its presentation can be catastrophic [13].

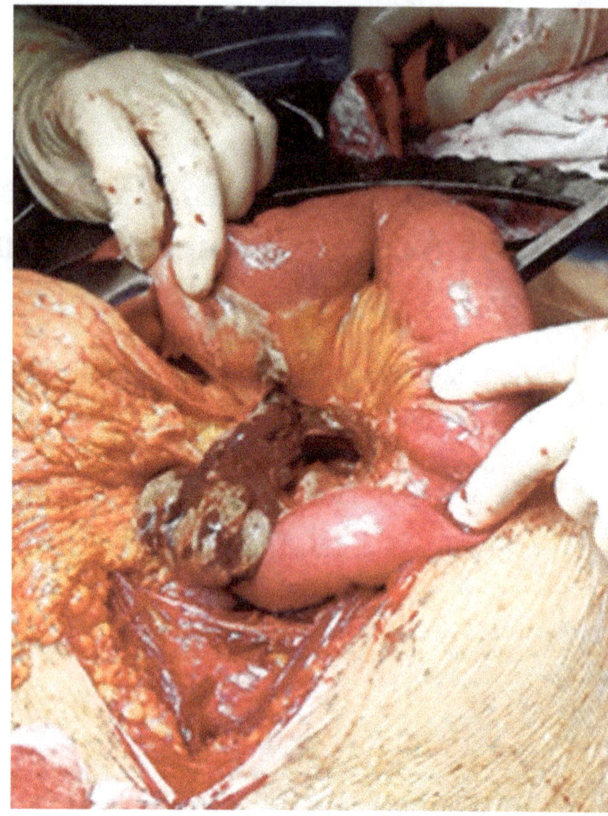

FIGURE 1: Distended and necrotic Meckel's diverticulum.

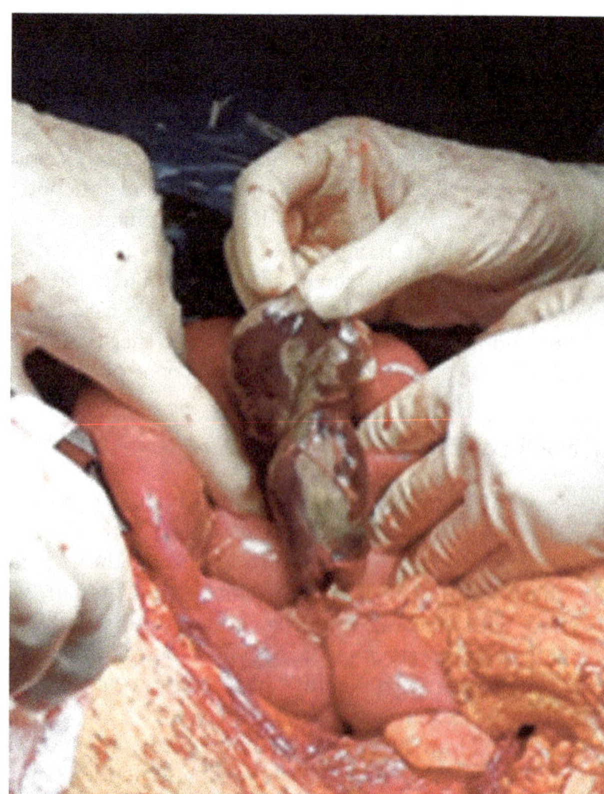

FIGURE 2: Perforation site of Meckel's diverticulum.

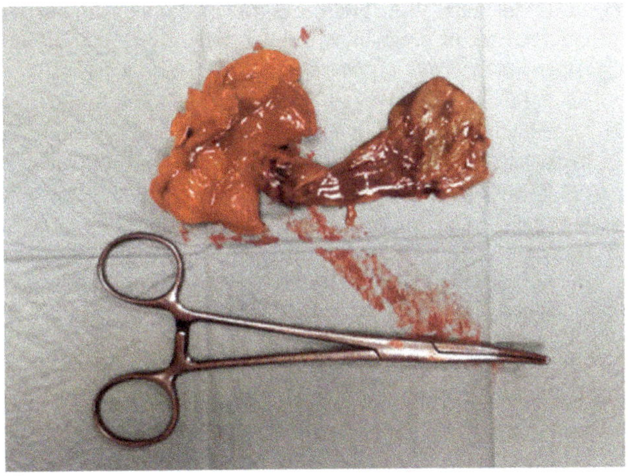

FIGURE 3: Meckel's diverticulum true dimensions (9 cm in length and 3 cm in diameter).

Ultrasound is often the first and most used diagnostic modality [6]. It is fast, noninvasive and involves no radiation; however, its sensibility is very limited as it is operator dependent and has limited field of view due to pregnant uterus. Computer tomography (CT) is usually the gold standard for diagnosis of several abdominal pathologies and can be utilized in pregnant women. Nevertheless, in a recent systematic review, CT had a very low diagnostic value (14.7%) [6] and exposes the fetus to radiation. MRI without gadolinium, if available, is a good alternative to CT because of its higher sensitivity and no radiation exposure [6, 14]. Technetium-99m (99mTc) pertechnetate, also known as a Meckel's scan, is a modality used to diagnose MD with good results, particularly in children. Although there are no reports of its use in this context, it is considered safe and might be a potential tool when suspecting MD. Overall, the role of imaging studies remains limited and the diagnosis remains one of clinical suspicion [5].

Management of MD usually involves an exploratory laparoscopy or laparotomy with surgical resection: either diverticulectomy or segmental bowel resection in case of ectopic tissue at the diverticular base, intestinal ischemia, or perforation at the diverticular base [14]. Laparoscopy has been performed in early pregnancy with no adverse fetal outcome [6]. A laparotomy may be more suitable in the third trimester given the larger uterus and the possible need of delivery. Although there is a report of one case managed with antibiotics and surgery performed only four months postpartum [15], conservative management failed in all other cases; therefore, it is not advisable because of the poor outcomes [6]. The optimal management of the incidentally discovered MD is not consensual; some authors advocate that given the high-risk complications and difficult diagnosis during pregnancy, prophylactic removal is reasonable [9], while others do not support it, arguing that leaving an incidentally detected MD in situ reduces the risk of postoperative complications without increasing late complications [16].

Regarding pregnancy, the rate of MD complication does not seem higher than in general population but the question remains as to whether is there any mechanism during pregnancy that might help the occurrence of complications. Can the growing uterus compress the bowel facilitating an obstruction/loop process? On the other hand, there seems to be a higher rate of perforation of MD during pregnancy, between 40.7% and 57% [5, 6], whereas in general population, the rate is 7% [9]. This might be due to not only the difficult diagnosis but also the reluctance to perform invasive exams and procedures, resulting in a delayed diagnosis [5]. Perforation of MD has been present in all cases of maternal death registered so far, although all of these occurred before 1973 [5].

Obstetric outcomes are difficult to evaluate due to the low number of cases. It has been reported a maternal mortality of 16%, fetal mortality of 13%, and incidence of preterm delivery of 25% [5]. According to a recent systematic review, that includes all cases registered between 1990 and 2021, the majority of cases occurred on the second (48.1%) and third trimester (48.1%), and only 3.7% happened on the first trimester [6]. In all 27 cases, the right preoperative diagnosis was correct in only 2 cases (7.4%). There were 10 cases of preterm delivery, 1 spontaneous late abortion at 20 weeks of gestation in a patient that presented with massive gastrointestinal bleeding, and 1 stillbirth at 24 weeks of gestation in a patient with a perforated MD; both of these could be attributable to delayed presentation or diagnosis. There were no cases of maternal death or other morbidities except for paralytic ileus [6].

Our case demonstrates the diagnostic challenge of an acute abdomen in pregnancy and the serious consequences that Meckel's diverticulum can have in pregnancy. The initial patient's evaluation was not easy considering a third trimester pregnancy and large uterus. The fact that the pain was more intense at the left abdominal quadrant was a confounding factor as well as the initial clinical improvement with antibiotics and analgesia. At first, the most likely diagnosis did not include MD but rather appendicitis and diverticulitis. Despite the general reluctance of performing radiation exams, we decided to do a CT scan at an early stage. Unfortunately, diagnostic imaging did not provide a clear diagnosis which reinforces the importance of clinical sense. Conservative management was attempted with no success as the clinical status continued to worsen. The clinical decision was obvious facing an acute abdomen and surgery was crucial to the resolution of the case. A multidisciplinary approach is fundamental in management of these cases [17]. From the obstetrical point of view, MD contributed to poor outcomes, specifically cesarean section performance, iatrogenic preterm delivery, and newborn prematurity.

4. Conclusion

Although extremely rare, Meckel's diverticulitis is an important cause of acute abdomen during pregnancy. Its diagnosis implies a high index of clinical suspicion and must be considered especially when causes like appendicitis seem less plausible. Perforation of MD is more frequent in pregnant women. Symptomatic MD is associated with poor outcomes in pregnancy; therefore, a continuous monitoring, multidisciplinary approach, and an early and active management considering surgery are essential.

Consent

Written informed consent was obtained from the subject of this case report prior to preparation of this manuscript.

Authors' Contributions

BF gathered the clinical information and wrote the manuscript report. All authors read and approved the final manuscript.

Supplementary Materials

(1) CARE guidelines with corresponding lines on the manuscript. (2) Original patient informed consent as it was different from Hindawi's consent ("if they use another form, they must provide a blank copy of the consent form on submission"). (3) Signed patient informed consent. *(Supplementary Materials)*

References

[1] S. Barber-Millet, J. B. Lledó, P. G. Castro, I. G. Gavara, N. B. Pla, and R. G. Domínguez, "Update on the management of non-obstetric acute abdomen in pregnant patients," *Cirugía Española (English Edition)*, vol. 94, no. 5, pp. 257–265, 2016.

[2] G. Augustin and M. Majerovic, "Non-obstetrical acute abdomen during pregnancy," *European Journal of Obstetrics & Gynecology and Reproductive Biology*, vol. 131, no. 1, pp. 4–12, 2007.

[3] I. Pandeva, S. Kumar, A. Alvi, and H. Nosib, "Meckel's diverticulitis as a cause of an acute abdomen in the second trimester of pregnancy: laparoscopic management," *Case Reports in Obstetrics and Gynecology*, vol. 2015, Article ID 835609, 12 pages, 2015.

[4] Y. S. Wong, S. Y. W. Liu, S. S. M. Ng et al., "Giant Meckel's diverticulitis: a rare condition complicating pregnancy," *The American Journal of Surgery*, vol. 200, no. 1, pp. 184-185, 2010.

[5] U. Rudloff, S. Jobanputra, M. Smith-Levitin, and E. Kessler, "Meckel's diverticulum complicating pregnancy," *Archives of Gynecology and Obstetrics*, vol. 271, no. 1, pp. 89–93, 2005.

[6] J. Y. J. Wong, M. Conroy, and N. Farkas, "Systematic review of Meckel's diverticulum in pregnancy," *ANZ Journal of Surgery*, vol. 91, no. 9, pp. E561–E569, 2021.

[7] J. Sagar, V. Kumar, and D. K. Shah, "Meckel's diverticulum: a systematic review," *Journal of the Royal Society of Medicine*, vol. 99, no. 10, pp. 501–505, 2006.

[8] J. Dumper, S. Mackenzie, P. Mitchell, F. Sutherland, M. L. Quan, and D. Mew, "Complications of Meckel's diverticula in adults," *Canadian Journal of Surgery*, vol. 49, no. 5, article 353, 2006.

[9] S. Huerta, A. Barleben, M. A. Peck, and I. L. Gordon, "Meckel's diverticulitis: a rare etiology of an acute abdomen during pregnancy," *Current Surgery*, vol. 63, no. 4, pp. 290–293, 2006.

[10] J. J. Choi, R. Mustafa, E. T. Lynn, and C. M. Divino, "Appendectomy during pregnancy: follow-up of progeny," *Journal of the American College of Surgeons*, vol. 213, no. 5, pp. 627–632, 2011.

[11] M. T. Coleman, V. A. Trianfo, and D. A. Rund, "Nonobstetric emergencies in pregnancy: trauma and surgical conditions," *American Journal of Obstetrics and Gynecology*, vol. 177, no. 3, pp. 497–502, 1997.

[12] C. S. Pitchumoni and B. Yegneswaran, "Acute pancreatitis in pregnancy," *World Journal of Gastroenterology: WJG*, vol. 15, no. 45, article 5641, 2009.

[13] S. Baggio, S. Garzon, A. Russo et al., "Fertility and reproductive outcome after tubal ectopic pregnancy: comparison among methotrexate, surgery and expectant management," *Archives of Gynecology and Obstetrics*, vol. 303, no. 1, pp. 259–268, 2021.

[14] Z. Ahmed, S. Chhabra, J. Kankaria, and R. K. Jenaw, "Meckel's diverticular perforation presenting as acute abdomen in the second trimester of pregnancy," *Case Reports*, vol. 2016, article bcr2016216643, 2016.

[15] J. Eisdorfer, N. T. Zinkin, and D. E. Rivadeneira, "Meckel's diverticulitis: a rare cause of abdominal pain during pregnancy," *ANZ Journal of Surgery*, vol. 88, no. 7-8, 2018.

[16] A. Zani, S. Eaton, C. M. Rees, and A. Pierro, "Incidentally detected Meckel diverticulum: to resect or not to resect?," *Annals of Surgery*, vol. 247, no. 2, pp. 276–281, 2008.

[17] V. La Rosa, G. Valenti, F. Sapia, G. Gullo, A. Maria, and C. Rapisarda, "Psychological impact of gynecological diseases: the importance of a multidisciplinary approach," *Journal Gynaecology Obstet*, vol. 30, pp. 23–26, 2018.

29

When the Uterus Competes for Perfusion: Management of a Pregnant Patient with Bypass Graft Occlusion

Sarah McGriff, Paige Percer, Iberia Sosa, Hector Mendez-Figueroa, Joseph L. Mills, and Manisha Gandhi

Baylor College of Medicine, Texas Children's Hospital, Houston, Texas, USA

Correspondence should be addressed to Paige Percer; ppercer84@gmail.com

Academic Editor: Erich Cosmi

Background. Peripheral arterial disease (PAD) in pregnancy has serious implications and requires multidisciplinary management. This becomes even more complicated in the setting of active disease and history of prior vascular grafts. *Case.* A woman presented with increasing left lower extremity pain at 18 weeks of gestation with a complex history of PAD and a previous bifurcated aorta-left femoral, -right iliac bypass. CT angiogram demonstrated known occluded bypass graft. A multidisciplinary team of providers developed guidelines for potential surgical intervention based upon clinical symptoms. *Conclusion.* Pelvic PAD can worsen in pregnancy in the setting of the enlarging uterus, which can potentially deplete perfusion of existing collateral vessels. Symptomatic approach to worsening disease provided an effective management strategy in this case.

1. Introduction

Pregnancy following aortic bypass or replacement grafting is uncommon, but has been previously reported [1–6]. Bypass grafts for arterial occlusive disease are often placed in an older population beyond typical child-bearing age. Overall, maternal and neonatal outcomes are favorable with careful management. A search of the literature revealed one case with expectant management of claudication with no permanent sequelae [4], and a single case of graft occlusion during pregnancy [5]. However, the patient with graft occlusion only had symptoms of claudication with physical activity and was successfully managed with antiplatelet therapy using aspirin. We present the management of a pregnancy in a patient with significant peripheral arterial disease (PAD) and an occluded graft from a previous aortic reconstruction that had severe rest pain and disability requiring increased anticoagulation.

2. Case

The patient is a 33-year-old woman gravida 5, para 3, abortion 1 with chronic hypertension and 3-year history of arterial thrombosis. At age 30, she underwent aortoiliac thrombectomy and bilateral femoral thrombectomies with repair, and was started on warfarin postoperatively. Fifteen months later, noncompliant with anticoagulation, she presented for severe back pain radiating down her legs bilaterally. A repeat CT angiogram revealed a left common iliac artery occlusion with thrombus in the infrarenal abdominal aorta with possible dissection flap above the bifurcation. She underwent aorta-left femoral and aorta-right iliac bypass with a bifurcated polytetrafluorethylene (PTFE) graft (Figure 1). Repeat hypercoagulable testing was negative, and she was discharged on warfarin treatment. The patient continued anticoagulation inconsistently. She presented multiple times over the following year complaining of lower extremity pain. Repeat CT angiograms demonstrated complete occlusion of both arms of the graft with normal runoff and patent pelvic collaterals.

Three years after her initial intervention, she was pregnant and established care with our maternal-fetal medicine practice at 13 weeks of gestation. Her obstetrical history included one prior spontaneous abortion, two term vaginal deliveries, and most recently a cesarean delivery at gestational week 28 due to preeclampsia with severe features. All previous pregnancies occurred prior to aortic reconstruction, and there was no history

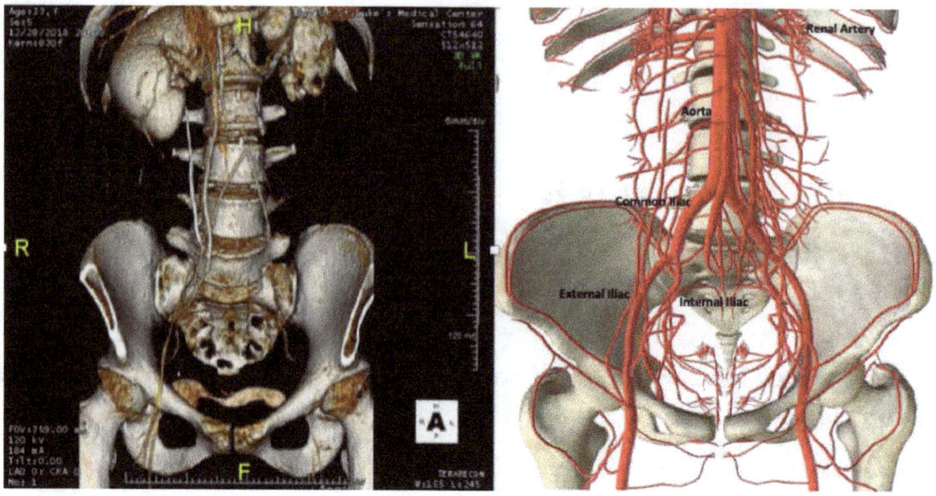

(a) (b)

FIGURE 1: Computed tomography angiogram of the abdomen, pelvis, and lower extremities with runoff (a). Computer generated pelvic vasculature demonstrating the stark difference (b).

of thrombotic disease with any pregnancy. The risk of the patient's gestation was reviewed in detail and included discussion of her grafts, disease burden, and anticoagulation requirements. She was offered termination of pregnancy but declined. She was prescribed therapeutic dose enoxaparin (1 mg/kg twice daily) and aspirin 81 mg daily for anticoagulation.

At 18 weeks of gestation, she presented with left leg pain and decreased sensation in the left lower extremity. Repeat CT angiogram showed no interval changes with apparent diversion of some collateral flow to the pregnant uterus. Urine drug screen was positive for cocaine. Due to worsening symptoms likely secondary to increased vascular demand of the gravid uterus and cocaine use, the patient was admitted and started on an unfractionated (UFH) heparin infusion.

After consulting vascular surgery, urgent surgical intervention was not offered as she had conserved sensation and motor function in lower extremities, there was increased likelihood that the gravid uterus would be a barrier to aortic reconstruction, and her occlusive disease appeared stable on repeat imaging. The vascular surgeons further assessed and recommended intervention only if worsening of blood flow, as defined by the loss of the patient's motor function in her lower extremities. If she reached that point, she would require axillofemoral bypass surgery. The goals of care were discussed, and the patient reported she was prepared to lose her leg before jeopardizing the pregnancy. She was discharged on therapeutic enoxaparin at 1 mg/kg twice daily and anti-factor Xa levels were followed monthly to adjust dose accordingly. Throughout the pregnancy, the patient was evaluated multiple times for increasing pain and required supportive care with wheelchair assistance and pain medications.

The patient presented at 31 weeks and 4 days of gestation with superimposed pre-eclampsia with severe features based on requirement of acute antihypertensives and persistent severe headache. Her CT head imaging was negative and she was transitioned to UFH. Her blood pressures stabilized and the headache resolved, but three days later the patient complained of a persistent headache refractory to medications and required increased dosing of her antihypertensive medications. Plans were made for delivery via repeat cesarean delivery. UFH was stopped 6 hours prior to delivery. The patient underwent an uncomplicated repeat cesarean delivery with bilateral tubal ligation with an estimated blood loss of 600 cc. She was managed in the intensive care unit in the immediate post-operative period and restarted on enoxaparin 1 mg/kg BID at 8 hours after delivery. The neonate weighed 1870 g with Apgar scores of 8 and 9 at 1 and 5 minutes, respectively.

Postoperatively, the patient did complain of some worsening left lower extremity pain, which was evaluated by vascular surgery. However, they determined there was no need for acute surgical intervention as the patient had preserved motor function and her pain was adequately controlled. She was discharged home on enoxaparin 100 mg BID and aspirin 81 g daily. Despite anticoagulation, she was readmitted 11 weeks after delivery with flank pain and found to have a left renal artery infarct and extension of the infrarenal aortic occlusion up to the level of the renal arteries. She was acutely treated with intravenous UFH. Her flank pain resolved and renal function remained within normal limits. However, her left leg pain progressively worsened and required an open surgical juxtarenal aortic thrombectomy and redo aorta-right common iliac,-left common femoral reconstruction with a bifurcated cryopreserved allograft spliced to an autogenous left femoral vein conduit (Figure 2). Prosthetic conduits were avoided because of her presumed hypercoagulable state and failure of previous prosthetic reconstruction.

3. Discussion

In this pregnant patient with complex arterial occlusive disease, we were able to successfully manage the pregnancy and the peripheral vascular disease with a multidisciplinary approach. Given that surgical management was more

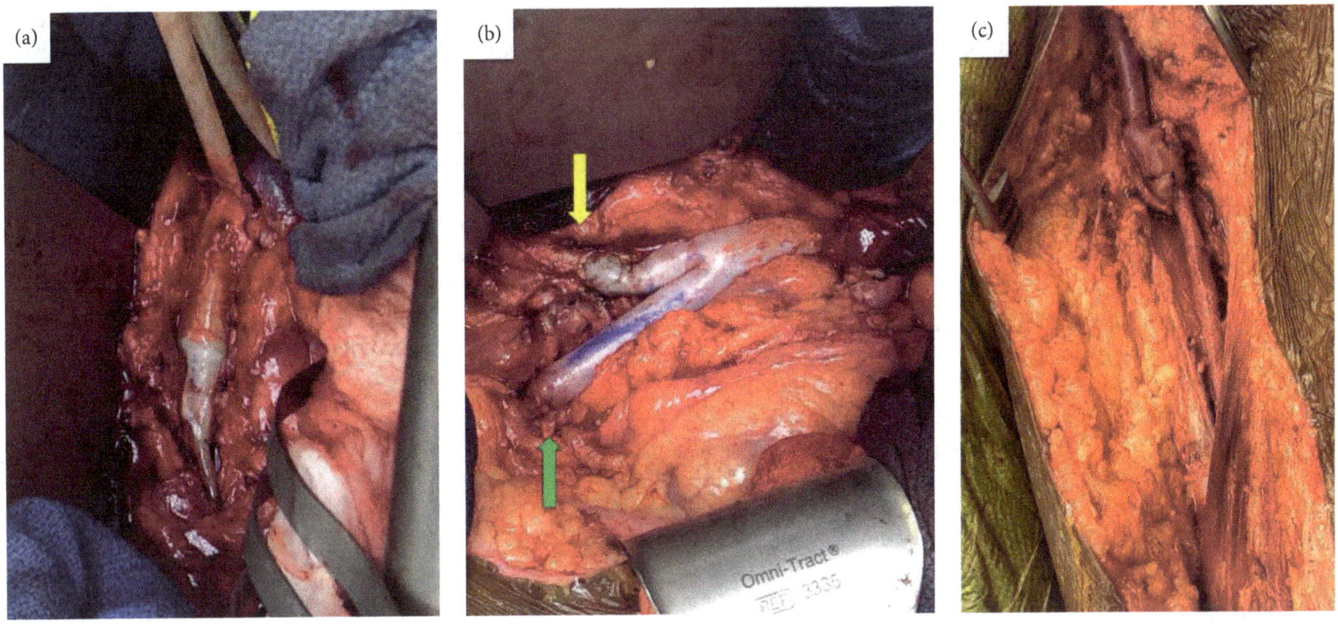

FIGURE 2: (a) Exposure of the infrarenal aorta and occluded PTFE graft. (b) Cryopreserved aorto-right common iliac allograft (yellow arrow) with left limb anastomosed to an autologous left femoral vein conduit (green arrow) to extend to left common femoral artery. (c) Left femoral vein conduit to left femoral bifurcation anastomosis.

complicated and less definitive due to her gravid uterus, the assessment of motor function was key. This motor function assessment gave our team objective data to assess her disease burden. In regard to the etiology of this patient's peripheral artery disease, we do not have a definitive answer, but suspect cocaine use as potential cause. There is evidence in the literature of limb ischemia and thrombosis in direct association with chronic cocaine use [7, 8].

No specific guidelines exist for maintaining the patency of vascular grafts in the obstetric population. Pregnancy is a known prothrombotic state and often exacerbates hypercoagulable disorders. Even with appropriate anticoagulation, the increased thrombotic risk may still not be mitigated. Multiple international obstetric guidelines recommend that women who have had a prior thrombotic event are prescribed prophylactic heparin throughout their pregnancy and at least 6 weeks postpartum [9, 10]. LMWH is recommended over unfractionated heparin (UFH) given its high bioavailability and ease of administration [11]. We generalized these recommendations to our patient, as any further arterial thrombi in the pelvic or collateral vasculature could result in devastating loss of limb or fetus.

The American College of Cardiology (ACC) and American Heart Association (AHA) developed guidelines for the management of patients with peripheral vascular disease, including revascularization [12]. However, these guidelines contain recommendations that might pose risk to the obstetrical population. Medications aimed at reducing cardiovascular risk factors or maintaining graft patency often have unknown effects or are contraindicated in pregnancy. Of the recommended medications, we prescribed aspirin as a secondary prophylaxis to our patient because it has been shown to prevent arterial thrombosis [12, 13]. Low dose aspirin was additionally indicated due to preeclampsia in her previous pregnancy [14].

Furthermore, surgeries that are recommended by the ACC/AHA for revascularization of aortoiliac occlusive disease are difficult to execute in pregnancy. The optimal timing for surgical intervention in pregnant women is during the second trimester, as the risk posed by anesthesia and surgery is the lowest. However, a challenge with concomitant aortic disease, is that the gravid uterus is too large and blocks the surgical site. According to the ACC/AHA guidelines, when all other interventions are contraindicated in severe aortoiliac disease, the only indicated surgery is axillofemoral bypass [12].

This case also had ethical implications in terms of maternal well-being. The ACC/AHA identified multiple risk factors for amputation in patients with chronic limb-threatening ischemia [12]. Of these, our patient had one: ischemic pain at rest. Our patient affirmed multiple times that she desired amputation over loss of pregnancy. However, not all women may have the same goals of care. Overall, patient compliance with the recommended treatment is essential. In this case, noncompliance with anticoagulation prior to pregnancy may have led to increased thrombotic burden. Cocaine use also likely led to increased vasoconstriction which resulted in increased symptoms. Lack of compliance can be due to a multitude of factors associated with numerous health system constraints, including lack of supportive resources during pregnancy and potential loss of the mother's health insurance after birth. Resources are currently being examined at a national level to address the care of women after pregnancy [15].

Management of pregnant patients with arterial occlusive disease and previous abdominal vascular grafts is challenging due to the demands of the gravid uterus competing for collateral vasculature. Limited surgical access to the area due to the gravid uterus can lead to potentially devastating outcomes, including loss of limb and/or the fetus. A multidisciplinary approach is required to balance the complex medical management of these patients, along with clarifying maternal goals of care. Conservative management is generally recommended with anticoagulation and plan for surgical intervention only in cases of true limb-threatening acute ischemia. In this patient, symptoms failed to improve after pregnancy and redo aorto-iliofemoral reconstruction was performed after delivery when the uterus was no longer enlarged and engorged.

Additional Points

Teaching Points. (1) Motor function deficits can help guide the need for intervention in a patient with complex peripheral arterial disease. (2) Timing of delivery in a pregnancy complicated by peripheral artery disease and bypass grafts needs to be individualized. (3) A multidisciplinary team approach including vascular surgery, hematology, maternal fetal medicine, anesthesiology, and neonatology is recommended to optimize both maternal and neonatal outcomes.

References

[1] T. Manotaya and C. Manothaya, "Pregnancy after removal of abdominal aortic aneurysm," *Obstetrics and Gynecology*, vol. 47, no. 1, pp. 12S–14S, 1976.

[2] D. A. Ott, S. Rothchild, and A. J. Springer, "Resolution of infertility, conception, and successful delivery after abdominal vascular reconstruction," *Texas Heart Institute Journal*, vol. 10, no. 3, pp. 279–282, 1983.

[3] P. J. Bradley-Watson, "Pregnancy after aortofemoral bypass grafting in a diabetic patient," *American Journal of Obstetrics and Gynecology*, vol. 161, no. 1, pp. 200–201, 1989.

[4] N. Khandanpour, T. A. Mehta, M. Adiseshiah, and F. J. Meyer, "Are aortic stent grafts safe in pregnancy?," *Case Reports in Radiology*, vol. 2015, Article ID 190878, 3 pages, 2015.

[5] R. Nakae, S. Matsuzaki, T. Egawa-Takata, K. Mimura, T. Kanagawa, and T. Kimura, "Pregnancy management for a patient with graft occlusion after right iliac artery bypass surgery," *Journal of Obstetrics and Gynaecology Research*, vol. 41, no. 6, pp. 979–984, 2015.

[6] N. Miyasaka, M. Egawa, M. Isobe, Y. Inoue, and T. Kubota, "Ostetrical mandagement of patients with extra-anatomic vascular bypass grafts due to takayasu arteritis," *Journal of Obstetrics and Gynaecology Research*, vol. 42, no. 12, pp. 1864–1869, 2016.

[7] J. C. Chen, Y. N. Hsiang, D. C. Morris, and W. B. Benny, "Cocaine-induced multiple vascular occlusions: a case report," *Journal of Vascular Surgery*, vol. 23, no. 4, pp. 719–723, 1996.

[8] W. Zhou, P. H. Lin, R. L. Bush, L. Nguyen, and A. B. Lumsden, "Acute arterial thrombosis associated with cocaine abuse," *Journal of Vascular Surgery*, vol. 40, no. 2, pp. 291–295, 2004.

[9] Committee on Bulletins Obstetrics American of Obstetricians and Gynecologists, "Practice bulletin No 132: antiphospholipid syndrome," *Obstetrics and Gynecology*, vol. 120, no. 6, pp. 1514–1521, 2012.

[10] S. M. Bates, I. A. Greer, I. Pabinger, S. Sofaer, and J. Hirsh, "Venous thromboembolism, thrombophilia, antithrombotic therapy, and pregnancy," *Chest*, vol. 133, no. 6, pp. 844S–886S, 2008.

[11] "ACOG practice bulletin no. 196: thromboembolism in pregnancy," *Obstetrics and Gynecology*, vol. 132, no. 1, pp. 243–248, 2018.

[12] A. T. Hirsch, Z. J. Haskal, N. R. Hertzer et al., "ACC/AHA 2005 practice guidelines for the management of patients with peripheral arterial disease (lower extremity, renal, mesenteric, and abdominal aortic)," *Circulation*, vol. 113, no. 11, 2006.

[13] T. E. Warkentin, "Aspirin for dual prevention of venous and arterial thrombosis," *New England Journal of Medicine*, vol. 367, no. 21, pp. 2039–2041, 2012.

[14] D. L. Rolnik, D. Wright, L. C. Poon et al., "Aspirin versus placebo in pregnancies at high risk for preterm preeclampsia," *New England Journal of Medicine*, vol. 377, no. 7, pp. 613–622, 2017.

[15] K. P. Tully, A. M. Stuebe, and S. B. Verbiest, "The fourth trimester: a critical transitional period with unmet maternal health needs," *American Journal of Obstetrics and Gynecology*, vol. 217, no. 1, pp. 37–41, 2017.

Osler-Weber-Rendu Disease Uncovered by Preeclampsia in a Case Report

Jamal Ouachaou,[1] Hamza Mimouni,[1] Mohammed Maarad,[1] Yassine Mellagui,[1] Asmae Oulad Amar,[2] Houssam Bkiyar,[1] Imane Kamaoui,[2] and Brahim Housni[1]

[1]*Intensive Care Unit, Mohammed VI University Hospital Center, Faculty of Medicine and Pharmacy of Oujda, Mohammed I University, Oujda, Morocco*
[2]*Radiology Department, Mohammed VI University Hospital Center, Faculty of Medicine and Pharmacy of Oujda, Mohammed I University, Oujda, Morocco*

Correspondence should be addressed to Jamal Ouachaou; ouachaoujamal@gmail.com

Academic Editor: Maria Grazia Porpora

Osler-Weber-Rendu disease (OWRD), called hereditary hemorrhagic telangiectasia, is an uncommon genetic illness with the dominant autosomal transmission. It cannot be easily or quickly diagnosed because of both its infrequency and its various associated symptoms. As far as its symptoms are concerned, the patient experiences recurring epistaxis, mucocutaneous telangiectasia, and arteriovenous malformations that can lead to severe undesirable symptoms. In our case, we report a 32-year-old female that was diagnosed with postpartum preeclampsia and whose paraclinical examinations showed that she suffers from hereditary hemorrhagic telangiectasia disease. Management of OWRD includes systematic diagnosis of visceral arteriovenous malformations (AVMs) in regular intervals, measures to prevent complications, and symptomatic treatment.

1. Introduction

Hereditary Rendu-Osler disease (MRO) or hereditary hemorrhagic telangiectasia is a form of vascular dysplasia involving hemorrhagic symptoms, cutaneous mucosal telangiectasia, and visceral shunts with arteriovenous defects. It is pregnancy that contributes to the proliferation and growth of VAM. What causes this disease is the vessels' disorder (vasculogenesis), disruptive angiogenesis, and vessels' regulation (homeostasis). The basic lesion is the distension of the distal vessels (telangiectasia) which is marked by a hemorrhagic tendency when it is cutaneous or mucous. On the other hand, when located in an organ, this type of lesion is reflected in the installation of an arteriovenous shunt between the arterioles and the venules, which are dependent on the viscera where the lesion is installed [1].

This report describes the case of a 32-year-old woman who got diagnosed with postpartum preeclampsia and suffers from stem and sublingual telangiectasia. The investigations showed the presence of the liver's subcapsular hematoma and arteriovenous malformations in pulmonary and hepatic areas.

2. Observation

Our patient is a 32-year-old female from a low social class and married for 7 years. She has already lost her fetus after 34 AW 4 years ago, and she had already undergone miscarriage after 16 AW 2 years ago. One year after, she suffered from epistaxis two times, and she was put in medical reanimation after 15 days following her pregnancy. She gave birth to her baby boy vaginally. The progression of the disease was noticed two days after the installation of headache in helmets with epigastric pain in irradiating strips towards the right hypochondrium.

The physical examination revealed a high blood pressure that reaches TA = 150/80 mmHg in the right limb and 155/90 mmHg in the left one, FC = 90 bpm, labstix: 2

proteinuria crosses, and stable in respiration. Moreover, the patient has epigastric sensitivity and telangiectasia in both the trunk and the sublingual area. Table 1 presents the main biological results;

In the aforementioned table, the postpartum preeclampsia' diagnosis was noted.

An abdominal ultrasound scan was conducted to look for a subcapsular hematoma of the liver that returned in favour of a hypoechogenic lesion in segments VII and II of the liver and which was complemented by an angioscanner that showed vascular abnormalities in the lung and the liver (Figures 1 and 2). Encephalic MRI is positive.

Oesophagogastroduodenoscopy was conducted in favour of the following:

(i) erythematous and nodular antritis

(ii) Antral millimetric telangiectasia lesion that bleeds

(iii) Telangiectasic lesions scattered in both the bulb and the duodenum

Treatment is based on treating preeclampsia using oral antihypertensives (nicardipine 50 mg 2x/day) and proton pump inhibitors per bone 40 mg/day.

The patient's situation was improved after two days of treatment in that the pain disappeared.

Table 1: The main biological results.

Creatinine (μmol/L)	30
Urea (mmol/L)	2
Proteinuria of 24 h g/L	232
ASAT	55
ALAT	45
Lipase	61
Hemoglobin (g/dL)	9.7
Platelet (G/L)	277
Prothrombin rate (%)	66
Fibrinogen (g/L)	3.8

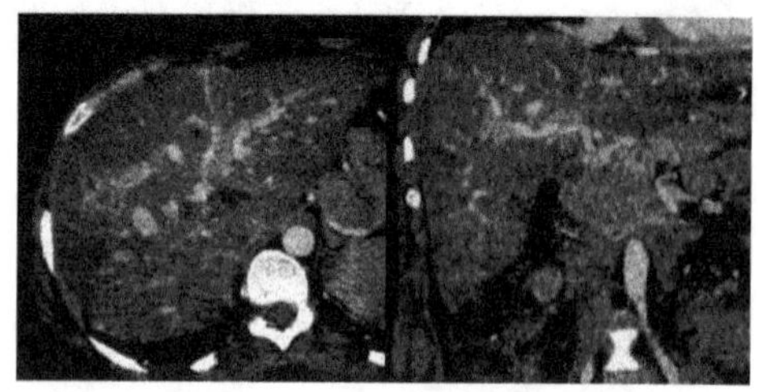

Figure 1: The transversal and sagittal section of the CT scan shows arteriovenous disorders in the liver.

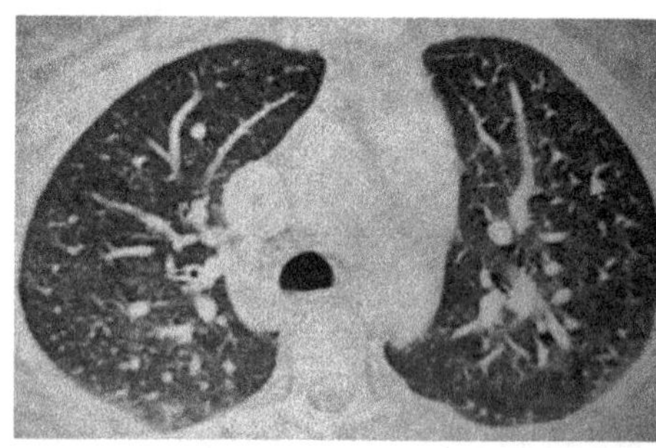

Figure 2: The transversal section of the CT scan shows arteriovenous pulmonary disorders.

3. Discussion

One of the first pioneers who had initiated the talk about this disease is the French dermatologist Henri Rendu in 1896. Following his discovery, in 1902, the Canadian doctor, William Osler, had elaborated on it more. Then, another English dermatologist called Frederick Parkes Weber provided enough information on it in 1907. In 1909, the American doctor named Hanes renamed this disease with HHT that stands for hereditary hemorrhagic telangiectasia.

Osler-Weber-Rendu disease is a multisystemic vascular dysplasia. The diagnosis is clinically based on the presence of spontaneous and recurrent epistaxis (occurring in the absence of blood coagulation disorders), multiple telangiectasias (lips, mouth, fingers, and nose), visceral sites, and prior presence in the family history that are relative to the first degree of the disease. According to the diagnostic criteria of the Curacao Consensus Conference (Table 2), the diagnosis of ORM is regarded as positive when at least three of the criteria are present [2]. The diagnosis of ORM is suspected when two criteria are observed, including the presence of pulmonary arteriovenous malformations.

Pulmonary arteriovenous abnormalities of ORM are more common among women (sex ratio 1.5 : 1). Since the predominance of the disease is age-related, their penetrance increases over the life cycle. There are about 10% of pulmonary arteriovenous defects that are identified during childhood or adolescence, and then, its rate increases starting from the second decade to approximately 30% [3].

About 70% of pulmonary AVMs are part of the ORM. They are more often multiple (35-65% of cases) [3–6] and bilateral [7]. Also, they would be more often related to neurological complications than isolated MAVPs that occur in the absence of an MRO.

3.1. Liver Arteriovenous Malformations.

3.1. Liver Arteriovenous Malformations. Liver disease is prevalent in 41-78% patients suffering from ORM, but the majorities show no symptoms [8, 9].

There are three shunt types that can occur together. For instance, there are shunts between the hepatic artery and the hepatic vein, the hepatic artery and the portal vein, and the portal vein and the hepatic vein.

These intrahepatic shunts are responsible for the development of cardiac dysfunction, portal hypertension, and biliary ischemia. The best test that can be conducted to screen hepatic AVMs is abdominal Doppler ultrasound or hepatic MRI [10].

3.2. Special Cases of Pregnant Women. To be pregnant while suffering from ORM is risky even if there are no pregnancy-related complications for most cases. For any patient

TABLE 2: Curaçao Diagnostic Criteria, 1997 [11].

Epistaxis
Spontaneous, repeated, and irregular nasal bleeding which can cause to chronic anemia
Telangiectasias
Terminal dilations of blood vessels or lesions, cutaneous (located on the lips, fingers, face, hands, and feet) and mucous (inner surface of the lips, tongue, palate, nasal, and digestive mucosa)
Family affectedness
The existence of at least one of the parents who suffer from the first degree of MRO. Due to the dominant autosomal aspect, this criterion is confirmed in more than 86% cases. Penetrance is almost complete at the age of 50. There are many variations in expressivity ranging from neonatal to asymptomatic adult forms
Arteriovenous abnormalities (AVM)
The visceral disease can replace one of the three previous signs in the positive diagnosis. The location of the MAVs can be as follows: (i) Pulmonary, 30-50% of patients (ii) Hepatic, 30-80% of patients (iii) Neurological, 8-25% of patients (iv) In the digestive system

desiring to become pregnant, she should receive multidisciplinary preconception guidance and screening tests especially if the patient is diagnosed with Osler rendering disease.

Different types of procedures can be offered to patients depending on the degree and frequency of epistaxis. For instance, FLOSEAL hemostatic foam, used in local application, has shown positive results and decreases the use of more invasive treatments [12]. Selective embolization, arterial ligation, endonasal coagulation of telangiectasias using Nd:YAG or KTP lasers, and bipolar electrical cauterization are sort of procedures that are often involved. In the case of severe epistaxis, performing skin transplantation (Saunders' operation) or closing the nasal cavities (Young's operation) can be recommended.

The treatment of hormones using estrogen-progestin or antiestrogen (tamoxifen) is proposed in some cases but remains controversial, especially in the case of men and postmenopausal women due to their undesirable effects [13].

Bevacizumab which is an anti-angiogenic treatment for some tumors, and tranexamic acid which is an antifibrinolytic, have shown some usefulness in reducing the frequency and severity of epistaxis in ORM, but are not yet used in clinical practices [14, 15].

In our case study, the patient exhibited neglected epistaxis and is presented in a postpartum preeclampsia table. The clinical investigation shows signs of telangiectasia preeclampsia. Other paraclinical examinations were in favour of arteriovenous liver and lung malformations. However, encephalic MRI has shown no abnormalities.

In our example, the patient is asymptomatic and the treatment was symptomatic.

After a six-month control of the patient's situation, it has been found that she has experienced two episodes of epistaxis treated symptomatically (tranexamic acid 500 mg 3x/day). The clinical examination found that there is the persistence of sublingual and trunk telangiectasia without extension.

4. Conclusion and "Take-Away"

MRO is marked by spontaneous epistaxis, mucocutaneous telangiectasia, and visceral arteriovenous defects (lung, liver, digestive tract, and brain).

The therapy includes a screening of visceral arteriovenous malformations and treatments to prevent their complications.

5. Patient's Perspective

The patient expressed her satisfaction with the treatment and was connected to the hepatic gastroenterology consultation for possible medical follow-up.

References

[1] H. Plauchu, G. Brunet, A. Bideau, and J. M. Robert, "La maladie de Rendu-Osler," *Concours médical (Paris)*, vol. 114, no. 29, pp. 2469–2476, 1992.

[2] C. L. Shovlin, A. E. Guttmacher, E. Buscarini et al., "Diagnostic criteria for hereditary hemorrhagic telangiectasia (Rendu-Osler-Weber syndrome)," *American Journal of Medical Genetics*, vol. 91, no. 1, pp. 66-67, 2000.

[3] K. L. Swanson, U. B. Prakash, and A. W. Stanson, "Pulmonary arteriovenous fistulas: Mayo Clinic experience, 1982-1997," *Mayo Clinic Proceedings*, vol. 74, no. 7, pp. 671–680, 1999.

[4] R. I. White Jr., A. Lynch-Nyhan, P. Terry et al., "Pulmonary arteriovenous malformations: techniques and long-term outcome of embolotherapy," *Radiology*, vol. 169, no. 3, pp. 663–669, 1988.

[5] D. E. Dines, R. A. Arms, P. E. Bernatz, and M. R. Gomes, "Pulmonary arteriovenous fistulas," *Mayo Clinic Proceedings*, vol. 49, no. 7, pp. 460–465, 1974.

[6] M. Moussoutas, P. B. Fayad, M. M. Rosenblatt et al., "Pulmonary arteriovenous malformations: Cerebral ischemia and neurologic manifestations," *Neurology*, vol. 55, no. 7, pp. 959–964, 2000.

[7] J. D. Puskas, M. S. Allen, A. C. Moncure et al., "Pulmonary arteriovenous malformations: therapeutic options," *The Annals of Thoracic Surgery*, vol. 56, no. 2, pp. 253–258, 1993.

[8] S. Singh, K. L. Swanson, M. A. Hathcock et al., "Identifying the presence of clinically significant hepatic involvement in hereditary haemorrhagic telangiectasia using a simple clinical scoring index," *Journal of Hepatology*, vol. 61, no. 1, pp. 124–131, 2014.

[9] A. A. S. Ianora, M. Memeo, C. Sabbà, A. Cirulli, A. Rotondo, and G. Angelelli, "Hereditary hemorrhagic telangiectasia: multi-detector row helical ct assessment of hepatic involvement," *Radiology*, vol. 230, no. 1, pp. 250–259, 2004.

[10] M. E. Faughnan, V. A. Palda, G. Garcia-Tsao et al., "International guidelines for the diagnosis and management of hereditary haemorrhagic telangiectasia," *Journal of Medical Genetics*, vol. 48, pp. 73–87, 2011.

[11] C. L. Shovlin and M. Letarte, "Hereditary haemorrhagic telangiectasia and pulmonary arteriovenous malformations: issues in clinical management and review of pathogenic mechanisms," *Thorax*, vol. 54, no. 8, pp. 714–729, 1999.

[12] L. Warner, J. Halliday, K. James, and J. de Carpentier, "Domiciliary floseal prevents admission for epistaxis in hereditary hemorrhagic telangiectasia," *The Laryngoscope*, vol. 124, no. 10, pp. 2238–2240, 2014.

[13] J. J. Jameson and D. R. Cave, "Hormonal and antihormonal therapy for epistaxis in hereditary hemorrhagic telangiectasia," *The Laryngoscope*, vol. 114, no. 4, pp. 705–709, 2004.

[14] S. Chen, T. Karnezis, and T. M. Davidson, "Safety of intranasal bevacizumab (avastin) treatment in patients with hereditary hemorrhagic telangiectasia-associated epistaxis," *The Laryngoscope*, vol. 121, no. 3, pp. 644–646, 2011.

[15] S. Gaillard, S. Dupuis-Girod, F. Boutitie et al., "Tranexamic acid for epistaxis in hereditary hemorrhagic telangiectasia patients : a European cross-over controlled trial in a rare disease," *Journal of Thrombosis and Haemostasis*, vol. 12, no. 9, pp. 1494–1502, 2014.

Two Cases of Ectopic Pregnancy Mimicking Gestational Trophoblastic Disease

Haruka Suzuki, Yoshitsugu Chigusa, Junzo Hamanishi, Masaki Mandai, and Eiji Kondoh

Department of Gynecology and Obstetrics, Kyoto University, 54 Shogoin Kawahara-cho, Sakyo, Kyoto 606-8507, Japan

Correspondence should be addressed to Eiji Kondoh; kondo@kuhp.kyoto-u.ac.jp

Academic Editor: Kyousuke Takeuchi

A well-known typical feature of ectopic pregnancy is an evident gestational sac structure outside of the uterus. However, some cases show atypical appearance that is described as a heterogeneous hypervascular mass. We report two cases of ectopic pregnancy that presented heterogeneous findings mimicking gestational trophoblastic diseases but were correctly diagnosed as ectopic pregnancies on MRI. The first case was an interstitial pregnancy in which the patient underwent surgical treatment. The second case was a cesarean scar pregnancy that was treated conservatively but showed spurious enlargement of pregnancy-related lesions after the treatment. Both cases lacked myometrial invasion on MRI, and the patients were diagnosed with ectopic pregnancies. Invasive findings on MRI may discriminate ectopic pregnancy from trophoblastic tumors and avoid unnecessary hysterectomy.

1. Introduction

Ectopic implantation occurs in approximately 1–2% of all pregnancies. Fallopian tube pregnancy accounts for 90% of ectopic pregnancies. Other unusual implantation sites include the uterine cervix, interstitium, ovary, abdominal cavity, and cesarean scar tissue [1]. Magnetic resonance imaging (MRI) is a useful diagnostic modality for detection of an ectopic pregnancy. Typically, an extrauterine gestational sac (GS) is exhibited as a high-intensity cystic structure surrounded by a thick wall on T2-weighted images and is enhanced in the early phase [2]. However, not all cases of ectopic pregnancy show these typical image findings.

We report two cases of ectopic pregnancy that presented heterogeneous findings mimicking gestational trophoblastic disease (GTD) on MRI.

2. Case 1

A 40-year-old, gravida 5, para 2 patient with a history of two spontaneous miscarriages and one right tubal pregnancy treated with laparoscopic right salpingectomy consulted our hospital with a complaint of amenorrhea over the previous 7 weeks and 3 days. She had mild lower abdominal pain, and her vital signs were stable. The serum human chorionic gonadotropin (hCG) β level was 63,557 mIU/ml, which indicated pregnancy. Transvaginal ultrasonography (TV-USG) did not show a GS, but an eccentric, 38-mm heterogeneous mass was detected in the uterine interstitium. MRI was performed at 7 weeks and 5 days of pregnancy, and a heterogeneously enhanced hypervascular mass was identified on the right side of the uterine fundus (Figures 1(a)–1(c)). The mass measured 52 mm, which was larger than a GS at the corresponding estimated gestational age. An ectopic pregnancy was primarily suspected, but the possibility of GTD was also considered because of the atypical images and the size of the mass. She did not desire fertility preservation, and an abdominal hysterectomy was performed on the same day. The macroscopic contents of the mass included a villous component, an embryo, and a blood clot (Figures 1(d) and 1(e)). The crown-rump length (CRL) of the embryo was 10 mm, which corresponded to 7 weeks of pregnancy. Histopathologic examination showed normal villi. The final diagnosis was interstitial pregnancy. The postoperative course was uneventful, and she was discharged on postoperative day 7.

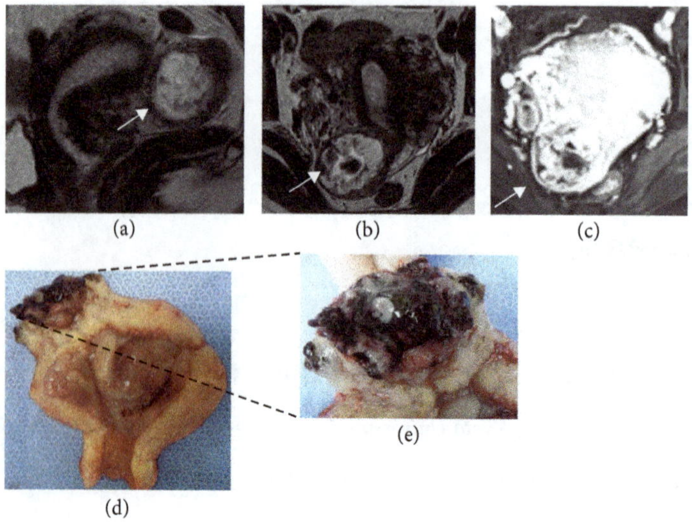

FIGURE 1: MR image performed at 7 weeks and 5 days in case 1 shows an interstitial pregnancy. A heterogeneously-enhanced hypervascular mass is identified on the right side of the uterine fundus. The mass measures 52 mm, which is larger than a GS at the corresponding estimated gestational age. Arrows indicate the pregnancy-associated lesion. (a) A sagittal T2-weighted MR image. (b) An axial T2-weighted MR image. (c) An enhanced axial MR image. (d) Gross pathology of the uterus and the pregnancy-related tissue. (e) An enlarged view of the implantation site.

3. Case 2

A 38-year-old, gravida 3, para 2 patient with a history of 2 cesarean sections was referred to our department and hospitalized at 8 weeks and 3 days of pregnancy due to a suspected cesarean scar pregnancy. The hCG β level was 228,454 mIU/ml. TV-USG showed the GS with a live fetus on the cesarean scar of the uterus. The CRL was 19.3 mm. MRI findings also confirmed a cesarean scar pregnancy. The patient requested termination, but she wanted fertility preservation and decided to undergo medical treatment. Methotrexate and potassium chloride were locally injected under ultrasonic guidance at 9 weeks and 2 days of pregnancy.

One month after treatment, the serum hCG β level had decreased to 1,506 mIU/ml. However, TV-USG revealed a hypervascular lesion in the uterus. Enhanced MRI showed a strongly enhanced hypervascular mass that was larger than that before the treatment (Figure 2). Sequential GTD was suspected because of the heterogeneous change and growth of the mass, but an invasive finding such as a fluffy appearance of tumor burden was absent on MRI; thus, the patient underwent careful follow-up. The lesion continued to grow gradually as shown on serial MRI on days 67 and 95; however, the size of the enhanced lesion did not change, and the enlarged part was considered to be a hematoma. The serum hCG β level continued to decrease. Menstruation restarted on day 120, necrotic tissue was extruded from the uterus on day 133, and the serum HCG β level became negative (<0.5 mIU/ml) on day 146. MRI was performed on day 165 and showed no residual disease in the uterus. There was no atypical bleeding or abdominal pain during the observation period. The final diagnosis was cesarean scar pregnancy.

4. Discussion

The differential diagnosis of ectopic pregnancy and GTD by imaging features is sometimes difficult. GTD is a group of rare tumors that can originate in any product of conception. Although GTD in ectopic pregnancy is quite rare, Tasha reported that GTD was found in approximately 18 of 100 ectopic pregnancies [3]. GTD is visualized as a heterogeneously hyperintense tumor on MRI [4]. In some cases of ectopic pregnancy, particularly interstitial, cervical, or cesarean scar pregnancy, the pregnancy-related tissue shows an atypical appearance that is described as a heterogeneous hypervascular mass on USG and MRI [5, 6]. When a hematoma exists around the mass, the size of the mass appears to be larger than that of the GS at the same gestational age. The embryo is obscured by the hematoma, which makes diagnosis difficult. The mass even shows spurious enlargement after medical treatment due to the formation of the hematoma [7]. This is probably because the muscle layer of the uterus stretches in an interstitial or cesarean scar pregnancy, which allows the formation of growing hematoma, whereas the fallopian tube tears easily in a tubal pregnancy. One of the differences between an ectopic pregnancy and GTD may be an invasive finding in the myometrium on MRI [4]. Actually, in our cases, the pregnancy-associated mass was heterogeneous and deceptively looked similar to ectopic GTD; however, the invasive findings were absent, and the radiologist correctly diagnosed them as ectopic pregnancies. In case 2, the ectopic lesion enlarged and showed heterogeneous change even after medical treatment, but the invasive finding was similarly absent. The reason why the lesion increased may be the expansion of hematoma in the residual villous tissue. As described, the lesion sometimes shows heterogeneous changes and grows in a nonmalignant

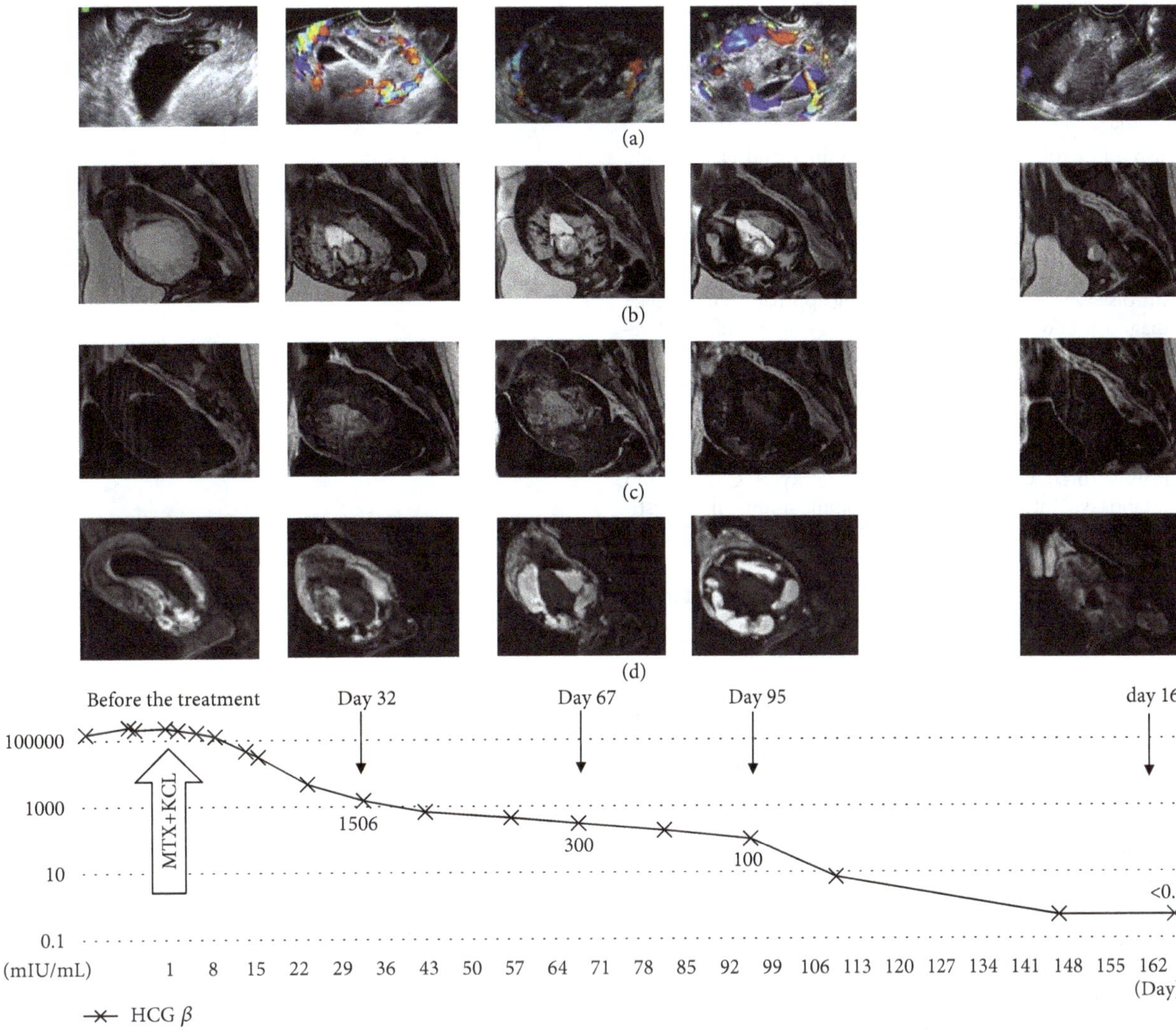

Figure 2: Serial images before and after medical treatment in case 2, a cesarean scar pregnancy, are shown. Transition of the serum hCG β level is shown by a graph of an exponential function. The lesion did not decrease in size and even increased despite a decrease in the serum hCG level. (a) TV-USG. (b) T2-weighted MR image. (c) T1-weighted MR image. (d) Enhanced MR image.

ectopic pregnancy; thus, it is important to assess the myometrial invasion on MRI.

The management differs for an ectopic pregnancy vs. ectopic GTD. For ectopic GTD, the management is usually a combination of surgical removal of the conceptus and chemotherapy [8]. For an ectopic pregnancy, either surgical treatment or medical treatment is selected. Surgical treatment is conventionally chosen for an interstitial pregnancy and a cesarean scar pregnancy, but medical treatment has recently become more prevalent [9, 10]. When sufficient medical treatment is rendered in an ectopic pregnancy, the duration until the pregnancy-related tissue disappears varies from 1 to 6 months [10]. Some researchers report that the lesion vanishes before the serum hCG level becomes negative [11], while other researchers report that conversion to a negative serum hCG level occurs earlier [12]. In case 2, it took approximately 5 months until the remnant tissue was discharged. These findings indicate that even if the pregnancy-related tissue remains for an extended period or even shows growth after treatment in an ectopic pregnancy, it is possible to wait for a complete recovery with careful follow-up providing that the hCG level decreases and the patient's general status remains stable. To protect patients from overtreatment, additional studies are required to distinguish an ectopic pregnancy with confusing imaging features from GTD.

In conclusion, we reported two cases of ectopic pregnancy that posed difficulty in determining the differential diagnosis of GTD. MRI may lead to an accurate diagnosis of ectopic pregnancy and avoidance of unnecessary hysterectomy.

References

[1] D. M. Panelli, C. H. Phillips, and P. C. Brady, "Incidence, diagnosis and management of tubal and nontubal ectopic pregnan-

cies: a review," *Fertility Research and Practice*, vol. 1, no. 1, p. 15, 2015.

[2] K. Tamai, T. Koyama, and K. Togashi, "MR features of ectopic pregnancy," *European Radiology*, vol. 17, no. 12, pp. 3236–3246, 2007.

[3] I. Tasha, E. Kroi, A. Karameta, R. Shahinaj, and N. Manoku, "Prevalence of gestational trophoblastic disease in ectopic pregnancy," *Journal of prenatal medicine*, vol. 4, no. 2, pp. 26–29, 2010.

[4] S. Dhanda, S. Ramani, and M. Thakur, "Gestational trophoblastic disease: a multimodality imaging approach with impact on diagnosis and management," *Radiology Research and Practice*, vol. 2014, 842712 pages, 2014.

[5] M. Rheinboldt and S. Ibrahim, "Atypical presentation of a large interstitial pregnancy," *Emergency Radiology*, vol. 20, no. 3, pp. 251–254, 2013.

[6] T. E. Ackerman, C. S. Levi, S. M. Dashefsky, S. C. Holt, and D. J. Lindsay, "Interstitial line: sonographic finding in interstitial (cornual) ectopic pregnancy," *Radiology*, vol. 189, no. 1, pp. 83–87, 1993.

[7] G. Guzowski and P. Sieroszewski, "Invasive ultrasound in the management of cervical ectopic pregnancy," *European Journal of Obstetrics, Gynecology, and Reproductive Biology*, vol. 172, pp. 7–9, 2014.

[8] A. M. Gillespie, E. A. Lidbury, J. A. Tidy, and B. W. Hancock, "The clinical presentation, treatment, and outcome of patients diagnosed with possible ectopic molar gestation," *International Journal of Gynecological Cancer*, vol. 14, no. 2, pp. 366–369, 2004.

[9] A. Monteagudo, V. K. Minior, C. Stephenson, S. Monda, and I. E. Timor-Tritsch, "Non-surgical management of live ectopic pregnancy with ultrasound-guided local injection: a case series," *Ultrasound in Obstetrics & Gynecology*, vol. 25, no. 3, pp. 282–288, 2005.

[10] R. Pirjani, L. Bayani, and M. Shirazi, "Successful local and systemic medical treatment of cesarean scar pregnancy and a subsequent term pregnancy after treatment: a case series," *Iranian Journal of Reproductive Medicine*, vol. 13, no. 7, pp. 445–450, 2015.

[11] V. Dadhwal, D. Deka, B. Ghosh, and S. Mittal, "Successful management of live ectopic pregnancy with high beta-hCG titres by ultrasound-guided potassium chloride injection and systemic methotrexate," *Archives of Gynecology and Obstetrics*, vol. 280, no. 5, pp. 799–801, 2009.

[12] S. Petousis, C. Margioula-Siarkou, I. Kalogiannidis et al., "Conservative management of cervical pregnancy with intramuscular administration of methotrexate and KCl injection: case report and review of the literature," *World Journal of Clinical Cases*, vol. 3, no. 1, pp. 81–84, 2015.

32

A Successful Pregnancy Despite the Presence of an Intrauterine Fetal Bone Fragment

Evangelos Petrakis, Ioannis Chatzipapas, Ioannis K. Papapanagiotou , Panagiotis Fotinopoulos, Panagiota Siemou, Konstantinos Ntzeros, and Dimitrios Loutradis

1st Department of Obstetrics and Gynaecology, School of Medicine, National and Kapodistrian University of Athens, Alexandra General Hospital, Lourou and Vasilisis Sofias Avenue, 11528 Athens, Greece

Correspondence should be addressed to Ioannis K. Papapanagiotou; gpapamd@hotmail.com

Academic Editor: Maria Grazia Porpora

Objective. Intrauterine retention of fetal bones following a termination of a pregnancy is a rare complication. Among the few reported cases in literature, there has been no report describing the birth of a live fetus, despite the presence of an embryonic ossicle within the endometrial cavity. *Case Report.* A 28-year-old woman, with an obstetrical history of a miscarriage at the 19th week of gestation, underwent a diagnostic hysteroscopy for evaluation of pelvic pain and infertility, which revealed an intrauterine embryonic ossicle. The patient did not comply with our recommendations to undergo a surgical hysteroscopy. The patient's next visit was during her 9th week of gestation. She was followed up regularly at our Obstetrics Department. Her gestation was uneventful, while an elective caesarean section at the 39th week of gestation was performed. *Conclusion.* The present clinical case has demonstrated that achieving childbearing is possible, despite the requirement of removing such bone fragments.

1. Introduction

Intrauterine retention of fetal bones following a termination of a pregnancy in the second and third trimester of gestation is correlated with high rates of spontaneous miscarriages. It is a rare complication as it is observed in 0.15% [1] of the women undergoing diagnostic hysteroscopy for investigation of secondary infertility and a history of a recent termination of a pregnancy. Bony fragments usually imitate the role of intrauterine contraceptive devices (ICD) by stimulating the secretion of endometrial prostaglandins, thus resulting in secondary infertility. Once the bones are hysteroscopically removed, and if no coexisting infertility factors are present, normal fertility is restored in most of the cases. Thus, hysteroscopy, in these cases, is both diagnostic and therapeutic. Among the few reported cases in the literature, there has been no report describing the achievement of a pregnancy and the birth of a live fetus, despite the presence of an embryonic ossicle within the endometrial cavity.

2. Case Presentation

A 28-year-old woman (G1, P0, A1) visited the Outpatient Gynecological Department of our Hospital complaining about chronic pelvic pain and infertility problems. We evaluated her symptoms and proceeded to the appropriate laboratory and imaging examinations. Ultrasound as well as the mobile diagnostic hysteroscopy performed in the Outpatient Department revealed the presence of an intrauterine embryonic ossicle (Figures 1 and 2). On the other hand, laboratory examinations and patient's vital signs were all normal. Therefore, the patient was scheduled for a surgical hysteroscopy in 2 weeks, with a ultimate goal of removing the fetal bone fragment and restoring the physiological enviroment of the uterus. However, the patient did not comply with our recommendations.

Her obstetric history included a miscarriage at the 19th week of gestation due to placental abruption, one-year prior to her visit to our hospital. The patient declared undergoing

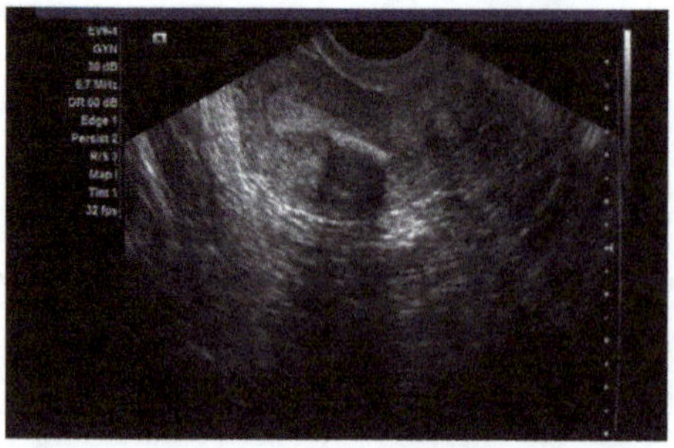

FIGURE 1: Transvaginal image of the uterus: intrauterine retention of fetal bone.

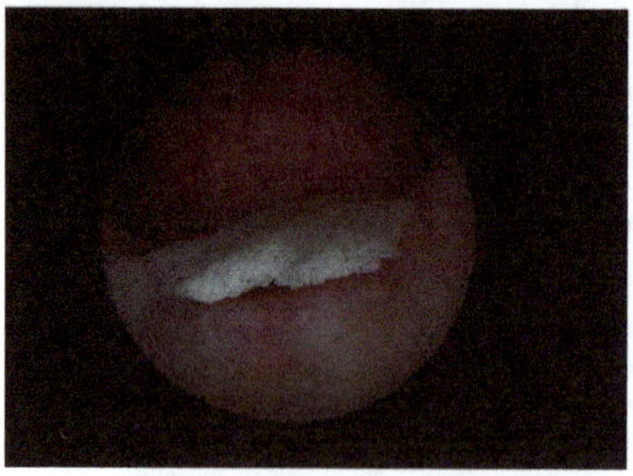

FIGURE 2: Hysteroscopy: intrauterine retention of fetal bone.

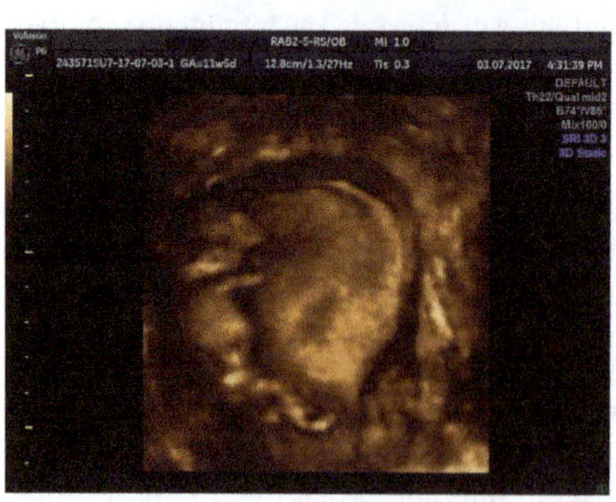

FIGURE 3: First trimester ultrasound: the concurrent presence of fetus and fetal bone.

an emergency surgical dilatation and curettage, due to heavy bleeding, in order to remove the fetal components.

Impressively, one year after our initial diagnosis, the patient visited our hospital during her 9th week of gestation. Transvaginal antenatal ultrasound examination revealed the following: fetal movement, crown rump length (CRL) of 26 mm, fetal heart rate of 170 bpm and the intrauterine fetal bone fragment. She was appropriately informed about the risk factors of her gestation and advised to have regular appointments at our Outpatient Obstetrics Department. Obstetric ultrasounds of the 1st, 2nd and 3rd trimesters, as well as the laboratory examinations were all physiological, despite the presence of the intrauterine ossicle (Figure 3).

The woman was admitted to the Hospital during her 39th week of gestation and an elective caesarean section was performed, due to her volition. A live and full-fledged fetus was delivered, weighing 3180 kilograms and with an Apgar score of 9 and 10 in the 1st and 5th minute respectively. Following the procedure, we observed formed bony tissue macroscopically in the placenta, therefore the placenta was sent for histopathological analysis (Figure 4). The report from the Pathology Department indicated the presence of placental components and calcium salt deposits as well as the intrauterine rendition of the fetal bone.

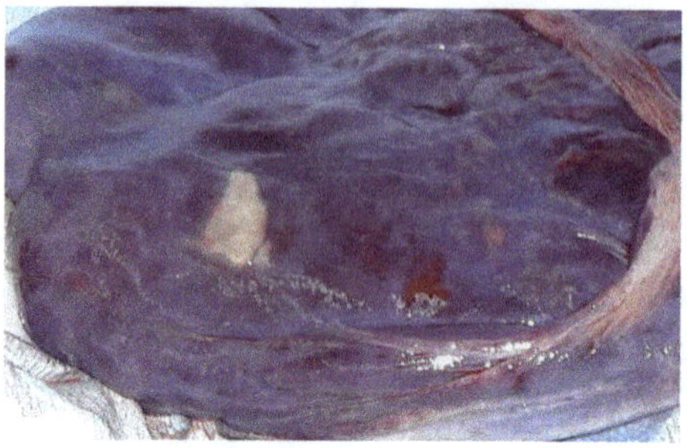

FIGURE 4: Formed bony tissue on the placenta.

3. Discussion

Miscarriage is the most common complication of pregnancy in the United States, occurring in 15–20% of clinically recognized pregnancies, or 750,000–1,000,000 cases annually [2]. The vast majority (60%) of miscarriages are due to aneuploidy, while other established causes of miscarriage include structural abnormalities in the uterus (such as fibroids or a uterine septum), thrombophilias (such as anti-phospholipid syndrome), endocrine disorders (such as hypothyroidism), and autoimmune disorders (such as anti-thyroid antibodies) [2].

Intrauterine retention of fetal bones is a rare complication observed after spontaneous miscarriages or abortions in the second and third trimester in patients undergoing surgical dilatation and curettage. It is found in 0.15% of patients undergoing diagnostic hysteroscopy [1]. However, the percentage of fetal bone fragments removed hysteroscopically in one prospective study, in patients undergoing infertility treatment, reached 11.9% [3]. Such a condition, of fetal bone retention in utero, can result in infertility (72.9%), menstrual abnormalities (30.3%), chronic pelvic pain (10.1%), vaginal bleeding (10.1%), vaginal discharge (4.5%) and dyspareunia (1.1%) [4–6].

Secondary infertility is the most major and frequent complication. Endometrial ossification may cause secondary infertility by three mechanisms: (a) prevention of implantation as a result of obliteration of the uterine cavity (mechanical effect); (b) prevention of implantation as a result of the chronic inflammatory effect of intrauterine bony fragments (intrauterine device-like effect); (c) and direct toxicity of osseous particles on the embryo (embryotoxicity). The extent of uterine involvement is one of the most crucial points determining the effects of endometrial ossification [7].

Ultrasound examination is the gold standard and the most frequently used diagnostic tool, establishing the diagnosis of endometrial ossification. Retained fetal bones appear sonographically as a single or multiple hyperechogenic bands with acoustic shadowing filling the cavity [7]. Transvaginal ultrasound surpasses other diagnostic tools as it is a noninvasive, painless, and relatively low cost method [8]. Furthermore, retained fetal bone fragments can be diagnosed by the presence of filling defects during hysterosalpingography or visualized directly during a hysteroscopy procedure. Although hysterosalpingography and hysteroscopy have traditionally been considered the gold standard methods for uterine evaluation, hysterosalpingography may be unable to detect over 40% of abnormalities of the uterine cavity, while hysteroscopy may overlook bone fragments embedded in the uterine wall [9]. Other diagnostic methods include dilation and curettage, endometrial biopsy, magnetic resonance imaging, and computed tomography [5]. However, histological examination is necessary for the definite diagnosis.

The differential diagnosis of endometrial ossification includes intrauterine contraceptive devices, foreign bodies, calcified submucous fibroids, Asherman syndrome or rare cases such as heterotopic bones. Echogenic endometrium is the most likely finding in these cases [6].

Hysteroscopic resection is the most frequently used method for the removal of bony fragments from the uterine cavity. Surgical treatment with hysteroscopy must be complemented by ultrasonographic guidance to ensure that bone fragments embedded within the myometrium are not missed [9]. In a publication, Dimirtas et al. suggested that dilatation and curettage should be combined with ultrasonography assistance in order to ensure that all abnormal tissue is removed [10]. It is well reported in literature, that in order to achieve high live birth rates and a spontaneous conception, bone fragments should be removed [9].

In conclusion, intrauterine retention of fetal ossicles after a spontaneous miscarriage or termination of pregnancy in the second and third trimester is correlated with secondary infertility. This situation requires the hysteroscopic removal of such bone fragments in order to enable physiological development of the fetus. However, the present clinical case has demonstrated that achieving childbearing is possible, despite the presence of fetal bone fragments within the endometrial cavity.

Consent

A written consent was also acquired from our patient.

References

[1] N. Makris, K. Stefanidis, D. Loutradis, K. Anastasiadou, G. Hatjipappas, and A. Antsaklis, "The incidence of retained fetal bone revealed in 2000 diagnostic hysteroscopies," *Journal of the Society of Laparoendoscopic Surgeons*, vol. 10, no. 1, pp. 76–77, 2006.

[2] J. Bardos, D. Hercz, J. Friedenthal, S. A. Missmer, and Z. Williams, "A national survey on public perceptions of miscarriage," *Obstetrics and Gynecology*, vol. 125, no. 6, pp. 1313–1320, 2015.

[3] B. J. Kazakov, I. M. Khankoev, and W. Pererva, "Results of hysteroscopic method of foreign body removal out of the uterus cavity," *The Journal of the American Association of Gynecologic Laparoscopists*, vol. 1, no. 4, p. S16, 1994.

[4] F. Bergauer, H. Meißner, K. Friese, and I. Mylonas, "Intrauterine fetal bone retention after late-term abortion by external force in the 20th week of pregnancy," *Archives of Gynecology and Obstetrics*, vol. 281, no. 3, pp. 569–570, 2010.

[5] M. C. Pereira, M. M. Vaz, S. P. Miranda, S. R. Araújo, D. B. Menezes, and F. das Chagas Medeiros, "Uterine cavity calcifications: a report of 7 cases and a systematic literature review," *Journal of Minimally Invasive Gynecology*, vol. 21, no. 3, pp. 346–352, 2014.

[6] R. Izhar, S. Husain, S. Tahir, and S. Husain, "Secondary infertility due to retained fetal bones diagnosed via saline sonography," *Journal of the College of Physicians and Surgeons Pakistan*, vol. 26, no. 10, pp. 861–862, 2016.

[7] D. Garg, G. Bekker, F. Akseirod, and D. M. Narasimhulu, "Endometrial osseous metaplasia: an unusual cause of infertility," *BMJ Case Report*, 2015.

[8] C. H. Phillips, C. B. Benson, E. S. Ginsburg, and M. C. Frates, "Comparison of uterine and tubal pathology identified by transvaginal sonography, hysterosalpingography and hysteroscopy in female patients with infertility," *Fertility Research and Practice*, pp. 1–20, 2015.

[9] W. D. Winkelman, M. C. Frates, J. H. Fox, E. S. Ginsburg, and S. Srouji, "Secondary infertility and retained fetal bone fragments," *Obstetrics and Gynecology*, vol. 122, no. 2 Part 2, pp. 458–461, 2013.

[10] O. Demirtas, H. Terzi, A. Kale, B. Sanibrahim, and O. T. Guler, "A rare and unexpected case of retained foetal bone after an unsafe abortion," *Journal of Pakistan Medical Association*, vol. 65, no. 10, pp. 1119–1121, 2015.

33

Successful Management of Complicated Uterine Displacement Caused by Unilateral Incarceration of the Bicornuate Uterus

Nozomi Ouchi, Yoshimitsu Kuwabara, Mirei Yonezawa, Ryuhei Kurashina, Tomoko Ichikawa, Rintaro Sawa, and Toshiyuki Takeshita

Department of Obstetrics and Gynecology, Nippon Medical School Hospital, 1-1-5 Sendagi, Bunkyo-ku, Tokyo, Japan

Correspondence should be addressed to Yoshimitsu Kuwabara; kuwa@nms.ac.jp

Academic Editor: A. O. Awonuga

Uterine incarceration is a serious complication of pregnancy, in which the gravid uterus becomes trapped in the posterior pelvis. When labor occurs, delivery does not progress, and the uterus may rupture. Therefore, preoperative diagnosis of uterine incarceration is important, and a caesarian section is indispensable except when the polarity of the uterus can be successfully restored. We report the case of a 35-year-old primipara with a complication of a bicornuate uterus who became pregnant after in vitro fertilization and embryo transfer. No abnormality was observed on regular checkups until the second trimester. At 28 weeks' gestation, the uterine cervix revealed marked dislocation, and, at 31 weeks, magnetic resonance imaging (MRI) revealed uterine cervix elongation and left horn incarceration. At 37 weeks' gestation, an elective cesarean section was performed. On laparotomy, the uterus was found to be markedly dislocated, and distended blood vessels were observed on the surface. Ultrasound examination was performed directly on the uterine wall to decide the incision site. After delivery of the baby, manual repositioning of the uterus revealed the unique concurrent clockwise rotation and retro-vertical deflection. Thus, we concluded that incarceration accompanied by a bicornuate uterus can cause complicated uterine displacement, and preoperative MRI and intraoperative ultrasound examination are useful for managing this condition.

1. Introduction

Uterine incarceration is a serious complication of pregnancy, reported to occur at a frequency of 1/3000-1/10000 per pregnancy [1–3]. In this condition, the gravid uterus becomes trapped in the posterior pelvis, which sometimes causes pelvic discomfort, lower abdominal or back pain, and dysuria [4]. However, asymptomatic uterine incarceration is considered extremely rare. Only 28 cases of this condition, which were initially diagnosed in the third trimester, were identified in the past 147 years according to a systematic search of English articles in EMBASE and PubMed [5].

When labor occurs, delivery does not proceed and uterine rupture may occur [6]. Therefore, preoperative diagnosis is important and caesarian section is indispensable except when the polarity of the uterus can be successfully restored. Deciding the uterine incision site is the most important, because inappropriate incision into the extended cervical canal, accompanied by incarceration, may cause cervical canal amputation and/or massive bleeding. We report a case of successfully managed uterine incarceration which showed complex uterine displacement, with retroflexion, as well as marked clockwise and vertical rotation, by trapping of the unilateral horn of the bicornuate uterus.

2. Case

A 35-year-old primipara visited our hospital because of a history of two miscarriages. Diagnostic screening tests revealed a retroverted bicornuate uterus and deficiency of *factor XII*, which may have been related to the previous recurrent abortion. Owing to secondary sterility, her third pregnancy was the result of in vitro fertilization and embryo transfer, and low-dose aspirin therapy was started after embryo transfer. In the first trimester, a gestational sac was detected on the right side of the uterine horn. At 18 weeks and 4 days of gestation, no abnormality in the fetal or placental position was detected by transvaginal ultrasonography.

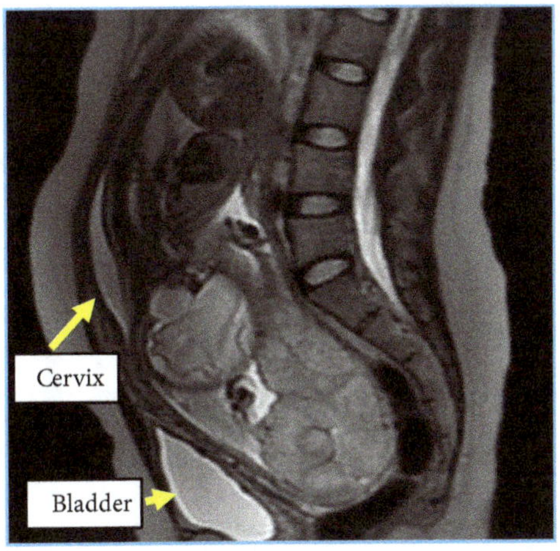

FIGURE 1: Magnetic resonance imaging scan at 31 weeks and 2 days of gestation.

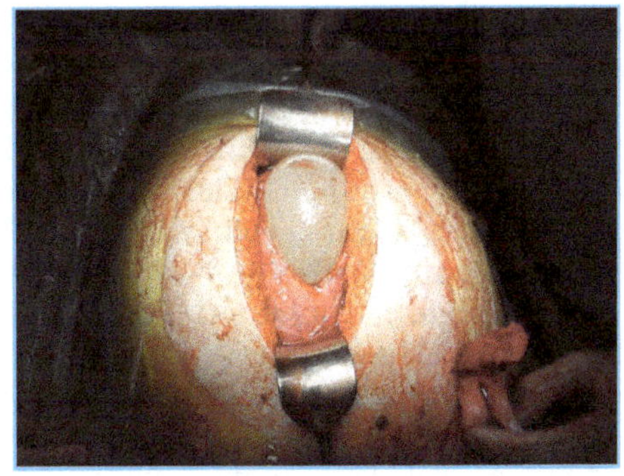

FIGURE 2: The uterus is cut vertically.

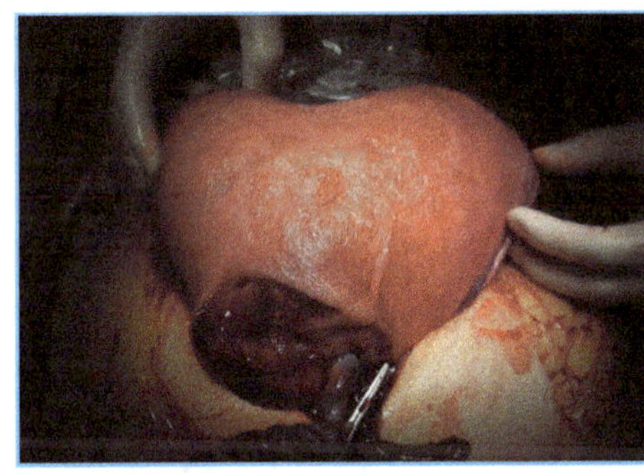

FIGURE 3: The uterus is repositioned after delivery of the baby.

At 28 weeks and 4 days of gestation, marked dislocation of the uterine cervix was suggested by speculum and internal genital examinations. On transvaginal ultrasound examination, the uterine cervix was difficult to detect, whereas the placenta was located on the maternal dorsal side, mimicking the placenta previa. At 31 weeks and 2 days of gestation, MRI was performed to assess the positions of the uterus, placenta, and fetus. The left side of the uterine horn containing a major part of the placenta showed marked retroversion and was trapped in the Douglas cavity. The uterine cervix showed elongation and was located behind the bladder. The fetus was on both sides of the uterine horn, showing a transverse position (Figure 1). This was considered a unique case of unilateral incarceration of the bicornuate uterus showing complicated uterine retroversion. She did not notice any characteristic symptoms such as abdominal pain or urinary retention throughout the gestational period. At 37 weeks and 3 days of gestation, an elective cesarean section was performed. On laparotomy, the uterus was markedly rotated, and distended blood vessels were observed on the surface. Ultrasound examination was performed directly on the uterine wall to check the fetal and placental positions. A vertical incision of the recognized uterine wall under the umbilical part of the abdominal wall was made (Figure 2), and a live male infant, weighing 2500 grams, was born. The uterus was repositioned manually, and a 45° clockwise and 90° retrovertical rotation was confirmed. Furthermore, the site of the uterine wall incision was located in the lower uterine segment transversely, which is the usual position for a normal cesarean section (Figure 3), and the distended blood vessels were identified as the uterine artery and vein.

3. Discussion

Uterine incarceration is known to be caused by uterine myoma, endometriosis, adhesion after intraperitoneal inflammation, or malformation of the uterus [2, 7]. Although there are a few reports on uterus incarceration complicated by a bicornuate uterus [8–10], the clinical characteristics of such cases remain unknown.

This case revealed a risk of complex displacement of the bicornuate uterus accompanied by concurrent rotation and deflection when a unilateral corn is trapped in the Douglas pouch. This is a novel point that has not been suggested in previous reports showing bilateral incarcerated corns of the bicornuate uterus. Because of marked displacement of the uterus accompanied by distended vessels on the surface, it appeared difficult to decide the uterine incision site just by setting it higher than usual, which is the standard strategy for cesarean section of an incarcerated uterus.

To manage this condition successfully, a two-stage setting of preoperative MRI and intraoperative ultrasound examination was helpful. The effectiveness of MRI in the diagnosis of uterine incarceration has been previously reported [1, 11]. In this case, the possibility of placenta previa or a low-lying placenta was accurately excluded by MRI, and it could also be predicted that only a unilateral corn was incarcerated in the Douglas pouch. On the other hand, it was difficult to make a surgical design for the uterine incision site at this point. From the laparotomy findings, it was still difficult to assess the anatomical displacement of the uterus accurately, and the appropriate incision site was finally determined by intraoperative ultrasound examination. To our knowledge, there are no reports concerning the usefulness of an intraoperative direct ultrasound examination at the time of caesarean section in the English literature. However, in some cases of anterior low-lying placenta or placenta previa, we have recognized that a direct intraoperative ultrasound examination is useful in determining the appropriate incision site to avoid placental parenchyma, and it is considered beneficial for reducing maternal bleeding and fetal blood loss. By taking advantage of this technique, the concurrent evaluation of macroscopic findings of the uterine surface and ultrasonographic findings of the intrauterine cavity enabled us to avoid amputation of the extended cervix and determine a safe incision site where the placenta does not exist.

Repositioning of the displaced uterus after delivery of the baby revealed that the site of the uterine wall incision was located in the usual lower uterine segment and that the distended blood vessels that were located in front of the operative field were arteriovenous and originally located in the parametrium of the uterus.

In conclusion, in the case of uterine incarceration complicated by a bicornuate uterus, it is important to remember that severe uterine displacement caused by complex rotation may exist. Preoperative MRI and intraoperative ultrasound examination are useful to manage this condition, especially to decide on the appropriate site for uterine incision during cesarean section.

References

[1] E. M. Gottschalk, J.-P. Siedentopf, I. Schoenborn, S. Gartenschlaeger, J. W. Dudenhausen, and W. Henrich, "Prenatal sonographic and MRI findings in a pregnancy complicated by uterine sacculation: case report and review of the literature," *Ultrasound in Obstetrics & Gynecology*, vol. 32, no. 4, pp. 582–586, 2008.

[2] L. Lettieri, J. F. Rodis, D. A. McLean, W. A. Campbell, and A. M. Vintzileos, "Incarceration of the gravid uterus," *Obstetrical & Gynecological Survey*, vol. 49, no. 9, pp. 640–646, 1994.

[3] L. W. Hess, T. E. Nolan, R. W. Martin, J. N. Martin, W. L. Wiser, and J. C. Morrison, "Incarceration of the retroverted gravid uterus: Report of four patients managed with uterine reduction," *Southern Medical Journal*, vol. 82, no. 3, pp. 310–312, 1989.

[4] A. N. Sweigart and M. J. Matteucci, "Fever, sacral pain, and pregnancy: an incarcerated uterus," *West Journal of Emergency Medicine*, vol. 9, pp. 232–234, 2008.

[5] M. N. Singh, J. Payappagoudar, J. Lo, and S. Prashar, "Incarcerated retroverted uterus in the third trimester complicated by postpartum pulmonary embolism," *Obstetrics & Gynecology*, vol. 109, no. 2, pp. 498–501, 2007.

[6] M. C. Renaud, S. Bazin, and P. Blanchet, "Case condensations: Asymptomatic uterine incarceration at term," *Obstetrics & Gynecology*, vol. 88, no. 4, p. 721, 1996.

[7] J. M. Gibbons and W. B. Paley, "The incarcerated gravid uterus," *Obstetrics & Gynecology*, vol. 33, no. 6, pp. 842–845, 1969.

[8] H. Sadath, R. Carpenter, and K. Adam, "Uterine incarceration in a primigravid retroverted bicornuate uterus," *BMJ Case Reports*, vol. 2016, no. bcr2016215245, 2016.

[9] E. Laird, "Incarceration of a bicornuate retroverted gravid uterus presenting with bilateral uretric obstruction," *BJOG: An International Journal of Obstetrics & Gynaecology*, vol. 99, no. 11, p. 937, 1992.

[10] P. J. Keating, S. M. Walton, and P. Maouris, "Incarceration of a bicornuate retroverted gravid uterus presenting with bilateral ureteric obstruction," *BJOG: An International Journal of Obstetrics & Gynaecology*, vol. 99, no. 4, pp. 345–347, 1992.

[11] H. J. Van Beekhuizen, H. W. Bodewes, E. M. Tepe, H. P. Oosterbaan, R. Kruitwagen, and R. Nijland, "Role of magnetic resonance imaging in the diagnosis of incarceration of the gravid uterus," *Obstetrics & Gynecology*, vol. 102, no. 5, pp. 1134–1137, 2003.

34

Bali Belly: *Salmonella senftenberg* Found in an Infected Ovarian Endometrioma

P. D. M. Pathiraja[1] **Junaid Rafi,**[2] **Emily Woolnough,**[2] **and Anna Clare**[2]

[1]*Ministry of Health, Sri Lanka*
[2]*St John of God Midland Public and Private Hospitals, Australia*

Correspondence should be addressed to P. D. M. Pathiraja; madushan_pathi@yahoo.com

Academic Editor: Julio Rosa e Silva

Salmonella is an extremely rare cause of an infected endometrioma. We present a case of a 30-year-old immunocompetent woman presenting with fevers and abdominal pain, on a background of prior endometriosis. Initial antibiotic treatment for pelvic inflammatory disease failed, and the patient progressed to septic shock requiring surgical evacuation of an infected ovarian endometrioma. Microbiological samples from stool, ovary, and peritoneal fluid revealed infection with *Salmonella senftenberg*. The likely diagnosis was Salmonella enterocolitis with bacterial translocation to an ovarian endometrioma.

1. Case Report

A 30-year-old nulliparous woman presented to the emergency department with sudden onset of generalized lower abdominal pain, mild fever, and vomiting for one-day duration on a background of three days of diarrhea. She had associated generalized aches and headache. She had a past medical history of endometriosis. She was otherwise generally fit and well, worked in administration on a remote mine site, and had recently returned from a holiday in Bali. On assessment, her temperature was 37.9°C, and she was hemodynamically stable. An abdominal examination revealed tenderness over the suprapubic area. A vaginal assessment showed a normal sized uterus and severe right-sided adnexal tenderness with no abnormal discharge.

Her inflammatory markers were raised (white cell count 23×10^9/L, neutrophil 21×10^9/L, C-reactive protein 233 mg/L). A computed tomography of the abdomen (CT abdomen) and pelvis (Figure 1) showed a possible tubo-ovarian abscess secondary to an ovarian cyst or endometrioma $111 \times 118 \times 95$ mm in size. Her liver and renal function was normal. Endocervical swabs for chlamydia and gonorrhea polymerase chain reaction (PCR) were negative, and a high vaginal swab was sent for microbiology showed normal flora. Of note, a stool PCR was positive for Salmonella species; the significance of this was uncertain. The initial diagnosis was pelvic inflammatory disease, and she was treated with intravenous ceftriaxone, metronidazole, and azithromycin as per local guidelines. After three days of antibiotics, she was well and discharged with oral azithromycin to complete treatment for possible mild Salmonella enteritis. Follow-up in the gynecology clinic was planned to discuss the ongoing management of endometriosis.

However, four days later, she presented with an acute surgical abdomen and septic shock requiring inotropic support. The CT of the abdomen and pelvis revealed a large pelvic mass ($120 \times 130 \times 150$ mm in size) with copious free fluid in the pelvis and edematous bowel (Figure 2). She had an emergency laparotomy and drained 1500 ml of endometriotic fluid from the peritoneal cavity. There was inflammatory exudate present over the bowel wall, and when the endometrioma was laid open, it was noted to be purulent and malodourous. A peritoneal fluid was sent for culture and grew *Salmonella senftenberg*. A cystectomy of the endometrioma was performed, and histology of the cyst wall was compatible with endometriosis. Infectious disease consultation was

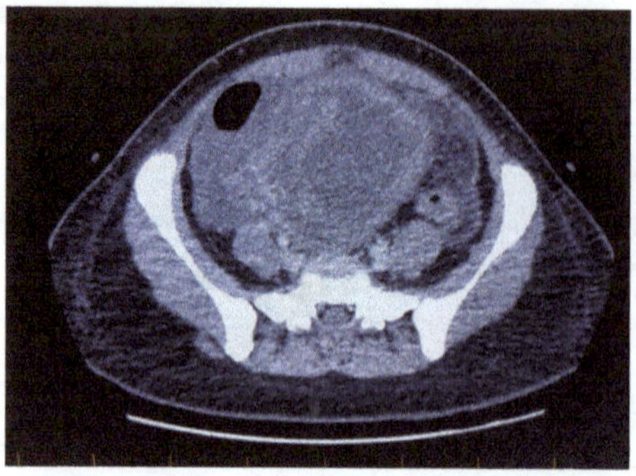

FIGURE 1: CT report of the abdomen and pelvis. Large pelvic mass which may be ovarian in nature. The fluid content of this cystic lesion is 24 HU in density. It has a thick irregular wall. There is generalized ascites and peritoneal induration.

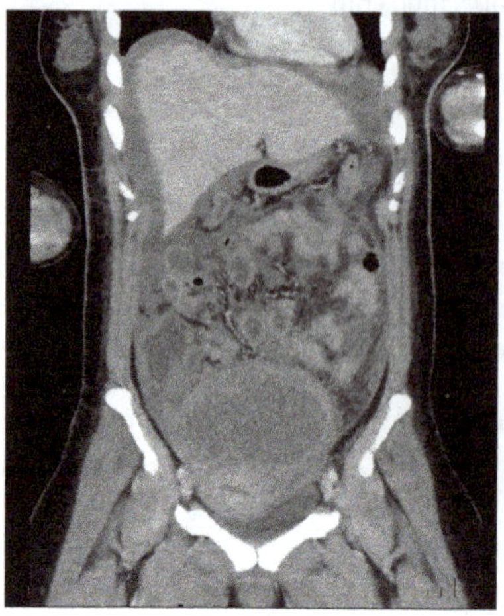

FIGURE 2: CT report of the abdomen and pelvis. There is a large cystic mass arising off the pelvis, which is complex in appearance. The wall is thick and irregular; this lesion has axial/transverse dimensions of 12.6 × 13.6 cm, with a sag/oblique long axis of 15.4 cm.

sought. She had nine days of intravenous antibiotics and was discharged on a three-week course of high dose oral ciprofloxacin, to which the organism was susceptible. The patient had recovered well on review in clinic.

2. Discussion

The Salmonellae are a family of gram-negative motile bacilli, of which two serotypes cause severe enteric fever—S. typhi and S. paratyphi. The remainder is collectively known as the nontyphoidal Salmonellae, and this includes Salmonella senftenberg. Enteric fever due to typhoidal Salmonella is a major global health problem, which causes 200000 deaths annually and further significant morbidity [1]. Patients with nontyphoidal Salmonella typically present with self-limiting gastroenteritis. Less than 5% of patients with Salmonella gastroenteritis develop bacteremia and distant spread.

Salmonella is transmitted via the fecal-oral route from contaminated food, most commonly poultry, milk, and eggs [2]. Direct animal contact and person-to-person transmission are rare. The incubation period for salmonellosis is 12–72 hours. The typical initial symptoms are fever, diarrhea, abdominal pain, and generalized myalgia.

Salmonella can breach the barrier of the intestinal cell wall through the process of phagocytosis and then enter macrophages through micropinocytosis. The microorganism then disseminates through the body via hematogenous spread and can metastasize to distant sites. These complicated disseminated cases require prolonged antimicrobial therapy.

The most common sites of secondary involvement are the bone, lung, heart, spleen, and kidney. Ovarian involvement is rare. In this case, a spread of infection to the ovaries could have been due to direct contact with inflamed bowel, through hematogenous spread or via ascending infection. Those with immunodeficiency conditions are at higher risk of aggressive and disseminated disease [3–5]. There have been previous case reports of Salmonella presenting during pregnancy with ovarian infection and mimicking a gynecological malignancy [6, 7].

A literature review revealed nearly thirty cases of ovarian involvement reported over the past five decades. *Salmonella enteritidis* and *Salmonella typhi* are the subtypes most frequently isolated from the ovary. *Salmonella senftenberg* infection in an ovary is unreported. In previous case reports, a wide range of antibiotics have been used for treatment, including cephalosporins, fluoroquinolones, and macrolides. Increasing rates of Salmonella resistance to fluoroquinolones are reported, particularly in Asian regions [8].

3. Conclusion

This case likely represents Salmonella enterocolitis with translocation to a preexisting endometrioma, leading to cyst rupture and septic shock. The case alerts the gynecologist that salmonella infection can manifest in multiple organ systems and highlights the importance of a broad differential diagnosis in a patient with a presentation of fevers and abdominal pain.

References

[1] J. A. Crump, S. P. Luby, and E. D. Mintz, "The global burden of typhoid fever," *Bulletin of the World Health Organization*, vol. 82, no. 5, pp. 346–353, 2004.

[2] J. A. Crump, M. Sjolund-Karlsson, M. A. Gordon, and C. M. Parry, "Epidemiology, clinical presentation, laboratory diagnosis, antimicrobial resistance, and antimicrobial management of invasive Salmonella infections," *Clinical Microbiology Reviews*, vol. 28, no. 4, pp. 901–937, 2015.

[3] M. K. Lalitha and R. John, "Unusual manifestations of salmonellosis—a surgical problem," *The Quarterly Journal of Medicine*, vol. 87, no. 5, pp. 301–309, 1994.

[4] A. Chao, A.-S. Chao, T.-H. Wang, L.-P. Liu, and C.-J. Wang, "Management of Salmonella ovarian abscess in a patient with systemic lupus erythematosus," *Fertility and Sterility*, vol. 92, no. 1, pp. 391.e1–391.e3, 2009.

[5] M. Inoue, N. Yanaihara, and A. Okamoto, "Salmonella ovarian abscess in a patient with rheumatoid arthritis (RA): a case

report with literature review," *Clinical and Experimental Obstetrics & Gynecology*, vol. 41, no. 4, pp. 465–467, 2014.

[6] I. D. Nuttall, P. D. Wilson, and B. K. Mandal, "A suppurative ovarian cyst in pregnancy due to Salmonella typhi," *Scandinavian Journal of Infectious Diseases*, vol. 12, no. 4, pp. 311-312, 1980.

[7] R. Kudesia and D. Gupta, "Pelvic Salmonella infection masquerading as gynecologic malignancy," *Obstetrics and Gynecology*, vol. 118, 2, Part 2, pp. 475–477, 2011.

[8] H. Y. Lee, L. H. Su, M. H. Tsai et al., "High rate of reduced susceptibility to ciprofloxacin and ceftriaxone among nontyphoid Salmonella clinical isolates in Asia," *Antimicrobial Agents and Chemotherapy*, vol. 53, no. 6, pp. 2696–2699, 2009.

35

Third Trimester Lower Extremity Lymphorrhea

Kaori Morimoto and Luke O'Rourke

Western University of Health Sciences College of Osteopathic Medicine Pacific Northwest, 200 Mullins Dr., Lebanon OR 97355, USA

Correspondence should be addressed to Luke O'Rourke; orourkeluke@gmail.com

Academic Editor: John P. Geisler

Introduction. Lower extremity edema is one of the most common complaints among pregnant patients. However, there is no literature mentioning weeping edema (i.e., lymphorrhea) in a pregnant woman who has no concordant underlying renal and/or cardiac pathology. There is also a lack of evidence and recommendations regarding the therapeutic benefit and safety profile of diuretic use to treat profound pregnancy-associated edema. Herein, we present the case of 32-year-old female who presented with a significant lymphorrhea during the third trimester without cardiac or renal comorbidity and was successfully treated with torsemide. *Case Report.* We report a case of a 32-year-old multigravida patient pregnant with her third child and has two living full-term children (G3P2003). Her pregnancy was complicated by obesity, smoking (vape), and previous history of fetal growth restriction. The patient presented for routine prenatal care at 9-week gestation. She was diagnosed with chronic hypertension at 19 weeks of pregnancy based upon systolic blood pressure > 140. Lifestyle modifications were recommended, but the patient did not comply. At her 31-week office visit, the patient presented with anasarca and clear, slightly viscous fluid seeping through the atraumatic skin of her lower extremities. Preeclampsia, renal, cardiac, vascular, and infectious complications were all ruled out. The patient responded positively to loop diuretic therapy. Torsemide was found to be far more beneficial than furosemide. The patient was induced at 37 weeks secondary to chronic hypertension requiring antihypertensive therapy. Delivery was uncomplicated. The patient gave birth to a healthy male with birth weight of 2,920 g via spontaneous vaginal delivery. *Discussion.* Pitting edema of lower limbs frequently occurs as a result of fluid overload and chronic venous insufficiency, and pregnancy is one of the known risk factors. Additionally, the blockage of lymphatic channel with the gravida uterus likely was the main contributing factor for her lymphorrhea. In this patient, the capillary hydrostatic pressure was likely accentuated due to hypertension, obesity, and vaping. Furosemide was minimally effective to alleviate her symptoms. Torsemide provided much more effective diuresis and symptom control. However, her symptoms persisted until delivery. *Conclusion.* Torsemide provided significant therapeutic benefit over furosemide in this patient without adverse maternal, fetal, or neonatal outcomes. Further study is needed to assess the safe use of loop diuretics in the pregnant population who suffers from significant lower extremity edema.

1. Introduction

Edema is one of the most common complaints during pregnancy due to increased hydrostatic pressure [1]. This can also contribute to the development of varicose veins in the lower extremity [2]. As the gravid uterus grows, the superficial lymphatic channels in the pelvic area can be obstructed [3]. In this patient, both factors along with chronic hypertension and regular vaping could have contributed to the manifestation of lymphorrhea in her lower extremity. The mechanism is discussed in detail in Discussion.

After ruling out the cardiac and renal causes, the patient was placed on furosemide based on the cardiologist's recommendation. In general, loop diuretics is used with caution during pregnancy as it is known to cross the placenta, and their effect on fetal development is largely unknown [4]. In this patient, torsemide was more effective than furosemide in symptomatic relief. There is no available literature comparing the efficacy of furosemide versus torsemide for the treatment of symptomatic edema and specifically in pregnant patients.

2. Case Report

The patient was a 32-year-old Caucasian female pregnant with her third child and had two living full-term children. She was initially seen in the office at 9 weeks and 3 days of gestation. Her initial medications included prenatal vitamin daily, docusate PRN, polyethylene glycol PRN, ondansetron PRN, and topical nystatin PRN. The patient's past medical history included obesity, irritable bowel syndrome, anxiety, nicotine abuse (vape), umbilical hernia, recurrent urinary tract infections, and nephrolithiasis. She had no prior history of hypertension or preeclampsia. Pertinent past pregnancy history included severe fetal growth restriction (FGR) and close interval pregnancy.

Initial prenatal laboratory panel results were benign. The patient's blood type was B positive. She passed the 1-hour oral glucose test at 28 weeks of gestation.

At 19 weeks of gestation, the patient was diagnosed with chronic hypertension secondary to elevated systolic blood pressure > 140. She was started on aspirin 81 mg daily for primary prevention of preeclampsia. She admitted to non-compliance with this recommendation. Her blood pressure remained around 120 s-140 s/70 s-80 s without medication until 31-week gestation.

Per patient report, her symptoms of the pedal and leg edema, extreme sensitivity to touch, and erythematous discoloration of the caudal half of the shins, consistent with stasis dermatitis, started around 30 weeks of gestation. Over the following days, the patient started noticing a small amount of fluid continuously seeping through the skin of her lower extremities. This rapidly progressed to the point that fluid was streaming down her legs, leaving a trail behind her. The fluid had the appearance of egg white (Figure 1, blue arrows) or water (Figure 2, white arrow). Figure 1 is obtained at home by the patient, and Figure 2 is obtained by the authors during the patient's office visit at 31-week and 4-day gestation with patient permission. As the fluid dehydrated on her skin, its viscosity increased and eventually left the white residue, as seen in Figure 1.

During her office visit at 31 weeks and 4 days of gestation, her blood pressure was 140/100. There was no warmth or tenderness on the affected area during the physical examination. She was treated with oral antibiotics, cephalexin, in case of underlying infection. Unfortunately, antibiotics were of no value in her symptomatic improvement. Over several weeks, it became clear that she did not have cellulitis. Leg elevation and wearing medical compression stockings were not helpful. The patient demonstrated no other classical symptoms of heart failure, nephrotic syndrome, liver failure, or DVT. Urine protein dip was negative, and preeclampsia was ruled out via normal 24-hour urine protein collection. However, due to significant discomfort and profound edema, the patient was admitted to Labor and Delivery for observation, as suggested by the Maternal-Fetal Medicine consultation.

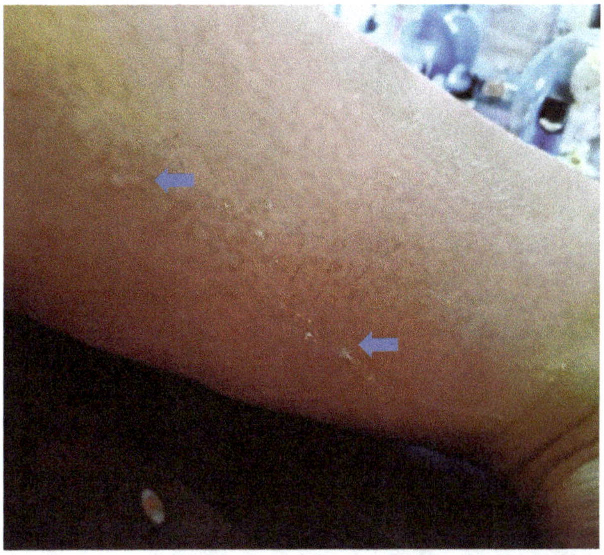

FIGURE 1: A photograph of the left calf taken by the patient at home. The blue arrows indicate the fluid seeping from the edema. The white residues are dried fluid.

Upon admission to the hospital, the patient received furosemide 20 mg orally per day for symptomatic relief. She had minimal diuresis with this intervention.

While admitted, urinalysis, comprehensive metabolic panel, and complete blood count results were all unremarkable. Well's score was zero. Brain natriuretic peptide level was 33. Fetal heart tones remained category one throughout her stay. Labetalol 200 mg orally twice a day was started for control of chronic hypertension. The patient remained afebrile and normotensive overnight and was discharged on the next day. Outpatient echocardiography showed normal cardiac anatomy and function.

The following week, at 32 weeks and 4 days of gestation, the patient was admitted again for the worsening weeping edema. Chest X-ray and bilateral lower extremity venous duplex ultrasound showed benign findings. However, mild bilateral inguinal lymphedema secondary was noted in the ultrasound report. Upon recommendation by Cardiology, the patient received torsemide 20 mg orally, and she responded with a marked increase in diuresis. Torsemide was remarkably more effective than furosemide for diuresis, edema reduction, and symptomatic relief for this patient. Upon discharge, the patient was started on torsemide 20 mg orally every other day, which she continued for the remainder of her pregnancy.

Throughout the remaining pregnancy, the patient had electrolyte monitoring, and she never required potassium supplementation. Additionally, twice weekly fetal nonstress tests, a weekly ultrasound to follow amniotic fluid index (AFI), and 4-week interval fetal growth ultrasounds were performed to monitor maternal and fetal health closely.

Fetal growth trajectory and amniotic fluid index were unaffected by diuretic use. All fetal nonstress tests were category I and reactive.

The patient reported continuous weeping edema until her delivery at 37-week gestation, but her symptoms were

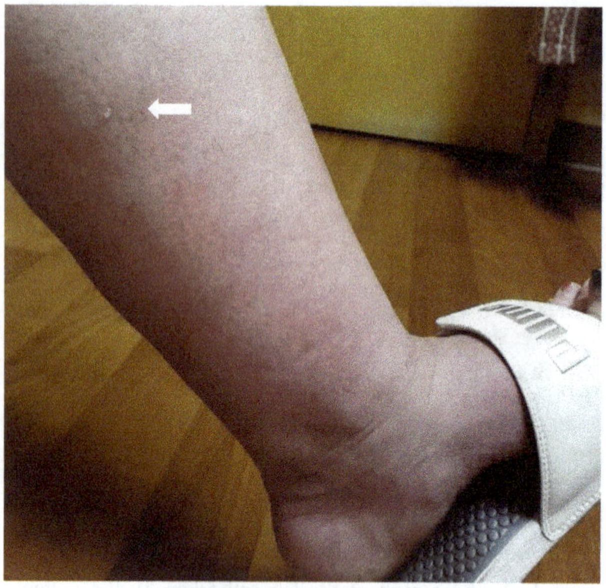

FIGURE 2: A photograph of the left calf taken by Kaori Morimoto during the prenatal visit. The patient was 31-week and 4-day gestation. Significant bilateral leg edema was noted along with the constant seeping indicated with the white arrow.

adequately managed so that she could adequately perform activities of daily living (ADLs) without profound discomfort, including caring for her other children.

The patient was induced by Pitocin administration for the indication of chronic hypertension on antihypertensive therapy at 37-week gestation. She successfully delivered a healthy 2,920 g male via spontaneous vaginal delivery after 11 hours of labor. Delivery and postpartum course were uncomplicated.

At the six-week postpartum appointment, her edema was resolved entirely. This suggests that the mechanical obstruction secondary to pregnancy was the likely primary cause of the patient presentation.

3. Discussion

Edema is one of the most common complaints during pregnancy. Approximately 70% of women present with clinical edema at some point during pregnancy. One of the common causes of lower extremity edema during pregnancy is an increase in hydrostatic pressure. As a normal physiologic change in pregnancy, total body water increases by 6 to 8 liters. Two-thirds of this fluid is extracellular, and one-third is stored interstitially [5].

Additionally, pregnancy is a risk factor for the development of venous insufficiency and varicosity in the lower extremity and iliac vessels. Varicose veins develop secondary to weakened blood vessel walls and incompetent valves. As the wall stretches, small balloons are formed and contribute to the stasis. While lower extremity vessels are the most vulnerable by gravity, vulvar, rectal, and internal iliac vessels can be affected due to the hemodynamic changes during pregnancy [2].

In its nonpregnant state, the uterus receives about 100 mL/min of blood, less than 3% of the total blood volume. On the other hand, the blood flow to the term uterus approaches 700 mL/min, about 16% of the cardiac output [6]. This increases the amount of blood flowing to the lower half of the body during the pregnancy. Additionally, the dynamic vascular remodeling of uterine vessels and cardiovascular changes accentuates the burden on the venous system.

The lower abdominal and superficial lower extremity lymphatics drain into the superficial inguinal nodes, followed by external iliac nodes, and eventually into the common iliac nodes [7]. Obstructions at any point of this channel can lead to significant lymphedema in the lower extremities and the abdomen. Because of this, lymphatic congestion can be seen during pregnancy secondary to direct compression of the lower extremity lymphatic system by the gravid uterus.

There is limited literature about lymphedema during pregnancy. However, two reported cases of reversible lower abdominal lymphedema in the third trimester showed tortuous dilatation of lymphatic channels, and biopsy confirmed that the obstruction of the lymphatic channels caused those dilatations [3]. Another reported case showed significant bilateral third-trimester leg lymphedema treated with kinesiotherapy [8]. Those symptoms were observed in our patient towards the end of her pregnancy. Additionally, our patient presented with fluid seeping through edematous tissues, which has never been reported previously in any literature.

The risk of vaping during pregnancy in comparison with smoking for humans is largely unknown. One study reported that smoking alters lipid homeostasis while vaping does not in a mouse model [9]. However, many animal studies report the direct toxicity of nicotine in the fetus' developing immune system, neural development, lung function, and cardiac function regardless of the delivery method [10]. Due to the lack of clear warning and addictive potential of nicotine, approximately 7% of women report vaping during pregnancy [11]. Smoking and vaping (e-cigarette use) are both associated with increased risk of hypertension in general. The risk of developing hypertension in people who smoke tobacco or vape regularly compared to those who do not is approximately 1.3 times higher. Furthermore, the risk increases with a combined use of both products to 1.8 times [12]. Therefore, chronic vaping in this patient was likely a contributing factor in developing chronic hypertension during this pregnancy.

Loop diuretics are not the first-line treatment of hypertension in pregnant women and need to be used with caution [4]. Furosemide is known to cross the placenta, and animal reproduction studies have shown adverse events in rat fetuses, including the perinatal growth restriction and subsequent decrease in kidney functions measured by creatinine and uric acid clearance rate [4, 13]. Additionally, the old study conducted by Sibai et al. suggests that a failure in plasma volume expansion at 20- to 25-week gestation may have a correlation with intrauterine fetal demise and intrauterine growth retardation. As shown in animal studies, furosemide decreases plasma volume rather quickly [14,

15]. For those reasons, furosemide was classified as a pregnancy category C drug in the old FDA categorization [4].

ACOG practice bulletin No. 203 lists antihypertensive medications safe during pregnancy. For oral agents, labetalol and nifedipine are most commonly used, followed by methyldopa and hydrochlorothiazide [16]. For chronic hypertension, daily low dose (81 mg) aspirin is recommended (level A), starting between 12 and 28 weeks of gestation [16].

In this patient, torsemide was far more effective than furosemide in edema reduction. The differences between furosemide and torsemide are summarized in the following three points. First, the half-life of torsemide is approximately 3.5 hours, while that of furosemide is 2 hours. Secondly, the bioavailability of oral torsemide is 80%, while that of furosemide is 47%. Lastly, torsemide is 80% metabolized via CYP2C9 in the liver, while furosemide is renally excreted. The onset of diuresis for both medications is within 1 hour [4, 17]. There is no available literature comparing the efficacy of furosemide versus torsemide for treating symptomatic edema in general, nor in pregnant patients.

Because of the lack of study and literature for pregnancy-related lymphorrhea and diuretic use, our case study provides valuable information for managing this rare condition.

4. Conclusion

Lower extremity edema is highly prevalent among pregnant women and can cause significant difficulties with ADLs. There is a lack of evidence and safety data regarding the use of diuretic therapy to treat the lower extremity edema during pregnancy. In this case, the patient had profound edema with fluid constantly seeping through the skin without any additional organ dysfunction. Her ADLs were significantly compromised by edema, which was successfully managed with loop diuretics. Torsemide was found to have a significant therapeutic benefit over furosemide in this patient. There were no adverse maternal, fetal, or neonatal effects demonstrated with loop diuretic use in the third trimester. Further study is needed to assess the safe use of loop diuretics in the pregnant population for the symptomatic relief of significant lower extremity edema.

Consent

The patient in this case report has provided verbal consent and permission for all images to be published and for the publication of potentially identifying information.

Authors' Contributions

KM and LO equally contributed to the writing of this case report. As the provider of this patient, LO provided the detailed history of this patient and her care. KM contributed through the literature search and review. Both authors read and approved the final manuscript.

References

[1] F. Tanveer and S. Shahid, "Frequency of lower extremity edema during third trimester of pregnancy," *S. Asian J. Med. Sci. (SAJMS)*, vol. 1, no. 2, pp. 41–43, 2015.

[2] R. M. Smyth, N. Aflaifel, and A. A. Bamigboye, "Interventions for varicose veins and leg oedema in pregnancy," *Cochrane Database of Systematic Reviews*, no. 10, article CD001066, 2015.

[3] B. R. Reed, S. Burke, M. Bozeman, L. E. Golitz, and J. C. Huff, "Lymphedema of the lower abdominal wall in pregnancy," *Journal of the American Academy of Dermatology*, vol. 12, no. 5, pp. 930–932, 1985.

[4] T. M. Khan, R. Patel, and A. H. Siddiqui, *Furosemide*, In: StatPearls. Treasure Island (FL): StatPearls Publishing, 2021, https://www.ncbi.nlm.nih.gov/books/NBK499921/.

[5] J. M. Davison, "Edema in pregnancy," *Kidney International. Supplement*, vol. 59, pp. S90–S96, 1997.

[6] S. Page and M. Rollins, "Physiology and Pharmacology of Obstetric Anesthesia," in *Pharmacology and Physiology for Anesthesia (Second Edition)*, pp. 732–751, Elsevier, 2019.

[7] P. L. Williams and R. Warwick, *Gray's anatomy*, Saunders Co, Philadelphia, 1980.

[8] K. Korabiusz and A. Katarzyna, "Lymphedema during pregnancy - case study," *Journal of Education, Health and Sport*, vol. 7, no. 6, pp. 397–407, 2017.

[9] G. Li, Y. L. Chan, B. Wang, S. Saad, B. G. Oliver, and H. Chen, "Replacing smoking with vaping during pregnancy: impacts on metabolic health in mice," *Reproductive Toxicology*, vol. 96, pp. 293–299, 2020.

[10] J. R. Whittington, P. M. Simmons, A. M. Phillips et al., "The use of electronic cigarettes in pregnancy: a review of the literature," *Obstetrical & Gynecological Survey*, vol. 73, no. 9, pp. 544–549, 2018.

[11] B. Kuehn, "Vaping and pregnancy," *Journal of the American Medical Association*, vol. 321, no. 14, p. 1344, 2019.

[12] C. R. Miller, H. Shi, D. Li, and M. L. Goniewicz, "Cross-sectional associations of smoking and E-cigarette use with self-reported diagnosed hypertension: findings from wave 3 of the population assessment of tobacco and health study," *Toxics*, vol. 9, no. 3, 2021.

[13] B. N. DuBois, J. Pearson, T. Mahmood, D. Nguyen, K. Thornburg, and G. Cherala, "Perinatal growth restriction decreases diuretic action of furosemide in adult rats," *European Journal of Pharmacology*, vol. 728, pp. 39–47, 2014.

[14] K. W. Hinchcliff, K. H. McKeever, and W. W. Muir 3rd., "Furosemide-induced changes in plasma and blood volume of horses," *Journal of Veterinary Pharmacology and Therapeutics*, vol. 14, no. 4, pp. 411–417, 1991.

[15] B. H. Ali, G. A. Alhadrami, and A. K. Bashir, "Furosemide-induced changes in plasma and blood volume of camels (Camelus dromedarius)," *Journal of Veterinary Pharmacology and Therapeutics*, vol. 20, no. 6, pp. 483–486, 1997.

[16] American College of Obstetricians and Gynecologists' Committee on Practice Bulletins-Obstetrics, "ACOG Practice Bulletin No. 203: Chronic Hypertension in Pregnancy," *Obstetrics & Gynecology*, vol. 133, no. 1, pp. e26–e50, 2019.

[17] T. Kanderi and P. Vaitla, *Torsemide*, In: StatPearls Treasure Island (FL): StatPearls Publishing, 2021, https://www.ncbi.nlm.nih.gov/books/NBK559175/.

36

Spontaneous Heterotopic Pregnancy Associated with Massive Intraperitoneal Haemorrhage and a Normal Heart Rate, Illustrating the Concept of Relative Bradycardia

Charles Gallaher,[1] Farshad Tahmasebi,[2] Ahmad Sayasneh,[2] and Gautam Mehra[2]

[1]*Emergency Department, St Helier Hospital, Wrythe Ln, Sutton, Carshalton SM5 1AA, UK*
[2]*Obstetrics and Gynaecology, Guy's & St Thomas' NHS Foundation Trust, Westminster Bridge Rd, London SE1 7EH, UK*

Correspondence should be addressed to Charles Gallaher; charlesgallaher@doctors.org.uk

Academic Editor: Giovanni Monni

A 28-year-old, 9 and a half weeks pregnant (spontaneous conception) multigravida presented with abdominal pain and vaginal bleeding. On examination, her abdomen was diffusely tender, particularly in the right iliac fossa, though guarding was absent. Transabdominal and transvaginal ultrasonography demonstrated a viable intrauterine pregnancy and large-volume intraperitoneal haemoperitoneum; the right ovary could not be identified. The patient became hypotensive with decreased responsiveness, yet her heart rate remained normal. She proceeded to surgery where a ruptured right tubal ectopic pregnancy was identified and right salpingectomy was performed. Estimated blood loss was 3900ml. Postoperative recovery was uneventful. Ultrasound 3 days after surgery demonstrated a viable intrauterine pregnancy of gestational age 9 weeks + 1 day. The patient remains well. Her anomaly scan at 20 weeks and 6 days showed normal growth, amniotic fluid, and Dopplers with no obvious structural defects. She is currently 27 weeks pregnant and will be rescanned at 36 weeks.

1. Introduction

Across the world, health professionals are trained to estimate severity of haemorrhage in accordance with the clinical criteria set out in the American College of Surgeons Advanced Trauma Life Support® (ATLS®) classification of haemorrhage [1]. This classifies haemorrhage into 4 classes (classes I-IV) based on clinical signs and is described in the text as "a useful tool for estimating the percentage of acute blood loss." Class I haemorrhage is defined as up to 15% blood volume loss; class II haemorrhage = 15-30% blood volume loss; class III haemorrhage = 30-40% blood volume loss; and class IV haemorrhage = more than 40% blood volume loss.

According to the ATLS® classification of haemorrhage, class IV haemorrhage – which for a 70kg patient refers to blood volume loss of >2000ml – is associated with the following:

(i) heart rate > 140 beats per minute (bpm)

(ii) decreased systolic blood pressure

(iii) decreased pulse pressure

(iv) respiratory rate > 35 breaths per minute

(v) negligible urine output

(vi) confusion and lethargy

We present a case where, with one exception (heart rate was 112 bpm on first arrival in the emergency department), a patient with severe intraperitoneal haemorrhage remained persistently normocardic, with a heart rate of around 70 bpm, until after anaesthesia had been induced.

The MBRRACE-UK confidential enquiry into maternal deaths (2016) highlights the significance of early diagnosis of ectopic pregnancy to reduce maternal mortality [2]. The diagnosis and treatment of ectopic pregnancy can be challenging, especially when this presents atypically following tubal rupture in a spontaneous heterotopic pregnancy which in itself is rare.

2. Case Presentation

A 28-year-old multigravida (gravida 2, para 1), weighing approximately 90kg, presented at 9 and a half weeks with an 18-hour history of severe right iliac fossa pain, associated with brownish vaginal discharge, dysuria, diarrhoea, light-headedness, and feeling shivery. She was afebrile and did not complain of shoulder tip pain.

Past obstetric and gynaecological history included one full-term caesarean section; there was no history of tubal or other gynaecological surgery, sexually transmitted disease, endometriosis, or subfertility treatment, nor was there a history of intrauterine contraceptive device or progestogen-only contraceptive use.

Past medical history was otherwise unremarkable. The patient was on no regular medications and was an ex-smoker, and social history was otherwise unremarkable.

On examination, the patient looked to be in pain. Her abdomen was diffusely tender, particularly in the right iliac fossa. There was no loin tenderness, no abdominal guarding, and no rebound tenderness. Pelvic examination revealed right adnexal tenderness and cervical excitation; on speculum examination, the cervix was closed and brownish discharge was noted.

Vital signs from first assessment by the ambulance service onwards are displayed in Table 1.

2.1. Investigations. Urine dip was positive for protein (+), blood (++++), ketones (+++), leucocyte esterase (+), and qualitative beta-human chorionic gonadotrophin (beta-hCG).

Venous blood gas on arrival in the emergency department (ED) showed pH 7.419 (7.350-7.450), partial pressure of carbon dioxide (pCO2) 3.97 kPa, base excess (BE) -4.5 mmol/L, corrected bicarbonate ($cHCO3^-$) 20.7 mmol/L, lactate 1.8 mmol/L (0.4-2.2 mmol/L), glucose 6.9 mmol/L (3.3-6.1 mmol/L), haemoglobin (Hb) 128 g/L (120-150 g/L), and haematocrit (Hct) 0.397 (0.360-0.470).

Laboratory blood tests on arrival in ED were as follows: total white cell count 14.1 $x10^9$/L (4.0-11.0 $x10^9$/L), neutrophils 11.1 $x10^9$/L (1.5-7.0 $x10^9$/L), Hb 130 g/L, Hct 0.375, sodium 138 mmol/L (135-145 mmol/L), potassium 4.0 mmol/L (3.5-5.0 mmol/L), creatinine 48 μmol/L (45-84 μmol/L), albumin 39 g/L (40-52 g/L), C-reactive protein 9 mg/L (0-4 mg/L), serum beta-hCG 133,561 IU/L, and HIV antibody screen negative.

On bedside transabdominal gynaecological ultrasound scan, performed in the ED approximately 2 hours after arrival, a 3.5cm intrauterine gestational sac was noted.

Formal gynaecological transabdominal ultrasound scan and Focused Assessment for Free Fluid (FAFF) ultrasound scan were performed on the early pregnancy unit approximately 3.5 hours after arrival in the ED, and showed a moderate amount of free fluid in the upper abdomen. Heterogeneous, avascular material was noted in the adnexa, in keeping with haemoperitoneum. The right ovary could not be identified, the left ovary appeared normal. An intrauterine gestational sac was noted.

Transvaginal ultrasound scan was performed immediately afterwards and showed a viable intrauterine pregnancy, with gestational sac 140mm, and crown-rump length 9mm. The adnexa was difficult to assess.

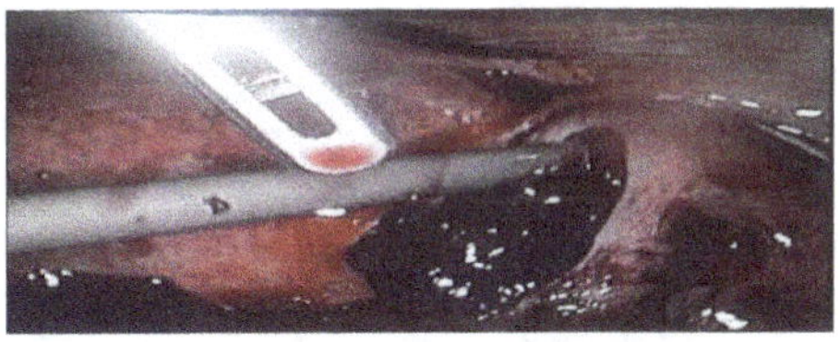

(a)

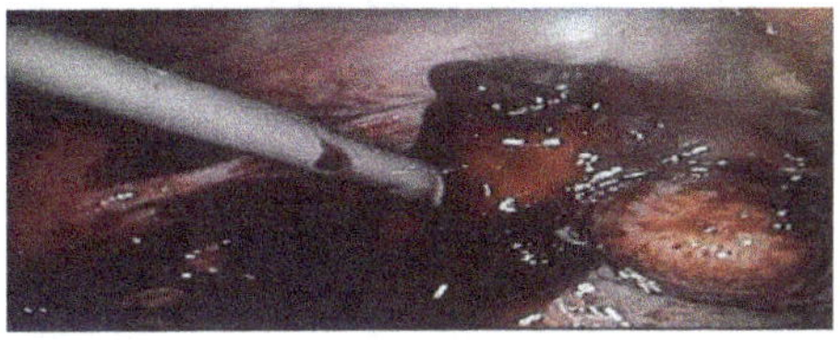

(b)

FIGURE 1: Ruptured right ectopic pregnancy.

Arterial blood gas on high flow oxygen via nonrebreathe mask was performed when the patient became acutely unwell immediately following the above scan, and showed pH 7.403, pCO2 3.78 (4.67-6.00), pO2 35.86, BE -6.4, $cHCO3^-$ 19.2, lactate 1.5, glucose 6.4, Hb 102 g/L, and Hct 0.315 (0.350-0.500).

2.2. Differential Diagnosis. Haemoperitoneum was diagnosed, with a differential diagnosis of either a ruptured spontaneous heterotopic pregnancy or a bleeding haemorrhagic corpus luteal cyst.

2.3. Treatment. In the scanning room on the early pregnancy unit, 4 hours after arrival in the ED, the patient complained of worsening, predominantly right-sided pain, and dizziness. She was re-examined and found to be cold and clammy with increased abdominal distension but no guarding. Vital signs recorded at the time were oxygen saturations of 100% on 2 litres of oxygen via nasal cannulae, heart rate of 76 bpm, and blood pressure of 90/59 mmHg. The patient became less responsive and the hospital medical emergency team was summoned. Intravenous crystalloid fluids had deliberately been withheld until this point in keeping with a hypotensive resuscitation strategy.

The patient was taken to the operating theatre where anaesthesia was induced approximately 6 hours after the patient's arrival in the ED. Having surgeons with advanced laparoscopic skills available, the decision was made to proceed with laparoscopic surgery (in most cases, surgeons might proceed with laparotomy).

Laparoscopic right salpingectomy and peritoneal lavage were performed (Figures 1(a) and 1(b)). Two units of red blood cells were transfused.

Summary of operative findings and procedures is as follows:

(i) Left ovary/tube normal

Table 1: Observations/vital signs.

Time	1105	1120	1150	1230	1230	1255	1320	1445	1450	1505	1720	1745
Location of patient	On scene	En route to hospital	Emergency department	Emergency department	Emergency department	Emergency department	Emergency department	Early pregnancy unit	Early pregnancy unit	Early pregnancy unit	Early pregnancy unit	Anaesthetic room
Respiratory rate (breaths per minute)	20	20	16	25	N/R	16	16	N/R	20	N/R	21	N/R
Oxygen saturation in air (%)	100	100	99	97	N/R	100	100	94	98	N/R	N/R	N/R
Heart rate (bpm)	70	70	112	69	N/R	71	69	71	62	73	82	86
Blood pressure (mmHg)	108/71	106/61	115/59	93/57 (right)	94/61 (left)	105/68	101/79	100/63	117/72	97/68	102/68	108/62
Colour	Normal	Normal	N/A	N/A	N/A	N/A	N/A	N/A	N/A	N/A	N/A	N/A
Conscious level	Alert	Alert	Alert	Alert	Alert	Alert	Alert	Alert	Alert	Alert	Alert	N/R
Blood sugar level (mmol/L)	5.7	5.7	N/A	N/A	N/A	N/A	N/A	N/A	N/A	N/A	N/A	N/A
Temperature (°C)	36.5	N/R	36.1	35.6	N/R	35.2	36.2	N/R	N/R	36.2	36.7	N/R
Pain score (0-10 scale)	10	8	N/A	N/A	N/A	N/A	N/A	N/A	N/A	N/A	N/A	N/A
National Early Warning System (NEWS) score	N/A	N/A	2	6	U	U	1	U	U	U	U	U

Key
N/A = not applicable (colour not routinely recorded on NEWS chart; blood sugar level not routinely recorded on NEWS chart; pain score not routinely recorded on NEWS chart; NEWS score only used in hospital).
N/R = not recorded.
U = Unable to calculate due incomplete documentation of observations.

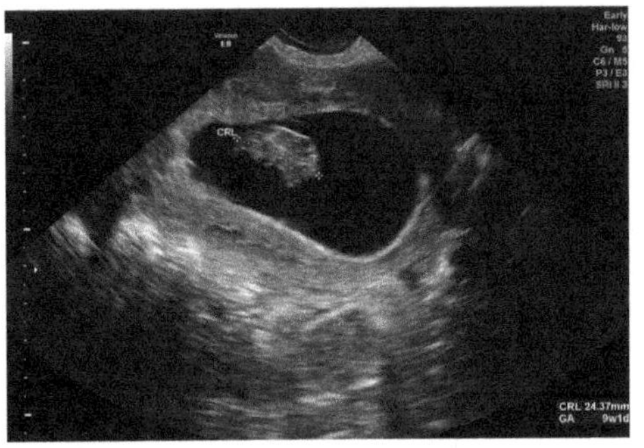

FIGURE 2: Intrauterine pregnancy demonstrated by transvaginal scan.

(ii) Right tube engorged with rupture at isthmo-ampullary junction with extruding trophoblastic tissue and active bleeding from site of rupture

(iii) 3900ml haemoperitoneum with large clots in pelvis, paracolic gutters, and upper abdomen

(iv) Right tubal ectopic located and right salpingectomy performed

(v) Robinson's drain inserted to allow remaining blood to drain

2.4. Outcome and Follow-Up. Postoperative recovery was uneventful. Hb and haematocrit reached a nadir of 76 g/L and 0.226 2 days after surgery (Hb and haematocrit were 130g/L and 0.375 on arrival in the ED, and 2 units of red cells were transfused intraoperatively); this time lag is in keeping with the known delayed fall in Hb after haemorrhage.

Formal early pregnancy ultrasound scan performed 3 days post-operatively showed a viable intrauterine pregnancy of gestational age 9 weeks + 1 day (Figure 2).

The patient was discharged from hospital 3 days after surgery, with a plan for a follow-up ultrasound scan in 2 weeks' time and iron supplementation.

Despite being critically ill with massive blood loss, her intrauterine pregnancy has developed normally. She is currently 27 weeks pregnant. Her routine dating and anomaly scans (performed at 12 weeks + 6 days and 20 + 6 days, respectively) demonstrated normal growth, amniotic fluid index, and uterine artery Dopplers.

She is to have early ultrasonography in future pregnancies.

3. Discussion

Heterotopic pregnancy—dizygotic twins, where one implants in the endometrial lining of the uterus and one outside of this location (i.e., ectopically)—is rare in spontaneous pregnancies (figures of approximately 1 in 4000 to 1 in 30,000 pregnancies are commonly quoted) [3–6]; it is far commoner if assisted reproductive technologies are used, with an incidence of approximately 1% [7, 8].

Barring pregnancies where assisted reproductive technologies have been used (where risk is disproportionately high), risk factors for heterotopic pregnancy are the same as for ectopic pregnancy [9, 10]. Our patient had no known risk factors except for being an ex-smoker.

What is particularly noteworthy about this case is the failure of the patient to mount a sustained tachycardia, despite massive intraperitoneal blood loss of nearly 4 litres.

This physiological response to haemorrhage runs counter to the above-described ATLS® principles, which are widely taught and internalised by health professionals across the world. A short-cut review was performed using 8 separate PubMed keyword searches, as follows:

(1) "heterotopic pregnancy tachycardia"

  (i) 3 search results, 1 relevant paper

(2) "heterotopic pregnancy bradycardia"

  (i) 1 search result, 1 relevant paper

(3) "ectopic pregnancy tachycardia"

  (i) 95 search results, 7 relevant papers

(4) "ectopic pregnancy bradycardia"

  (i) 27 search results, 3 relevant papers

(5) "relative bradycardia haemorrhage" (includes results for "relative bradycardia hemorrhage")

  (i) 43 search results, 3 relevant papers

(6) "relative bradycardia abdom∗"

  (i) 43 search results, 1 relevant paper

(7) "relative bradycardia shock"

  (i) 47 search results, 1 relevant paper

(8) "paradoxical bradycardia"

  (i) 158 search results, 6 relevant papers

All bar 3 relevant papers had abstracts available, and all these abstracts were in English. One French-language paper with an English abstract was analysed in detail. The papers comprised single case reports, (sometimes large) case series, retrospective chart reviews, and retrospective analyses of trauma registries. No relevant experimental studies were found.

Precise definitions of "relative bradycardia" (also known as "paradoxical bradycardia") vary. Quantitative definitions include

(i) HR <90 bpm with systolic BP < 90mmHg [11] and

(ii) HR <100 bpm with systolic BP < 100mmHg [12].

Qualitative definitions include "the inability of the heart to respond to shock with tachycardia"[11] and "hypotension and the lack of a tachycardic response"[13].

Jansen described relative bradycardia as a sign of acute intraperitoneal bleeding in 1978 [14]. He presented 4 cases of women with intraperitoneal bleeding of pelvic origin who demonstrated relative bradycardia, becoming symptomatically hypotensive with a pulse rate of <80 bpm. It is posited that the observed relative bradycardia is due to reflex, parasympathetically mediated vasomotor disturbance in response to irritation of the peritoneum by recently shed blood (hence the frequently observed syncope and presyncope in cases of acute intraperitoneal haemorrhage of wide-ranging aetiologies). Jansen concluded that the phenomenon of relative bradycardia in acute intraperitoneal haemorrhage potentially causes diagnostic difficulty and disproportionately severe hypotension.

Snyder, in a retrospective chart review of 154 patients with documented ectopic pregnancy, found that, of 20 patients with systolic BP ≤90mmHg, 11 (55%) had a HR <100 bpm [15]. The quantity of haemoperitoneum did not correlate with the observed haemodynamic response. Again, a parasympathetic reflex response was thought to explain the inappropriately slow heart rate for the degree of hypotension. This theory is supported by Oberg and Thoren, who correlated increased activity in vagal cardiac afferent nerves with the appearance of reflex bradycardia during severe haemorrhage [16].

Mathlouthi et al. examined the correlation between vital signs and haemoperitoneum in ruptured ectopic pregnancy on a retrospective sample of 32 patients [17]. Mean maximum HR was 81.5 bpm (range: 70-140 bpm), with a mean systolic BP of 109mmHg (range: 70-150mmHg) for a mean haemoperitoneum of 694ml (range: 100-2000ml). Correlation between vital signs and volume of haemoperitoneum was poor. Hypotension was associated with blood loss of at least 1280ml. In only two cases were hypotension and tachycardia seen together, and correlation between tachycardia and hypotension was poor.

Somers, Spears, Maynard, and Syverud present a case of heterotopic pregnancy with relative bradycardia [18]. Cobb describes a similar case of ectopic pregnancy [19].

Several papers describe a similar relative bradycardia concept in the context of trauma [11, 20–22].

Clearly, failure to recognise the association of intraperitoneal haemorrhage with relative bradycardia may have patient safety implications. Fortunately, our patient recovered well, but the sheer volume of haemoperitoneum found at laparoscopy raises concerns that had her surgery been performed later, her outcome may not have been positive.

Other authors to have commented on this potential patient safety issue include Sucov, Deveau, Feola, and Sculli, who present a case of heterotopic pregnancy where diagnosis was delayed, "potentially because of lack of tachycardia associated with the hypotension"[9]. Adams and Greene report 5 cases of intraperitoneal haemorrhage in young healthy women associated with hypotension and lack of tachycardia [13]. They comment that this may delay definitive treatment by confusing the clinical picture.

Hick, Rodgerson, Heegaard, and Sterner, in a retrospective chart review of 51 cases of ectopic pregnancy, found that patients with normal vital signs had a 20% chance of having class IV blood loss at surgery, lending further support to the above patient safety concerns [23].

At first glance, it is perhaps hard to credit that our patient suffered such massive blood loss, given that her Hb on arrival was 130g/L and reached a nadir of 76g/L. However, the observed figure of 3900ml for measured blood loss is similar to predicted blood loss based on previous data. Lata et al. measured the fall in Hb/haematocrit associated with bleeding in obstetric patients [24]. Based on their data, a fall in Hb of 1g/L in obstetric patients results from every 47ml of blood loss. Our patient had a fall in Hb of 54g/L after being transfused 2 units. Given that 1 unit of red cells should increase Hb by 6g/L in a 90 kg female, the true fall in Hb is estimated at 66g/L [25]. This corresponds to a theoretical blood loss of 3100ml. However, our patient's large body habitus means that she is likely to have exhibited a smaller drop in Hb for a given volume of blood loss, raising the theoretical blood loss value for a given Hb drop further. The authors therefore believe that the observed 3900ml actual blood loss figure is likely to have been reasonably accurate.

Finally, it should not be forgotten that, in heterotopic pregnancy, maternal hypotension occurring during acute haemorrhage from rupture of the ectopic pregnancy may compromise perfusion to the intrauterine pregnancy. Färkkilä and Laitinen report a case of heterotopic pregnancy where ectopic rupture at 19 weeks' gestation led to hypotension-induced brain damage in the intrauterine fetus, resulting in elective termination of this pregnancy [26].

In conclusion, whilst tachycardia is a useful clinical sign of haemoperitoneum when present, its absence should not reassure the clinician that large-volume haemoperitoneum is not present, particularly when normocardia is coupled with relatively low blood pressure. Implications for the diagnostic and therapeutic algorithm are significant; the urgency of the need for emergency surgical intervention may be no less in a normocardic patient than in a markedly tachycardic one.

Consent

The patient has given written consent to the inclusion of material pertaining to herself. She acknowledges that she cannot be identified through the paper and that she has been fully anonymised.

References

[1] *Advanced Trauma Life Support (ATLS) Student Course Manual*, American College of Surgeons, Chicago, USA, 9th edition, 2012.

[2] M. Knight, M. Nair, D. Tuffnell, J. Shakespeare, S. Kenyon, and J. J. Kurinczuk, *Saving Lives, Improving Mothers' Care - Lessons learned to inform maternity care from the UK and Ireland Confidential Enquiries into Maternal Deaths and Morbidity 2013–15*, on behalf of MBRRACE-UK, Ed., Oxford: National Perinatal Epidemiology Unit, University of Oxford, 2017.

[3] R. W. DeVoe and J. H. Pratt, "Simultaneous intrauterine and extrauterine pregnancy," *American Journal of Obstetrics & Gynecology*, vol. 56, no. 6, pp. 1119–1126, 1948.

[4] R. Maymon and A. Shulman, "Controversies and problems in the current management of tubal pregnancy," *Human Reproduction Update*, vol. 2, no. 6, pp. 541–551, 1996.

[5] A. Habana, A. Dokras, J. L. Giraldo, and E. E. Jones, "Cornual heterotopic pregnancy: Contemporary management options," *American Journal of Obstetrics & Gynecology*, vol. 182, no. 5, pp. 1264–1270, 2000.

[6] C. M. Farquhar, "Ectopic pregnancy," *The Lancet*, vol. 366, no. 9485, pp. 583–591, 2005.

[7] D. Molloy, W. Deambrosis, D. Keeping, J. Hynes, K. Harrison, and J. Hennessey, "Multiple-sited (heterotopic) pregnancy after in vitro fertilization and gamete intrafallopian transfer," *Fertility and Sterility*, vol. 53, no. 6, pp. 1068–1071, 1990.

[8] Practice Committee of American Society for Reproductive Medicine, "Medical treatment of ectopic pregnancy: a committee opinion," *Fertility and Sterility*, vol. 100, no. 3, pp. 638–644, 2013.

[9] A. Sucov, L. Deveau, P. Feola, and L. Sculli, "Heterotopic pregnancy after in vitro fertilization," *The American Journal of Emergency Medicine*, vol. 13, no. 6, pp. 641–643, 1995.

[10] K. Talbot, R. Simpson, N. Price, and S. R. Jackson, "Heterotopic pregnancy," *Journal of Obstetrics & Gynaecology*, vol. 31, no. 1, pp. 7–12, 2011.

[11] D. Demetriades, L. S. Chan, P. Bhasin et al., "Relative bradycardia in patients with traumatic hypotension," *Journal of Trauma - Injury Infection and Critical Care*, vol. 45, no. 3, pp. 534–539, 1998.

[12] D. Thompson, S. L. Adams, and J. Barrett, "Relative bradycardia in patients with isolated penetrating abdominal trauma and isolated extremity trauma," *Annals of Emergency Medicine*, vol. 19, no. 3, pp. 268–275, 1990.

[13] S. L. Adams and J. S. Greene, "Absence of a tachycardic response to intraperitoneal hemorrhage," *The Journal of Emergency Medicine*, vol. 4, no. 5, pp. 383–389, 1986.

[14] R. P. S. Jansen, "Relative bradycardia: a sign of acute intraperitoneal bleeding," *Australian and New Zealand Journal of Obstetrics and Gynaecology*, vol. 18, no. 3, pp. 206–208, 1978.

[15] H. S. Snyder, "Lack of a tachycardic response to hypotension with ruptured ectopic pregnancy," *The American Journal of Emergency Medicine*, vol. 8, no. 1, pp. 23–26, 1990.

[16] B. Öberg and P. Thorén, "Increased activity in vagal cardiac afferents correlated to the appearance of reflex bradycardia during severe hemorrhage," *Acta Physiologica Scandinavica*, vol. 80, pp. 22-23, 1970.

[17] N. Mathlouthi, I. Ghodbane, O. Slimani et al., "Correlation between vital signs and hemoperitoneum in ruptured ectopic pregnancy," *La Tunisie Médicale*, vol. 90, no. 11, pp. 784–788, 2012.

[18] M. P. Somers, M. Spears, A. S. Maynard, and S. A. Syverud, "Ruptured heterotopic pregnancy presenting with relative bradycardia in a woman not receiving reproductive assistance," *Annals of Emergency Medicine*, vol. 43, no. 3, pp. 382–385, 2004.

[19] T. L. Cobb, "Orthostatic tachycardia and ectopic pregnancy: Normal pulse rate in the presence of massive hemorrhage," *Annals of Emergency Medicine*, vol. 11, no. 10, pp. 589-590, 1982.

[20] J. S. Vayer, J. V. Henderson, R. F. Bellamy, and A. R. Galper, "Absence of a tachycardic response to shock in penetrating intraperitoneal injury," *Annals of Emergency Medicine*, vol. 17, no. 3, pp. 227–231, 1988.

[21] E. J. Ley, A. Salim, S. Kohanzadeh, J. Mirocha, and D. R. Margulies, "Relative bradycardia in hypotensive trauma patients: A reappraisal," *Journal of Trauma - Injury Infection and Critical Care*, vol. 67, no. 5, pp. 1051–1054, 2009.

[22] M. S. Rana, U. Khalid, and S. Law, "Paradoxical bradycardia in a patient with haemorrhagic shock secondary to blunt abdominal trauma," *BMJ Case Reports*, 2010.

[23] J. L. Hick, J. D. Rodgerson, W. G. Heegaard, and S. Sterner, "Vital signs fail to correlate with hemoperitoneum from ruptured ectopic pregnancy," *The American Journal of Emergency Medicine*, vol. 19, no. 6, pp. 488–491, 2001.

[24] L. Rajoria, A. Verma, N. Hooja, S. Hemani, K. Verma, and R. Moolchandani, "Active management of third stage of labour in low resource setting: sublingual misoprostol or intramuscular oxytocin," *Indian Journal of Medical Case Reports*, vol. 2, no. 3, pp. 42–46, 2013.

[25] G. Liumbruno, F. Bennardello, A. Lattanzio, P. Piccoli, and G. Rossetti, "Recommendations for the transfusion of red blood cells," *Blood Transfusion*, vol. 7, no. 1, pp. 49–64, 2009.

[26] A. Färkkilä and L. Laitinen, "Heterotopic pregnancy during the second trimester is a severe complication of pregnancy," *Duodecim*, vol. 132, no. 8, pp. 730–733, 2016.

37

Primary Amenorrhea, Aplastic Uterus and a Functional Vagina: A Rare Case of Mayer-Rokitansky-Küster-Hauser Syndrome

Gregory W. Kirschen[1] **and Natalie Semenyuk**[2]

[1]*Medical Scientist Training Program, Stony Brook Medicine, USA*
[2]*Albert Einstein College of Medicine, Montefiore Medical Center, USA*

Correspondence should be addressed to Natalie Semenyuk; nsemenyuk@montefiore.org

Academic Editor: Kyousuke Takeuchi

Background. Müllerian agenesis, also known as Mayer-Rokitansky-Küster-Hauser syndrome (MRKHS), a failure of female urogenital development, typically results in a completely stenotic or rudimentary dimple vagina, both of which are generally nonfunctional in adulthood without mechanical dilation or surgical reconstruction. *Case.* A 20-year-old Tanner stage V heterosexual woman with normal sexual function since coitarche presented with a chief complaint of primary amenorrhea. She was found to have aplastic uterine buds, absent endometrium/cervix, normal ovaries, and an unusually well-developed lower vagina, a rare presentation of MRKHS. We discuss mechanisms by which the anomaly may have arisen. *Summary & Conclusion.* This case thus expands the clinical presentation of MRKHS to include a normal appearing vagina with intact sexual function from first sexual encounter, raising interesting questions about the basic underlying embryology.

1. Introduction

The Müllerian ducts are paired tubes abutting the urogenital ridge that give rise to the upper portion of the female reproductive tract. Failure of proper development of the upper female urogenital tract results in a wide spectrum of anatomical abnormalities of the gynecological and urological systems. Müllerian agenesis, also known as Mayer-Rokitansky-Küster-Hauser syndrome (MRKHS), represents a failure of urogenital development with an estimated incidence of 1/4500 live female births, characterized by absence or aplasia of the uterus, cervix, and/or upper vagina without or with associated urological and other organ system involvement (MRKHS type I versus type II, respectively) [1].

Depending on the particular structures affected and the severity of involvement, such abnormalities may be detected at birth or may go clinically unnoticed until there is absence of menarche or complaints of dyspareunia/sexual dysfunction with attempted sexual activity [2]. Vaginal agenesis during embryological development often leads to complete absence of the vagina if not the remnant of a small vaginal dimple in adults [2]. Here, we report an unusual case of MRKHS in an otherwise healthy, previously sexually active woman who presented at age 20 with primary amenorrhea and was found to have aplastic uterine buds, absent endometrium, and absent cervix, but with a well-developed lower vagina with intact sexual function. This case highlights a unique variant of MRKHS with a normal appearing vagina and intact sexual function without any medical or surgical intervention, expanding the clinical presentation of this condition.

Informed consent was obtained from the patient to use her medical information for this case report.

2. Case

A 20-year-old woman from Honduras presented on 3/20/2018 with her adoptive mother for a normal gynecological annual exam with a chief complaint of never having a menstrual period. She had lacked access to gynecological care in Honduras and had thus never been previously evaluated by a gynecologist. Her first sexual encounter was at age 17 and she reported having penetrative vaginal intercourse on a few occasions, although she was not currently sexually active at the time of evaluation. Previous sexual history included one

Table 1: Biochemical evidence of female phenotype.

Serum marker	Patient value (ng/mL)	Reference range (ng/mL)
Estriol	208.1	43.8—211.0 (Luteal phase)
Follicle-stimulating hormone	1.6	1.7—7.7 (Luteal phase)
Luteinizing hormone	4.8	1.0-11.4 (Luteal phase)
Testosterone (total)	27	8—48
Anti-Müllerian hormone	2.57	1.23-11.51 (females 20-25 years)

male partner, condom use for protection against sexually transmitted infections, and good sexual function. Importantly, she had never experienced poor sexual satisfaction or dyspareunia. Her known family history was limited but was significant for a cousin who had also never had a menstrual period and a maternal grandmother who had had a brain tumor of unspecified type. She took no medications, and her only allergy was penicillin, with no reaction documented. She denied tobacco or illicit drug use and used alcohol occasionally. She denied any breast lumps, masses, nipple discharge, breast pain, excessive facial/body hair, abdominal/pelvic pain, genital lesions, rashes, or pruritus.

On physical exam, her vital signs were within normal limits and her body mass index (BMI) was 25.51. She was alert and oriented and in no acute distress. Neck was without lymphadenopathy or thyromegaly. Breasts were well-developed with no masses, tenderness, or discharge, Tanner stage V. Abdomen was soft and nontender. Gynecological exam showed no lesions and normal adult female pubic hair pattern, Tanner stage V. The cervix was unable to be palpated or visualized. The uterus was notpalpable and no adnexal masses were appreciated. The vagina was normal in appearance, measured 8 cm, was two fingerbreadths in diameter, and was without bleeding or discharge. The urethra was normal in appearance. The patient was cooperative, with appropriate mood and affect.

In light of the patient's presentation, transabdominal/transvaginal ultrasound was performed on 3/22/2018, which revealed bilateral remnant uteri with no endometrium appreciated (Figure 1). The right remnant of the uterus was more prominent compared to the left. The cervix was not imaged. Follicle-containing ovaries were imaged transvaginally and transabdominally and were normal in size and appearance bilaterally, definitively excluding the presence of testes and effectively ruling out congenital androgen insensitivity syndrome (CAIS). There were no ovarian cysts or masses imaged. No fluid was appreciated in the cul de sac.

A follow-up MRI of the pelvis without and with contrast performed on 4/4/2018 demonstrated absence of the cervix, bilateral homogeneous enhancing uterine buds within the pelvis measuring 3.0 × 1.7 × 2.3 cm on right, 2.9 × 1.7 × 2.6 cm left. The upper one-third of the vagina was absent, while the lower two-thirds were present. The right ovary was of normal size, measuring 2.8 × 1.4 × 1.6 cm, and with multiple normal ovarian follicles. The left ovary was also of normal size measuring 2.1 × 1.5 × 1.9 cm, with multiple normal ovarian follicles and 1 cm left corpus luteum. Trace physiological free fluid was identified. No enlarged lymph nodes were noted. The bladder was unremarkable. The urethra was notable for 2 adjacent tiny cystic structures abutting the right posterior aspect of the external urethral meatus measuring 0.6 cm and 0.3 cm, respectively, most compatible with tiny Skene gland cysts. Together, the findings of primary amenorrhea, normal ovaries and female secondary sexual characteristics, and aplasia of the uterus with absence of the cervix and upper one-third of the vagina, were consistent with a diagnosis of MRKHS.

A subsequent biochemical analysis was performed to further support the diagnosis of MRKHS. Levels of estriol, follicle-stimulating hormone (FSH), luteinizing hormone (LH), total testosterone, and anti-Müllerian hormone (AMH) were all within normal limits, again consistent with the diagnosis of MRKHS (Table 1). The patient declined karyotype analysis due to financial limitations.

Because of the well-known association between MRKHS and anatomical abnormalities of the urological system [2], a renal ultrasound was performed on 4/20/2018, which demonstrated normal bilateral kidneys, no evidence of hydronephrosis, and no evidence of contour deforming mass or shadowing renal calculus. Bilateral ureteral jets were demonstrated on color Doppler, and no distal hydroureter was seen. Thus, our patient displayed characteristics of MRKHS type I.

Upon hearing the diagnosis, our patient was anxious, especially with regard to future reproductive prospects; however she was counseled for 45 minutes with her stepmother/guardian present regarding the implications of the diagnosis and reproductive options such as use of a surrogate to carry a pregnancy for her. She expressed gratitude at the end of the encounter for the information and services provided and was offered follow-up as needed.

Upon last follow-up (August, 2018), the patient was doing well at age 21, living with her supportive stepmother, and not sexually active.

3. Summary & Conclusion

MRKHS represents a spectrum of urogenital anomalies arising from failure of the upper female reproductive tract (Müllerian duct derivatives) to properly form during embryogenesis. In cases of MRKHS type I, patients exhibit varying degrees of congenital aplasia of the uterus and upper vagina, without extragynecological involvement and with normal secondary sexual characteristics [2]. Cases of

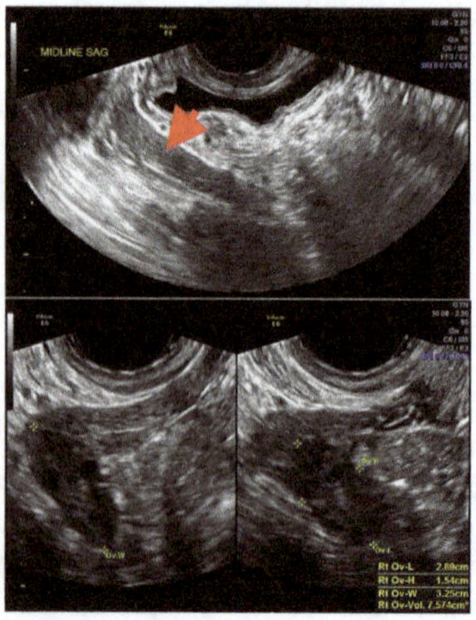

FIGURE 1: Ultrasound demonstrating bilateral aplastic left (top) and right (bottom) hemiuteri with normal-sized ovaries.

MRKHS type II involve renal, vertebral, auditory, and/or cardiac defects in addition to the aforementioned gynecological anomalies.

Regardless of subtype, the majority of patients afflicted by MRKHS exhibit vaginal aplasia, with a rudimentary vaginal dimple measuring between 1 and 4 cm that, untreated, may preclude penile-vaginal intercourse or lead to sexual dysfunction and/or dyspareunia [2–4], although not in all cases. It is important to point out that many women with MRKHS or CAIS report adequate sexual function, including penile-vaginal intercourse, at baseline, and nonsurgical or surgical approaches may be of benefit only to select candidates who experience sexual dysfunction attributable to an anatomical abnormality [5]. Likewise, a woman's actual vaginal length may be a poor surrogate for sexual experience, and practitioners should not assume that a short vaginal length implies inadequate sexual function. Rather, women may perceive that their vaginas are "too small," which may lead to psychological stress that must be addressed by the provider but which may not accurately reflect potential for satisfying sexual experience [5]. Management for those who do desire intervention is aimed at improving sexual function and ranges from nonsurgical to surgical, including serial vaginal dilation (first-line) and surgical neovagina construction (second-line) [6]. Treatment of these women must focus on psychological preparedness for sexual activity and any fears or anxiety that the women may suffer. As one of the reviewers pointed out, there are two valuable resources that practitioners taking care of patient with MRKHS should be aware of, the support group BEAUTIFUL YOU (https://www.beautifulyoumrkh.org) and Accord Alliance (https://www.accordalliance.org), an organization that lists a number of support groups for people affected by disorders of sexual development. We will counsel our patient about these resources, and we encourage others to do the same.

Here, we report a case of a woman with MRKHS with a well-formed lower vagina and satisfactory sexual function since onset of first intercourse and with a sexual history of only a handful of previous penetrative sexual encounters, whose only complaint was primary amenorrhea. One limitation of our report is that we did not have access to a vaginal length before onset of intercourse and are thus unable to state unequivocally whether sexual intercourse played a role in vaginal expansion, although we feel this possibility is less likely given her sexual history. In addition, we were unable to confirm the patient's karyotype, which would have provided further support of the diagnosis of MRKHS over CAIS, although presence of pubic hair, sonographic and MRI evidence of ovaries, and normal female hormonal profiles in the absence of a formed uterus and upper vagina all favor MRKHS (Figure 1 and Table 1). Nevertheless, clinical features and imaging, particularly MRI, which was also obtained in this case, are sufficient to make the diagnosis of MRKHS [7]. However, in equivocal cases unlike ours, a karyotype should be obtained to confirm the diagnosis.

In any case, we hypothesize that in our patient's case, the urogenital sinus, responsible for giving rise to the lower two-thirds of the vagina, may have undergone unusually extensive proliferation during the 4th and 5th months of embryonic life, giving rise to a more elongated and well-canalized vagina than what would typically develop. This could compensate for the contraction and stenosis that would otherwise occur in the face of an aplastic upper vagina (uterovaginal primordium). While most cases of MRKHS are sporadic, a subgroup of patients has been shown to harbor mutations in *WNT* family genes [8]. Given the well-established role of WNT signaling in cellular proliferation, dysregulation of this pathway in our patient may have contributed to her phenotype, although this remains unknown at present. One historical feature consistent with a genetic cause of MRKHS is the patient's relative who also exhibited primary amenorrhea. However, further evaluation and work-up would have been necessary to confirm the diagnosis in her relative, and genetic testing of either of these women could potentially reveal an underlying polymorphism or mutation (though this can be costly).

As an alternative explanation, our patient may have undergone a more prolonged period of lower vaginal growth during embryogenesis than typically occurs, compensating for upper reproductive tract aplasia. The normal resting adult human vagina is known to vary in linear length of ~40-100 mm, although the precise genetic or environmental factors determining this final length remain to be completely understood [9]. Perhaps cases like the one we present will serve to spark new interest in revisiting the complex embryological processes underlying female reproductive tract development.

In summary, here we present an atypical case of MRKHS with a well-developed lower vagina in the absence of a cervix and aplastic uterine buds, in a sexually active woman with no sexual dysfunction. This case demonstrates that vaginal agenesis/dimpling and poor sexual function are not requisite features of MRKHS, providing evidence that contradicts traditional views of Müllerian development.

Abbreviations

MRKHS: Mayer-Rokitansky-Küster-Hauser syndrome
MRI: Magnetic resonance imaging.

Acknowledgments

The work was supported by National Institutes of Health (NIH) Grant 1F30MH110103 (to GWK). Albert Einstein College of Medicine, Montefiore Medical Center is covering the cost of the publication.

References

[1] M. Folch, I. Pigem, and J. C. Konje, "Mullerian agenesis: Etiology, diagnosis, and management," *Obstetrical & Gynecological Survey* , vol. 55, no. 10, pp. 644–649, 2000.

[2] K. Morcel and L. Camborieux, "Programme de Recherches sur les Aplasies," *Orphanet Journal of Rare Diseases*, vol. 2, p. 13, 2007.

[3] E. Bean, T. Mazur, and A. Robinson, "Mayer-Rokitansky-Küster-Hauser Syndrome: Sexuality, Psychological Effects, and Quality of Life," *Journal of Pediatric & Adolescent Gynecology*, vol. 22, no. 6, pp. 339–346, 2009.

[4] J.-L. Brun, G. Belleannée, N. Grafeille, A.-F. Aslan, and G. H. Brun, "Long-term results after neovagina creation in Mayer-Rokitanski-Kuster-Hauser syndrome by Vecchietti's operation," *European Journal of Obstetrics & Gynecology and Reproductive Biology*, vol. 103, no. 2, pp. 168–172, 2002.

[5] J. Dear, S. M. Creighton, G. S. Conway, L. Williams, and L. M. Liao, "Sexual experience before treatment for vaginal agenesis: a retrospective review of 137 women," *Journal of Pediatric and Adolescent Gynecology*, 2018.

[6] N. Callens, G. De Cuypere, P. De Sutter et al., "An update on surgical and non-surgical treatments for vaginal hypoplasia," *Human Reproduction Update*, vol. 20, no. 5, pp. 775–801, 2014.

[7] M. Govindarajan, R. S. Rajan, A. Kalyanpur, and Ravikumar, "Magnetic resonance imaging diagnosis of Mayer-Rokitansky-Kuster-Hauser syndrome," *Journal of Human Reproductive Sciences*, vol. 1, no. 2, pp. 83–85, 2008.

[8] S. Ledig and P. Wieacker, "Clinical and genetic aspects of Mayer–Rokitansky–Küster–Hauser syndrome," *medizinische genetik*, vol. 30, no. 1, pp. 3–11, 2018.

[9] K. T. Barnhart, A. Izquierdo, E. S. Pretorius, D. M. Shera, M. Shabbout, and A. Shaunik, "Baseline dimensions of the human vagina," *Human Reproduction*, vol. 21, no. 6, pp. 1618–1622, 2006.

The Sigmoidal Pregnancy: A Rare Entity Complicated by an Inappropriate Medical Intervention

Antoine Naem,[1] **Baraa Ahmad**,[1,2] **and Bashar Al-Kurdy**[1,2]

[1]*Faculty of Medicine of Damascus University, Damascus, Syria*
[2]*University Hospital of Obstetrics and Gynecology of Damascus, Damascus, Syria*

Correspondence should be addressed to Antoine Naem; antoine.naem@gmail.com

Academic Editor: Loïc Sentilhes

The abdominal ectopic pregnancy is very rare and accounts for less than 1% of all ectopic gestations. Due to the lack of clinical suspicion, many obstetricians confuse it with other diseases and manage it inappropriately. Here, we are reporting the case of a 41-year-old woman that was referred to our hospital because of severe vaginal bleeding caused by multiple uterine perforations during the dilatation and curettage. Her medical history was significant for constipation and a misdiagnosis of incomplete abortion. Upon the surgical exploration, a big amount of blood clots was taken out, and a fetus with his placenta inserted into the sigmoid colon were observed. The uterus and the sigmoid colon were resected. Ultimately, the patient recovered uneventfully. To the best of our knowledge, this is the third case of pure sigmoidal pregnancy and the first one to reach an advanced gestational age.

1. Introduction

The abdominal pregnancy is a rare form of ectopic gestations which occurs once in 10,000 live births [1] and accounts for less than 1% of ectopic pregnancies [2]. It is defined by the placental implantation into the peritoneal cavity, excluding the fallopian tubes, ovaries, and the interligamentous space. Primary abdominal pregnancy refers to the direct implantation of the fertilized ovum into the parietal or visceral peritoneum without previous attachments to the reproductive tract. Whereas the secondary abdominal pregnancy is the result of tubal abortion or the rupture of an intrauterine pregnancy into the peritoneal cavity. In general, the most common site of ectopic pregnancies is the fallopian tube as it accounts for 97% of the ectopic localizations. However, the posterior cul-de-sac seems to be the most common site of the primary abdominal pregnancy [2]. The ectopic pregnancy is a serious obstetric emergency that requires special medical attention as its maternal mortality rates can reach 20% [3]. The high mortalities could be attributed to the intensive hemorrhage provoked by separating the placental tissue from its insertion [4]. The variety of unspecific symptoms often hardens the diagnosis. The patients' complains usually range from acute abdominal pain and vaginal bleeding to mild pain and breast discomfort [5]. The diagnostic key of the abdominal pregnancy is the high clinical suspicion at the first place. In addition, the correlation between β-HCG levels and the radiologic imaging methods is crucial to achieve the diagnosis. Here, we present a rare case of a sigmoidal abdominal pregnancy that was misdiagnosed previously as incomplete abortion and complicated by several iatrogenic uterine perforations. To the best of our knowledge, this is the third sigmoidal pregnancy in literature and the first to reach 18 weeks of gestational age.

2. Case Presentation

A 41-year-old G1P0 woman was referred to the emergency department of our hospital because of severe vaginal bleeding. As the patient was unconscious, her medical history was taken from her accompanying sister. The patient's history was significant for 18 weeks of amenorrhea and positive pregnancy tests, in addition to constipation and a misdiagnosis of incomplete abortion. As a result of the wrong diagnosis, an external obstetrician performed a dilatation and curettage (D&C) that ended up in perforating the uterus. Upon the

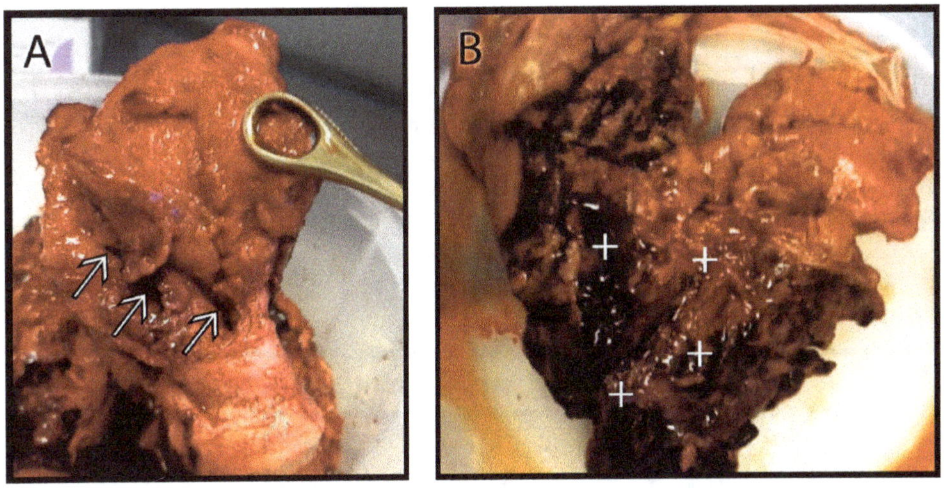

(a) (b)

FIGURE 1: (a) The resected uterus. Note the large perforations on its right wall (white arrows). (b) The resected sigmoid colon with the placental insertion (+). Note the aggressive placental invasion of the sigmoid colon provoking severe malformation.

clinical examination, the patient looked pale, her pulse was weak, her heart rate was 140 beats per minute, and her blood pressure was 80/40 mmHg. The transabdominal ultrasonography showed an empty heteromorphic uterus and excessive amount of free intra-abdominal fluid. Therefore the diagnosis of a perforated uterus was confirmed, and a ruptured ectopic pregnancy was suspected. The patient was moved immediately to the operating room to perform an emergent exploratory laparotomy and resuscitated with 6 full-blood units and 5 plasma units. A Pfannenstiel incision was made; the abdominal muscles and fascia were dissected. Upon reaching the peritoneal cavity, a big amount of blood clots was taken out and a fetus with his placenta inserted exclusively into the sigmoid colon were observed. The uterus was perforated in different locations on the contralateral side of the placental insertion. In addition, ileal and appendicular injuries were also observed. So the diagnosis of an abdominal pregnancy was achieved intraoperatively. The fetus was taken out, and the internal iliac arteries were ligated to reduce the hemorrhage. A hysterectomy was done due to the multiple large defects of the uterine wall. Regarding the wide placental insertion on the sigmoid colon and the potential risk of inducing additional hemorrhage by dissecting it, a sigmoidectomy was considered as the ultimate management. Therefore, the incision was dilated longitudinally superior to the umbilicus, and the sigmoid colon was resected (Figure 1). The descending colon was isolated, and a skin colostomy was made.

Finally, the intestinal injury was repaired before skin closure. The operation lasted for 7 hours. The patient's vital signs returned to their normal limits after the surgery and she was stable during the eight days of follow-up. The pathologic examination of the resected specimen showed the presence of normal chorionic villi invading the sigmoid wall (Figure 2). However, due to the D&C, the endometrium was not fully evident when the uterus was examined microscopically. The endometrial remnants showed Arias-Stella reaction in the endometrial glands.

3. Discussion

The abdominal pregnancy occurs when the conceptus implants within the peritoneal cavity far from the ovaries, fallopian tubes, and the interligamentous space. The fertilized ovum seems to be able to implant exclusively into the parietal or visceral peritoneum and occasionally into islands of endometriosis [6]. The abdominal ectopic pregnancy is subdivided into primary and secondary. Primary abdominal pregnancy happens when the blastocyst implants directly into the peritoneal cavity without previous attachments to the uterus or fallopian tubes. While secondary abdominal pregnancy is the result of tubal abortion or the rupture of an intrauterine pregnancy with subsequent implantation in the abdomen. In 1942, Studdiford created three criteria to differentiate between these two types of pregnancy, which are "1) The two ovaries and tubes are normal without any evidence of recent or remote tubal injury. 2) The absence of any evidence of a uteroperitoneal fistula. 3) The presence of a pregnancy related exclusively to the peritoneal surface and early enough to eliminate the possibility of primary tubal nidation" [7]. Obviously, diagnosing the primary abdominal pregnancy using the mentioned criteria is based on eliminating any chance of a previous tubal or ovarian pregnancy. However, these criteria still have its limitations in categorizing the abdominal pregnancies. As noticed, the first two criteria tend to determine the uterine and tubal validity through gross inspection. The macroscopic examination carries a low diagnostic value because it might fail to detect a precedent primary tubal nidation. In addition, the microscopic evidence of a primary tubal pregnancy even when the tube appeared normal grossly was reported in the literature [6]. Therefore, the most confident way to investigate the tubal and uterine validity is the pathologic examination. However, this is not fully accepted recently, because the general intentions are now tending to preserve the maternal fertility when possible; making the uterus and tubes unavailable for the pathologic examination.

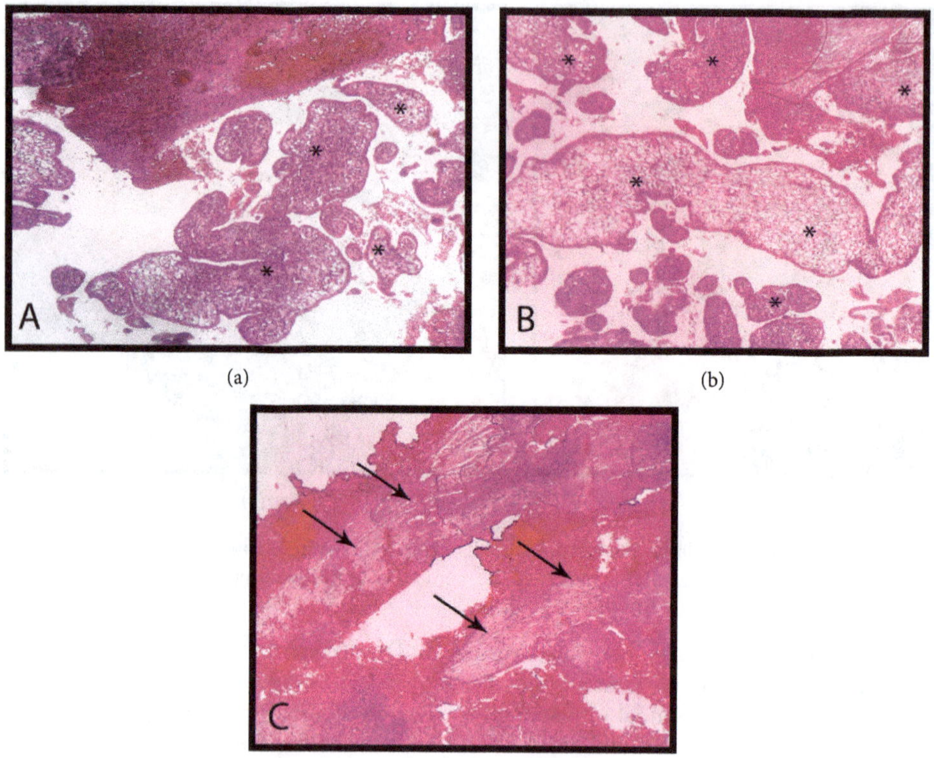

(a) (b) (c)

Figure 2: The pathologic appearance of the resected specimen stained in hematoxylin and eosin. (a, b) Chorionic villi (*) invading the sigmoid wall. (c) The intensive hemorrhage within the sigmoid wall between its smooth muscle layers (arrows) that was provoked by the ectopic placental insertion.

Another limitation of the Studdiford criteria is the unreliability of the gestational age to differentiate between primary and secondary abdominal pregnancies. When the ovum starts its mitotic activity, its nutritional requirements increase. Therefore, losing the placental blood supply by the separation of the developing placenta may harm the embryo and lead to its death, which is inconvenient with achieving a secondary abdominal implantation [8]. On this basis, we suggest that the secondary implantation after complete tubal abortion should happen also at an early gestational age and that contradicts the third criterion of Studdiford. Some authors considered the retention of the placental blood supply in the incomplete abortion an important survival factor for achieving a secondary implantation [6]. By taking the previous reasons in consideration, excluding the tubal abortion upon investigating its three forms that were described by Caspi and Sherman is highly recommended for categorizing the abdominal pregnancies [8]. In our case, we could not confirm the pregnancy type as we were unable to isolate the fallopian tubes due to the intense adhesions that were found within the abdomen.

The most common locations of the abdominal pregnancy are the posterior cul-de-sac, the mesosalpinx, and the omentum [2]. In fact, there are several reasons that make the sigmoid colon an elected implantation site, such as its intraperitoneal localization and the presence of the sigmoid mesocolon that may be prolonged in some patients making it closer to the ovaries. However, the small number of sigmoidal pregnancies could be explained by the relatively low vasculature of the sigmoid colon that may not meet the conceptus nutritional needs. Interestingly, altered defecating habits like increased defecating frequency [9] or constipation [10, 11] were noted to be exclusive to the abdominal pregnancy where chorionic villi invade the sigmoidal wall. This could be explained either by the inflammatory irritation caused by the implantation that increases the bowel motility or by damaging the myenteric plexus (Auerbachian plexus) causing localized ileus and a subsequent bowel obstruction. Therefore, these symptoms may refer to a sigmoidal pregnancy in patients with ectopic pregnancy of unknown location.

However, the high correlation between radiologic imaging methods and the laboratory pregnancy test is crucial to diagnose the abdominal pregnancy. In general, transvaginal ultrasonography and transabdominal ultrasonography are the most favorable initial imaging techniques [12]. When the β-HCG serum levels are elevated, with the presence of an empty uterus and adnexa, a pan-abdominal ultrasonographic scan is advisable. Occasionally, the computed tomography scan could be also used. In emergent cases, the presence of an empty uterus with free intra-abdominal fluid, accompanied by amenorrhea or elevated β-HCG serum levels above the discriminating zone, is a great indication of performing an exploratory laparotomy. Whether it is laparoscopy or laparotomy depends on the surgeon's experience and patient's stability. It is noteworthy that the negativity of the β-HCG test cannot exclude the diagnosis because more than 1% of the ectopic pregnancies may not have elevated β-HCG levels [13].

As the massive bleeding from the implantation site remains the major cause of maternal death [4], many authors have applied impressive hemostatic techniques to control the hemorrhage. The electric cauterization is a simple method to control the hemorrhage, but thermal injury could be provoked to the adjacent organs when the placental insertion is vast. Therefore, at early pregnancy, the vasopressin injection within and around the gestational sac is a good technique to minimize the hemorrhage after resecting the conceptus [14]. Whereas at advanced stages, applying the gelatin-thrombin matrix [15] is more suitable because it avoids the side effects that might be caused by the high dosage of the injected vasopressin. However, the early detection of the sigmoidal pregnancy minimizes the risks of the surgical procedure, and the gestational sac could be removed more easily using the traditional surgical methods [9, 11].

4. Conclusion

The primary abdominal pregnancy is a rare clinical finding that may be encountered once in a lifetime, but when it's encountered, it should be dealt with firmly. Although the majority of patients present with unspecific symptoms, the altered defecating habits like constipation may hide a sigmoidal pregnancy behind. The good correlation between the ultrasonographic findings and the β-HCG levels is crucial to achieve the diagnosis. However, the entire abdomen should be scaned by either ultrasonography or computed tomography scan. The management should be minimally invasive and well planned in order to prevent the massive hemorrhage that may cost the patient her life. In emergencies, performing an exploratory laparotomy or laparoscopy combined with less traumatic hemostatic technique is favorable. Finally, when the D&C is needed, it should be delayed until the patient is stable again.

Abbreviations

D&C: Dilatation and curettage
β-HCG: Beta subunit of the human chorionic gonadotropin.

Consent

Written patient consent was taken before reporting her case.

Acknowledgments

We would like to thank Dr. Abdallah Mohammad and Dr. Alia Al-Aitouni for providing the pathologic reports and images.

References

[1] H. K. Atrash, A. Friede, and C. J. Hogue, "Abdominal pregnancy in the United States: frequency and maternal mortality," *Obstetrics and Gynecology*, vol. 69, 3 Part 1, pp. 333–337, 1987.

[2] D. L. Fylstra, "Ectopic pregnancy not within the (distal) fallopian tube: etiology, diagnosis, and treatment," *American Journal of Obstetrics and Gynecology*, vol. 206, no. 4, pp. 289–299, 2012.

[3] C. Patel, J. Feldman, and C. Ogedegbe, "Complicated abdominal pregnancy with placenta feeding off sacral plexus and subsequent multiple ectopic pregnancies during a 4-year follow-up: a case report," *Journal of Medical Case Reports*, vol. 10, no. 1, 2016.

[4] R. Yildizhan, A. Kolusari, F. Adali et al., "Primary abdominal ectopic pregnancy: a case report," *Cases Journal*, vol. 2, no. 1, p. 8485, 2009.

[5] L. Wu, X. Jiang, and J. Ni, "Successful diagnosis and treatment of early splenic ectopic pregnancy: a case report," *Medicine (Baltimore)*, vol. 97, no. 17, article e0466, 2018.

[6] D. Cavanagh, "Primary peritoneal pregnancy; rationalization or established entity? Omental transference as an alternative explanation," *American Journal of Obstetrics and Gynecology*, vol. 76, no. 3, pp. 523–532, 1958.

[7] W. E. Studdiford, "Primary peritoneal pregnancy," *American Journal of Obstetrics and Gynecology*, vol. 44, no. 3, pp. 487–491, 1942.

[8] E. Caspi and D. Sherman, "Tubal abortion and infundibular ectopic pregnancy," *Clinical Obstetrics and Gynecology*, vol. 30, no. 1, pp. 155–163, 1987.

[9] S. Dubey, M. Satodiya, P. Garg, and M. Rani, "Primary abdominal pregnancy: a case report," *Journal of Clinical and DiagnostiC Research*, vol. 10, no. 11, pp. Qd04–QD06, 2016.

[10] I. S. S. Sarr, M. Faye, P. M. Faye, M. Seck, O. Ka, and M. Dieng, "Acute intestinal occlusion revealing abdominal pregnancy: a case study," *The Pan African Medical Journal*, vol. 31, p. 155, 2018.

[11] P. Ganeshselvi, D. Cherian, S. Champ, and N. Myerson, "Primary abdominal pregnancy implanted on the sigmoid colon," *Journal of Obstetrics and Gynaecology*, vol. 23, no. 6, p. 667, 2003.

[12] J. M. Cohen, J. C. Weinreb, T. W. Lowe, and C. Brown, "MR imaging of a viable full-term abdominal pregnancy," *AJR. American Journal of Roentgenology*, vol. 145, no. 2, pp. 407-408, 1985.

[13] E. Wong and S. O. Suat, "Ectopic pregnancy–a diagnostic challenge in the emergency department," *European Journal of Emergency Medicine*, vol. 7, no. 3, pp. 189–194, 2000.

[14] K. Hishikawa, T. Fukuda, H. Inoue et al., "Laparoscopic management of abdominal pregnancy with local injection of vasopressin solution: a case report," *American Journal of Case Reports*, vol. 17, pp. 637–640, 2016.

[15] R. Watrowski, A. Lange, and J. Mockel, "Primary omental pregnancy with secondary implantation into posterior cul-de-sac: laparoscopic treatment using hemostatic matrix," *Journal of Minimally Invasive Gynecology*, vol. 22, no. 3, p. 501, 2015.

Uterine Rupture on MRI Presenting as Nonspecific Abdominal Pain in a Primigravid Patient with 28-Week Twins Resulting in Normal Neurodevelopmental Outcomes at Age Two

Kathryn L. Ponder, Rosa Won, and Laurel Clymer

John Muir Medical Center, Walnut Creek, CA 94598, USA

Correspondence should be addressed to Kathryn L. Ponder; kathryn.ponder_md@johnmuirhealth.com

Academic Editor: Akihide Ohkuchi

Background. Uterine rupture is a rare occurrence that requires a high index of suspicion, particularly in a primigravid patient who presents prior to the onset of labor. Mortality rates are particularly high in primigravid patients. *Case.* A 36-year-old gravida 1, para 0 patient with dichorionic diamniotic twins presented at 28-weeks of gestation with abdominal pain. The pain was initially intermittent and felt to be musculoskeletal in origin. Ultrasound imaging after 3 days of worsening abdominal pain revealed extrauterine fluid, prompting an urgent MRI. MRI diagnosed the uterine rupture with hemoperitoneum and herniation of both amniotic sacs outside of the uterus, including one twin's torso and extremities, prompting emergency cesarean section. The premature twins required 2-month hospitalizations and had no neurodevelopmental impairments at 2-year follow-up. *Conclusion.* We present a unique case of rupture of an unscarred uterus in a primigravid patient prior to the onset of labor. Multiple gestation is a risk factor. This report adds to a handful of cases in which a history of endometriosis or extrauterine pelvic surgery was also present. The use of ultrasound and MRI to evaluate nonspecific abdominal pain led to the diagnosis and survival of both the mother and her premature twins.

1. Introduction

Uterine rupture is a rare occurrence (3-5.9 per 10,000 pregnancies) that requires a high index of suspicion, particularly in a primigravid patient who presents with nonspecific symptoms prior to the onset of labor [1, 2]. Here we discuss a primigravid patient with a history of endometriosis and extrauterine pelvic surgery presenting with abdominal pain in the setting of a dichorionic diamniotic twin pregnancy at 28 weeks of gestation. The patient's nonspecific symptoms and normal laboratory studies may have led to an initial delay in diagnosis; however, persistent symptoms and ultrasound imaging revealed a clue of extrauterine fluid, which prompted a stat MRI, diagnosis, and emergent intervention. This case demonstrates a rare presentation, occurring in an unscarred uterus and prior to the onset of labor. Between 3.1 and 12.9% of uterine ruptures in developed countries occur in an unscarred uterus (i.e., no history of cesarean section or hysterotomy) [2, 3]. Spontaneous uterine rupture in an unscarred uterus that occurs prior to the onset of labor is even rarer, representing only 13.6-16% of spontaneous cases [2, 4] and representing only 1.9% (4 out of 208 cases) [2] to 6.4% (3 out of 47 cases) [4] of all cases of uterine rupture. Maternal and perinatal mortality rates are particularly high in primigravid patients with spontaneous rupture compared to multigravid patients with a history of cesarean section [1–8].

Despite herniation of both intact amniotic sacs including the body of one twin into the peritoneal cavity, the patient and the resulting 28-week infants survived and did well. The infants were discharged after a 2-month hospitalization. They were evaluated in the High Risk Infant Follow-Up Clinic after discharge and had no neurodevelopmental impairments on the Bayley Scales of Infant and Toddler Development (Third Edition) and medical evaluation at 2 years of age. In this case, a high index of suspicion and the use of ultrasound and MRI to evaluate nonspecific abdominal pain resulted in the unique outcome of normal neurodevelopment in premature twins after uterine rupture.

2. Case Presentation

The patient was a 36-year-old U.S.-born woman of Indian ethnicity and high education level with a past medical history notable for endometriosis. Her surgical history was notable for 2 pelvic surgeries in the 2 years prior to her pregnancy. First she underwent removal of a large ovarian cyst, which began as a laparoscopy but converted to a laparotomy due to intestinal adhesions to the ovary and bleeding. The second procedure was a laparoscopic tubal ligation in the setting of hydrosalpinx that was uncomplicated. Sites of endometriosis and intestinal adhesions were noted intraoperatively but were not lysed at that time. She had no history of uterine surgery or dilation and curettage. Dichorionic diamniotic twins were conceived via in vitro fertilization (IVF), which involved uterine manipulation to the extent of an embryo transfer. At 13 weeks of gestation, she had a pulmonary embolus for which she was on enoxaparin sodium 80 mg subcutaneously twice a day. She had normal prenatal labs.

She was a gravida 1, para 0, at 28 weeks of gestation at the time of presentation. Three days prior to delivery she noted the new onset of left-sided abdominal pain described as intense "pressure." This initially subsided and then recurred the following day. One day prior to delivery she presented to triage of the Labor and Delivery floor with a chief complaint of worsening left-sided abdominal pain. She rated the pain as 9 out of 10 and described it as "sharp, shooting, spasm" in nature, from the left side of her rib cage down to her hip. The pain improved after a dose of hydrocodone-acetaminophen. She rated her pain as 6 out of 10 about 1 hour later. Complete blood count (CBC), electrolytes, and an AmniSure test were evaluated. The CBC showed a white blood cell count of $16.8 \times 10^{\wedge}3/\mu L$ (81% neutrophils, 14.7% lymphocytes), hemoglobin 10.4 g/dL, hematocrit 31.4%, and platelet count $215{,}000/\mu L$. Her glucose was 129 and albumin 2.7 with an otherwise normal electrolyte panel and liver function tests. A point of care AmniSure test for rupture of membranes was negative for amniotic fluid. Her other prenatal labs were all previously normal and she had no history of drug abuse. Vital signs were as follows: temperature 36.6°C, mild tachycardia with a heart rate of 120 beats per minute, respiratory rate 18-20, blood pressure 119/59, and SpO2 96-100%. The pain was felt to be most likely musculoskeletal in origin. She was sent home with a plan to follow up in the perinatologist's clinic the following morning at an appointment that had been previously scheduled.

In the perinatologist's office the following morning, she noted worsening abdominal pain. An ultrasound was performed, which showed an extrauterine fluid collection in the peritoneal cavity. She was given a dose of betamethasone and sent to the emergency department for a stat MRI of the abdomen and pelvis. In the emergency department her exam was notable for abdominal tenderness to palpation and guarding. She was otherwise alert and oriented with the following vital signs: temperature 37°C, heart rate 127 beats per minute, respiratory rate 20, and blood pressure 123/81. Fetal heart tracings were noted to be normal for age with moderate variability. No uterine contractions were present. She received a dose of IV morphine and IV fluids.

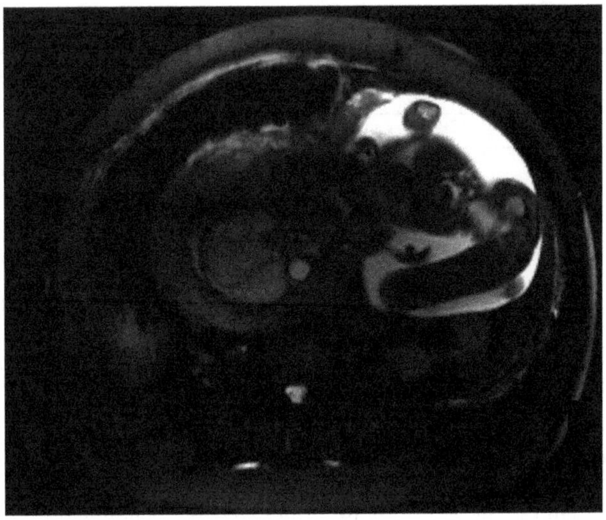

FIGURE 1: Lower portion of one fetus protruding out of the posterior aspect of the uterine fundus into the peritoneal cavity.

MRI of the abdomen and pelvis revealed a large defect within the left uterine wall with herniation of the body and extremities of one of the twins through the herniated defect. The head remained within the uterine cavity. A large portion of the intact amniotic sac of the second twin was also herniated through the uterine defect. There was moderate hemoperitoneum (Figure 1). Blood products were ordered in preparation for cesarean section. Her hemoglobin and hematocrit had decreased to 9 g/dL and 27.9% at the time of admission to the Labor and Delivery floor and 2 hours later, just prior to surgery, had decreased further to 8.2 g/dL and 25.1%.

2.1. Intervention. After imaging confirmation, the patient underwent emergency exploratory laparotomy and cesarean section through the uterine rupture at 28 weeks and 3 days of gestation. She received a 4 gram magnesium sulfate bolus for fetal neuroprotection and a dose of cefazolin at the start of the cesarean section. Intraoperatively, when the omentum was moved out of the way, an old blood clot was noted in the left upper side of the abdomen. The blood clot was removed and the amniotic sac was seen protruding into the peritoneal cavity from the site of the uterine rupture which was left lateral and cornual. The amniotic sac was ruptured and clear fluid was noted. The other twin's membrane was then seen and ruptured, again with clear fluid and delivered breech without difficulty, as the obstetrics team felt she could be delivered most quickly. Her cord was milked for autotransfusion of cord blood, clamped, and handed to the neonatology team. The second twin was immediately felt for. Her feet were grasped, the baby was delivered to the level of both scapulae, and the arms were sequentially swept across the chest. The fetal head was delivered via the Mauriceau–Smellie–Veit

Table 1: Bayley Scales of Infant and Toddler Development (Third Edition) Composite Scores at 2-year follow-up. Composite Scores classify whether the child's overall development is within the average range. The average range is considered to be 90 to 109.

	Subtest	Score	Range	Classification
Twin A				
	Cognitive	120	110-126	Superior
	Language	118	110-124	High Average
	Motor	103	95-110	Average
Twin B				
	Cognitive	120	110-126	Superior
	Language	138	128-143	Very Superior
	Motor	115	106-121	High Average

maneuver. The cord was milked for autotransfusion of cord blood and clamped, and she was handed to the awaiting neonatal resuscitation team. The placenta was delivered via massage. Pitocin was added to the IV fluids once the placenta was delivered. The uterus was cleared of all clots and debris with a moist laparotomy sponge. The uterine rupture site was closed with #1 Chromic suture in running-locked fashion. A second layer was also used to close the uterus with #1-0 Chromic suture in an imbricating fashion. One additional suture was required for another layer of closure. Two box stitches were needed for hemostasis. Excellent hemostasis was noted. There were adhesions of the bowel and bladder to the uterus which were not lysed given the complexity of the adhesions. The gutter and peritoneal cavity were copiously irrigated. Floseal was applied to the uterine closure. There was an estimated blood loss of 1000 mL during the procedure. The patient received 1000 mL of intravenous fluid and a unit of fresh frozen plasma intraoperatively.

2.2. Maternal Outcome. The patient remained in stable condition postoperatively. The postoperative course was complicated by anemia: several hours later on post-op day #1, her hemoglobin was as low as 6.3 g/dL, with a hematocrit of 19.3%, for which she received 2 units of packed red blood cells with normalization thereafter. She was placed on unfractionated heparin postoperatively due to her history of pulmonary embolism. She was discharged on postoperative day #3 on enoxaparin sodium 80 mg twice a day. Outpatient genetics consultation was obtained. Sequencing and deletion/duplication analysis of the COL3A1 gene was sent to evaluate for vascular Ehlers-Danlos Syndrome (type IV), which is associated with organ rupture, and was negative. Ultimately it was felt that the twin gestation may have placed her at higher risk as opposed to an underlying genetic condition.

2.3. Twin A Neonatal Course and Outcome. Twin A was a female with a birthweight of 1140 grams. She required 4 minutes of positive pressure ventilation (PPV) and then transitioned to Continuous Positive Airway Pressure (CPAP) with an Apgar score of 2 at 1 minute and 8 at 5 minutes. A capillary blood gas around 1 hour of life had a pH 7.31/pCO2 38.1/bicarb 18.7/ base deficit -6.4. She had Respiratory Distress Syndrome (RDS) and required nasal respiratory support for 2 weeks, but did not require oxygen support after that time. She was treated with caffeine for apnea of prematurity. A blood culture drawn at admission remained negative. She had a very small patent ductus arteriosus (PDA) on echocardiogram that remained until discharge. Head ultrasounds on day of life 9 and at 6 weeks of age were normal for age. She passed her newborn hearing screen. Her retinas were immature at the time of discharge, and noted to be mature at outpatient follow-up with no Retinopathy of Prematurity (ROP). She was hospitalized for 56 days and discharged at 36 weeks and 2 days adjusted age.

After her Neonatal Intensive Care Unit (NICU) discharge, she followed up with the cardiology clinic. A tiny PDA was still present on echocardiogram at 1 year of age, which did not require surgical correction. She followed up with the ophthalmology clinic annually for routine evaluations with normal vision. At 19 months adjusted age (21 months chronological age) she demonstrated typical development on the Clinical Linguistic and Auditory Milestone Scale (CLAMS) and the Cognitive Adaptive Test (CAT) of the Capute Scales. Her fine and gross motor skills were in a typical range for her adjusted age. At 26 months of age she was evaluated with the Bayley Scales of Infant and Toddler Development (Third Edition). She demonstrated "Above Average" Scaled Scores on the cognitive, expressive language, and receptive language portions and "Average" Scaled Scores for both gross motor and fine motor skills. Her Composite Scores were classified as "Superior" for cognition, "High Average" for language, and "Average" for motor skills (Table 1).

2.4. Twin B Neonatal Course and Outcome. Twin B was a female with a birthweight of 1115 grams. She required 7 minutes of PPV and then transitioned to CPAP in the delivery room with Apgar scores of 3 at 1 minute and 7 at 5 minutes. A capillary blood gas at 1 hour of life had a pH 7.33/pCO2 38/bicarb 19.7/base deficit -5.2. Her neonatal course was complicated by RDS, apnea of prematurity, and supraventricular tachycardia (SVT). She required intubation for 1 day with surfactant administration for RDS and then nasal respiratory support for 2 weeks. She was treated with caffeine for apnea of prematurity. A blood culture drawn at admission remained negative. She had 2 episodes of A-V reentrant SVT in the first week of life and another at 4 weeks of life, prompting cardiology consultation and digoxin treatment with no recurrent episodes. A head ultrasound on day of life 9 showed a tiny left choroid plexus cyst, a normal variant. A screening head ultrasound at 8 weeks of age showed resolution of the left choroid plexus cyst and new right choroid plexus cysts, also thought to be normal variants. There was no intraventricular or parenchymal hemorrhage and there was normal appearing periventricular white matter, consistent with a normal head ultrasound for her age. She passed her newborn hearing screen. Her retinas were immature at the time of discharge and noted to be mature at outpatient follow-up with no ROP. She was hospitalized for 60 days and discharged at 36 weeks and 6 days adjusted age.

After her NICU discharge, she followed up with the cardiology clinic with no recurrence of SVT. Digoxin was discontinued at 6 months of age. A small, hemodynamically insignificant PDA was still present but did not require surgical intervention. She followed up with the ophthalmology clinic annually for routine evaluations with normal vision. She followed up with feeding therapists and the gastroenterology clinic due to difficulty with feeding (emesis, oral aversion, and delayed gastric emptying). She was able to support her nutrition and growth with oral feedings and did not require a post-discharge feeding tube. Symptoms were improved by 2 years of age. At 19 months adjusted age (21 months chronological age) she demonstrated typical development on the CLAMS and the CAT of the Capute Scales. Her fine and gross motor skills were also in a typical range for her adjusted age. At 27 months of age she was evaluated with the Bayley Scales of Infant and Toddler Development (Third Edition). She demonstrated "Above Average" Scaled Scores on the cognitive, expressive language, receptive language, and fine motor portions and an "Average" Scaled Score for gross motor skills. Her Composite Scores were classified as "Superior" for cognition, "Very Superior" for language, and "High Average" for motor skills (Table 1).

3. Discussion

There are 3 major categories of uterine rupture: (1) presence of a uterine scar (history of cesarean section or hysterotomy), (2) trauma to an unscarred uterus (breech extraction, forceps, oxytocin, fundal pressure, and shoulder dystocia), and (3) spontaneous rupture of an unscarred uterus [4]. Most cases of uterine rupture in developed countries fall into the first category, which occur in the setting of a uterine scar. Only 3.1-12.9% of cases in developed countries fall into the second and third categories, which occur in the setting of an unscarred, intact uterus [2, 3]. This is in contrast to countries characterized as "less and least developed" by the United Nations, where most cases occur in an unscarred uterus [1]. Cases may be further subdivided based on whether they occur before or after the onset of labor. Uterine rupture that occurs both spontaneously and prior to the onset of labor is very rare, contributing to only 1.9-6.4% of uterine rupture cases overall [2, 4].

While both are rare, the spontaneous and traumatic types involving an unscarred uterus are associated with more catastrophic outcomes as far as maternal and perinatal morbidity and mortality [1, 2, 4]. Despite its rarity, uterine rupture accounts for about 5% of maternal deaths in the United States [4]. The risks of maternal hemorrhage requiring transfusion, intensive care unit admission, and hysterectomy are higher with an unscarred uterine rupture as compared to a uterine scar rupture [2]. Perinatal mortality rates associated with uterine rupture in less and least developed countries range from 74 to 92% [1], whereas rates of 8.7 to 11.7% are reported for developed countries [2, 3]. The risk of perinatal death is 3.8 times higher in the setting of an unscarred uterine rupture compared to a uterine scar rupture [2]. Population-based studies in more developed countries estimate that the incidence of uterine rupture is about 3 to 5.9 per 10,000 deliveries [1, 2]. A population-based study in the Netherlands reports an incidence of 5.1 per 10,000 pregnancies in women with a uterine scar [2]. For women without a uterine scar, the incidence is as low as 0.6 to 0.7 per 10,000 pregnancies [2, 9].

Besides a prior cesarean section, Zwart and colleagues note an increased risk for uterine rupture in women with epidural anesthesia, induction of labor, postterm pregnancy, non-Western immigrants, and advanced age [2]. In addition, other reports identify multiparity (particularly grand multiparity), placenta percreta, placental anomalies, prior uterine instrumentation, malpresentation, fetopelvic disproportion/macrosomia, version procedures, uterine anomalies, and history of gestational trophoblastic disease as risk factors to be considered [4, 9–12].

Multiple gestation, including twins, is a risk factor for uterine rupture which has been identified in numerous studies, as with this case [13, 14]. It is possible that this patient's previous extrauterine pelvic surgeries or endometriosis could have also contributed to the rupture. One other report indicates that out of 25 cases of rupture of an unscarred uterus, n = 1 had a history of another pelvic surgery and n = 2 had a history of endometriosis, as with the case we present [2]. Other possible contributing factors in the remaining cases in that report include a history of uterine instrumentation or manipulation (instrumental abortion, postpartum curettage, and hysteroscopy), history of ectopic pregnancy, and uterine fibroids. In 52% of cases with an unscarred uterus (n = 13), however, the authors do not identify any risk factors. The study does not include genetic testing for vascular Ehlers-Danlos Syndrome (type IV), a rare condition associated with organ rupture [15]. Analysis of the COL3A1 gene was negative for vascular Ehlers-Danlos Syndrome in our patient. The patient we present had a history of uterine manipulation to the extent of embryo transfer for IVF, but this has not been associated with rupture in any reported cases to our knowledge.

Other rare cases of spontaneous prelabor rupture of an unscarred uterus have been reported. These cases have included more catastrophic outcomes such as hysterectomy with perinatal mortality [6, 7] or both maternal and perinatal mortality [8]. The very preterm gestational age of the twins in this report adds to the rarity of the positive outcome. We identified only one other case of prolonged partial extrusion of a fetus from an unscarred ruptured uterus prior to labor with a good outcome from 1982, which was a singleton gestation [16]. Interestingly this occurred at a hospital located

15 miles away from our center. We did not identify any other reports with 2-year neurodevelopmental follow-up.

MRI imaging is an important tool in the diagnosis of uterine rupture, particularly in the setting of nonspecific abdominal pain in a patient with any of the previously mentioned risk factors. Advantages of MRI include the ability to visualize the uterine wall defect for a more definitive diagnosis, less operator dependence and less discomfort for a patient with abdominal pain compared to ultrasound, and no ionizing radiation with better visualization of soft tissues compared to CT scan [17]. Thus far, few reports aside from the case we have presented have described the associated MRI findings [17, 18].

4. Conclusion

We present a unique case of rupture of an unscarred uterus in a primigravid patient prior to the onset of labor. Multiple gestation is an important risk factor for uterine rupture. This report adds to a handful of other cases in which a history of endometriosis or extrauterine pelvic surgery was noted prior to an unscarred uterine rupture. A high index of suspicion and the use of ultrasound and MRI to evaluate nonspecific abdominal pain led to the diagnosis and survival of both the mother and her premature twins, with no neurodevelopmental impairments at 2 years of age.

Consent

Written informed consent was obtained from the patient for herself and her minors for publication of this case report and accompanying images.

Authors' Contributions

Kathryn L. Ponder prepared the manuscript and literature review, contributed to the medical care for the infants in the NICU, and administered the Capute Scales. Rosa Won performed the cesarean section and assisted with revisions of the manuscript. Laurel Clymer administered the Bayley Scales of Infant and Toddler Development (Third Edition) and assisted with revisions of the manuscript. All authors read and approved the final paper.

Acknowledgments

The authors would like to thank the patient and her family. Dr. Stephen Wells and Dr. Babak Edraki assisted with the cesarean delivery. Dr. Jeffrey Traynor was involved in the patient's postoperative obstetrical care and follow-up. The authors would also like to acknowledge the NICU staff. East Bay Newborn Specialists provided funding for the publication of this manuscript.

References

[1] G. J. Hofmeyr, L. Say, and A. M. Gülmezoglu, "WHO systematic review of maternal mortality and morbidity: the prevalence of uterine rupture," *BJOG: An International Journal of Obstetrics & Gynaecology*, vol. 112, no. 9, pp. 1221–1228, 2005.

[2] J. J. Zwart, J. M. Richters, F. Öry, J. I. P. De Vries, K. W. M. Bloemenkamp, and J. Van Roosmalen, "Uterine rupture in the Netherlands: a nationwide population-based cohort study," *BJOG: An International Journal of Obstetrics & Gynaecology*, vol. 116, no. 8, pp. 1069–1078, 2009.

[3] A. Kwee, M. L. Bots, G. H. Visser, and H. W. Bruinse, "Uterine rupture and its complications in the Netherlands: a prospective study," *European Journal of Obstetrics & Gynecology and Reproductive Biology*, vol. 128, no. 1-2, pp. 257–261, 2006.

[4] D. C. Schrinsky and R. C. Benson, "Rupture of the pregnant uterus: a review," *Obstetrical & Gynecological Survey*, vol. 33, no. 4, pp. 217–232, 1978.

[5] L. Posthumus and M. E. Donker, "Uterine rupture in a primigravid patient, an uncommon but severe obstetrical event: a case report," *Journal of Medical Case Reports*, vol. 11, no. 1, pp. 339–342, 2017.

[6] M. Misra, R. Roychowdury, N. C. Sarkar, and M. M. Koley, "The spontaneous prelabour rupture of an unscarred uterus at 34 weeks of pregnancy," *Journal of Clinical and Diagnostic Research*, vol. 7, no. 3, pp. 548-549, 2013.

[7] M. Guèye, M. Mbaye, M. D. Ndiaye-Guèye, S. M. Kane-Guèye et al., "Spontaneous uterine rupture of an unscarred uterus before labour," *Case Reports in Obstetrics and Gynecology*, vol. 2012, Article ID 598356, 3 pages, 2012.

[8] K. S. Gurudut, H. S. Gouda, S. C. Aramani, and R. H. Patil, "Spontaneous rupture of unscarred gravid uterus," *Journal of Forensic Sciences*, vol. 56, no. S1, pp. S263–S265, 2011.

[9] D. A. Miller, T. M. Goodwin, R. B. Gherman, and R. H. Paul, "Intrapartum rupture of the unscarred uterus," *Obstetrics & Gynecology*, vol. 89, pp. 671–673, 1997.

[10] K. M. Sweeten, W. K. Graves, and A. Athanassiou, "Spontaneous rupture of the unscarred uterus," *American Journal of Obstetrics & Gynecology*, vol. 172, no. 6, pp. 1851–1855, 1995.

[11] J. P. Neilson, T. Lavender, S. Quenby, and S. Wray, "Obstructed labour," *British Medical Bulletin*, vol. 67, pp. 191–204, 2003.

[12] S. Topuz, "Spontaneous uterine rupture at an unusual site due to placenta percreta in a 21-week twin pregnancy with previous cesarean section," *Clinical and Experimental Obstetrics & Gynecology*, vol. 31, no. 3, pp. 239–241, 2004.

[13] M. F. Mazzone and J. Woolever, "Uterine rupture in a patient with an unscarred uterus: a case study," *Wisconsin Medical Journal*, vol. 105, no. 2, pp. 64–66, 2006.

[14] C. M. Tarney, P. Whitecar, M. Sewell, L. Grubish, and E. Hope, "Rupture of an unscarred uterus in a quadruplet pregnancy," *Obstetrics & Gynecology*, vol. 121, pp. 483–485, 2013.

[15] M. L. Murray, M. Pepin, S. Peterson, and P. H. Byers, "Pregnancy-related deaths and complications in women with vascular Ehlers-Danlos syndrome," *Genetics in Medicine*, vol. 16, no. 12, pp. 874–880, 2014.

[16] D. B. Cotton, "Infant survival with prolonged uterine rupture," *American Journal of Obstetrics & Gynecology*, vol. 142, no. 8, pp. 1059-1060, 1982.

[17] K. M. Hruska, B. F. Coughlin, A. A. Coggins, and H. P. Wiczyk, "MRI diagnosis of spontaneous uterine rupture of an unscarred uterus," *Emergency Radiology*, vol. 12, no. 4, pp. 186–188, 2006.

[18] J. E. Hamrick-Turner, P. E. Cranston, and B. S. Lantrip, "Gravid uterine dehiscence: MR findings," *Abdominal Imaging*, vol. 20, no. 5, pp. 486–488, 1995.

40

Maternal Parvovirus B19 Infection Causing First-Trimester Increased Nuchal Translucency and Fetal Hydrops

Olivia Grubman, Farrah Naz Hussain, Zoe Nelson, and Lois Brustman

Department of Obstetrics and Gynecology, Mount Sinai West, Icahn School of Medicine at Mount Sinai, New York, NY 10019, USA

Correspondence should be addressed to Olivia Grubman; oliviagrubman@gmail.com

Academic Editor: Maria Grazia Porpora

This is a case report of a 31-year-old primigravida who was diagnosed with an asymptomatic acute parvovirus B19 infection in the second trimester of pregnancy and its suspected association with an increased nuchal translucency (NT) measurement. Parvovirus B19 is a single-stranded DNA virus that is cytotoxic to erythroid progenitor cells, causing inhibition of erythropoiesis. While maternal disease is usually mild, fetal infection can result in spontaneous abortion, aplastic anemia, nonimmune fetal hydrops, and fetal demise. This fetus had an increased NT of 3.2 mm at 11 weeks' gestation with a normal male karyotype and microarray analysis on chorionic villi sampling, in addition to a normal fetal echocardiogram at 15 weeks' gestation. The anatomy scan at 20 weeks' and 1-day gestation revealed fetal ascites, pleural effusion, and increased middle cerebral artery peak systolic velocity suspicious for fetal anemia. At this time, maternal serology for parvovirus was positive for IgM and IgG. Amniocentesis, cordocentesis, and intrauterine transfusion were performed. The amniocentesis revealed elevated parvovirus B19 DNA, quantitative PCR (2,589,801 copies/mL, reference range <100 copies/mL). The patient delivered a viable male fetus at 37 weeks' and 6-day gestation, without sequelae of the previously noted hydrops. Parvovirus B19 infection should be a consideration when evaluating increased NT and hydrops fetalis. It warrants close antepartum surveillance and possible intrauterine fetal transfusions. With prompt recognition, proper treatment, and surveillance, these patients can go on to achieve healthy term deliveries. Long-term outcomes of delivered infants require further study.

1. Case Presentation

A 31-year-old primigravida was referred to our Maternal Fetal Medicine practice after a routine first-trimester ultrasound at 11 weeks' gestation that revealed a nuchal translucency (NT) of 3.2 mm (Figure 1). The crown rump length measured 11 weeks two days, which was consistent with the patient's last menstrual period which placed her gestational age at 11 weeks. A chorionic villi sample (CVS) was performed at that time. Cytogenetic analysis from the chorionic villi showed a normal male karyotype of 46,XY. The results of the fluorescent in situ hybridization (FISH analysis), Noonan's panel, and microarray for aneuploidy testing were normal. Due to the elevated NT, the patient was referred for a fetal echocardiogram at 15 weeks and 5 days' gestation which revealed a regular atrial rhythm with no structural cardiac abnormalities. An early anatomy ultrasound at 16 weeks and 0 days' gestation was normal, with fetal size appropriate for gestational age and no evidence fetal anomalies.

A comprehensive anatomy scan at 20 weeks' and 1-day gestation revealed fetal ascites and a small pleural effusion (Figures 2, 3, and 4). No pericardial effusion was observed. The middle cerebral artery peak systolic velocity (MCA PSV) was elevated (1.95 multiples of the median (MoM)), which was suggestive of fetal anemia. At this time, routine serologic testing for herpes simplex virus (HSV), parvovirus, toxoplasmosis, and cytomegalovirus was performed. The patient underwent amniocentesis with polymerase chain reaction (PCR) testing for parvovirus, toxoplasmosis, cytomegalovirus (CMV), and adenovirus.

A follow-up fetal echocardiogram showed no structural cardiac abnormalities or rhythm abnormalities seen as a cause of hydrops. However, the fetus was noted to have scalp edema, worsening pleural effusion and ascites, and, now, a pericardial effusion. Fetal hemodynamics was normal,

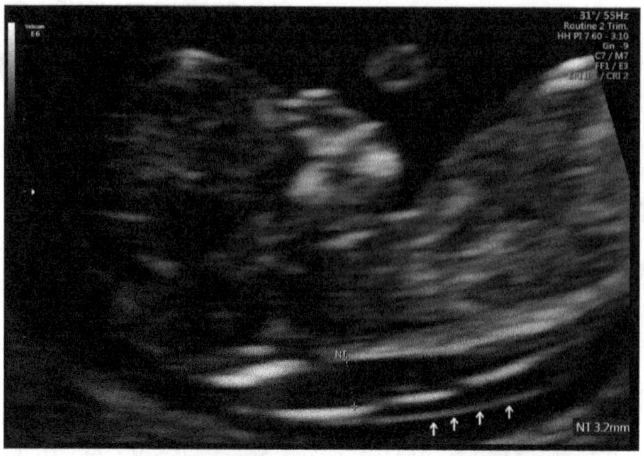

FIGURE 1: Nuchal translucency 3.2 mm.

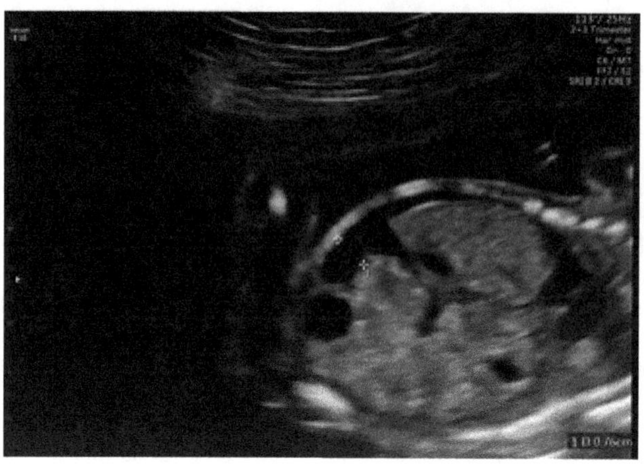

FIGURE 2: Anatomy ultrasound at 20 weeks' and 1-day gestation with fetal ascites.

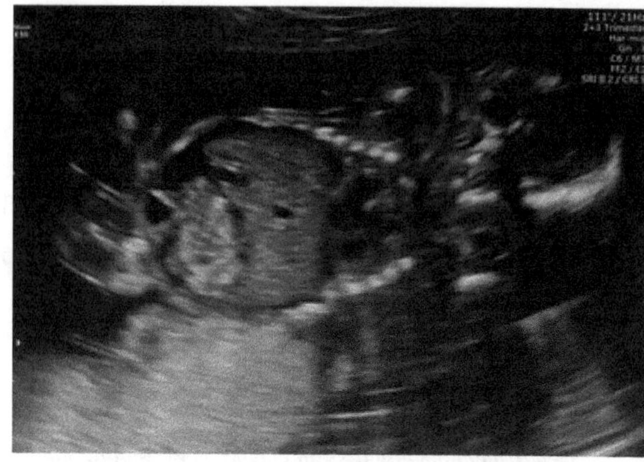

FIGURE 3: Anatomy ultrasound at 20 weeks' and 1-day gestation with fetal ascites.

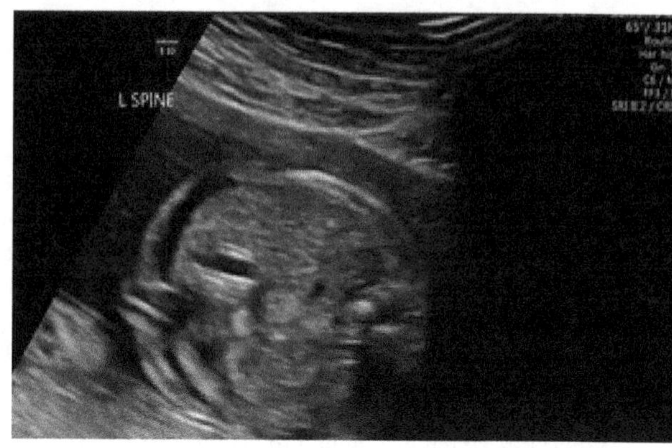

FIGURE 4: Anatomy ultrasound at 20 weeks' and 1-day gestation with fetal ascites.

including Doppler flow patterns in the umbilical artery and vein, ductus venosus and arteriosus, and middle cerebral artery. Fetal ascites was still present at 20 weeks and 2 days' gestation. The MCA PSV was elevated at 75 cm/second. Maternal parvovirus B19 IgG and IgM were elevated, with values of 5.3 and 2.4 (negative or equivocal <1.1), respectively. At this time, the patient recalled an upper respiratory illness at approximately 9 to 10 weeks' gestation. She denied rash, arthralgias, or knowledge of exposure to a child or an adult with symptoms consistent with a parvovirus infection. Given the above findings, the decision was made that day to perform an amniocentesis, a cordocentesis, and an intrauterine transfusion based on the presumptive diagnosis of fetal anemia secondary to an acute parvovirus infection. The fetal hematocrit was 10%, indicating anemia, and 12 cc of blood was transfused, raising the fetal hematocrit to 25%. At the end of the procedure, the MCA PSV was 45 cm/sec, with decreased systolic/diastolic (S/D) ratio of approximately 2.0.

At 20 weeks and 5 days' gestation, the results of the amniocentesis demonstrated elevated parvovirus B19 DNA, quantitative PCR (2,589,801 copies/mL, reference range <100 copies/mL). Fetal ascites persisted the following day at 20 weeks and 6 days' gestation. The MCA PSV was 42 cm/min. A cordocentesis revealed a fetal hematocrit of 24%, and an additional intrauterine transfusion was given for a total volume of 15 cc. The following week, there was no evidence of fetal ascites and the MCA PSV was normal. Subsequent maternal serologic testing for herpes simplex, cytomegalic, and toxoplasmosis virus was negative.

For the remainder of the second trimester, ultrasounds were performed every other week to assess fetal growth and MCA Doppler flow. Weekly antenatal surveillance was performed in the third trimester and was consistently reassuring.

At 37 weeks and 5 days' gestation, the patient was induced for gestational hypertension. She delivered a viable male fetus weighing 2880g at 37 weeks and 6 days. The neonatal Apgar scores were 8 and 9 at 1 and 5 minutes, respectively. At the time of this report, the infant is doing well and developing appropriately for 5 months of age.

2. Discussion

Our case report is one of few in the literature that suggests an association of an increased NT measurement with fetal anemia due to an asymptomatic parvovirus B19 infection in the mother. The fetal anemia was successfully treated, when diagnosed in second trimester, with fetal blood transfusions and subsequent prolongation of the pregnancy to term with no apparent sequelae.

Human parvovirus B19 is a small, nonenveloped, single-stranded DNA virus. It is disseminated by respiratory secretions or from hand to mouth contact. Other modes of transmission include transfusion of blood products and transplacental transfer. Also known as erythema infectiosum, parvovirus is a common childhood illness that is recognized by the classic bright facial rash or "slapped cheek rash." The virus generally affects children from age four to eleven. In addition to the facial rash, there is commonly a lacelike rash on the extremities and trunk. Conversely, adults generally do not present with a rash. Arthropathies are the most common symptom in adults, affecting up to 50% of pregnant women with acute B19 infection. Arthralgia including the hands, wrists, knees, and ankles can occur, lasting for one to two weeks [1]. It has been reported that 50-70% of pregnant women are immune to parvovirus B19, with the majority having no recollection of when they were infected. As with our patient, if infected with parvovirus in pregnancy, up to 70% of women will be asymptomatic.

The incidence of acute B19 infection in pregnancy is 3.3% to 3.8% [2, 3], with a transplacental transmission rate of approximately 30% [4]. Parvovirus infection that occurs during the first trimester has been associated with a 71% increased risk of fetal loss [5]. The fetal demise rate is up to 15% early in the second trimester and prior to 20 weeks. After 20 weeks, the rate of fetal demise decreases to about 2.3%, as the viral insult to the bone marrow is not as detrimental [2, 5]. It has been reported that fetal demise can occur up to 12 weeks after maternal infection in any trimester [6].

Parvovirus B19 replicates in red blood cell (RBC) precursors mainly in the bone marrow and fetal liver, which can result in hemolysis and RBC aplasia. Aplastic crisis in a fetus can lead to cardiac failure, nonimmune hydrops, and death. Parvovirus infects primarily the erythroid cell line and therefore can cause fetal anemia which can lead to cardiac failure with hydrops fetalis [7]. It is estimated that parvovirus accounts for 8% to 10% of nonimmune hydrops [2]. The suspected mechanism for the development of nonimmune hydrops fetalis involves the infection of fetal erythroid precursor cells with parvovirus, with subsequent erythroid hypoplasia. This then leads to severe fetal anemia, tissue hypoxia, and, eventually, a compensatory increase in cardiac output followed by heart failure [8]. Furthermore, it has been proposed that fetal death could also be due to myocarditis causing cardiac failure as a result of the affinity of the virus for cardiac tissue [9–11]. It has also been reported that the parvovirus B19 is toxic to the megakaryocytes, hepatocytes, and placental cells which could also attribute to a fetal demise [12].

There are few reports in the literature of increased NT associated with parvovirus [7, 12, 13]. Although an increased NT is not commonly associated with fetal infection, parvovirus B19 is the only infection that has a reported association with an increased NT [12]. Markenson et al. [14] reported a case in which they found an increased NT (3.7 mm) in a fetus with a normal karyotype, but parvovirus was detected in the amniotic fluid. In this case, the patient recalled that she was exposed to a child with a high fever and rash around 5 to 6 weeks' gestation. She went on to a delivery of a viable term male infant with redundant nuchal skin thickening. Another case found an NT (4.2 mm) and reversed a-wave in the ductus venosus (DV) during a first-trimester ultrasound. As with the prior case, the mother reported contact with children with erythema infectiosum and had positive serologic testing (IgG and IgM antibodies) for parvovirus B19. Unfortunately, in this case, a fetal demise occurred two weeks after diagnosis with parvovirus infection confirmed in the fetus based on immunocytochemical studies using specific antibodies [12]. Finally, Kempe et al. [7] report two cases with an increased NT, elevated MCA PSV, and cardiomegaly, all suspicious for fetal anemia in the first trimester. Maternal parvovirus infection was confirmed with a positive PCR. In each case, the fetus received a 3-mL umbilical vein transfusion of packed red blood cells. In one of the cases, three more intrauterine blood transfusions were necessary until the fetal hydrops resolved. There were good neonatal outcomes in both cases.

Based on the case reports above, although rare, acute parvovirus infection should be considered in the differential diagnosis, as an etiology for an increased NT. An early diagnosis can enable intervention via intrauterine blood transfusions, which can potentially cure hydrops fetalis. In our case, at the time of the finding of an increased NT in first trimester, the diagnosis of parvovirus infection was not considered and the patient's subtle history of upper respiratory symptoms was missed. If we had considered parvovirus as an etiology for an increased NT, the diagnosis could have been made earlier and, thus, the fetus could have been followed more closely with serial sonograms and Doppler studies.

As we have described, the management of fetuses with hydrops or anemia due to parvovirus B19 infection includes cordocentesis to assess fetal hemoglobin and reticulocyte count, and intrauterine fetal transfusion, if necessary. Furthermore, if the fetus is at or near term, delivery should be considered. A summary of 14 studies including 1436 cases of fetal parvovirus infection found a fetal survival rate of 82% with transfusion compared to a fetal survival rate of 55% for those who were not transfused [2]. Two to three transfusions may be required before resolution of the fetal hydrops or anemia, which usually takes place three to six weeks after the first transfusion. Recommended monitoring includes weekly ultrasonography and Doppler assessment to assess the MCA, which is a noninvasive method to measure a fetus at risk for anemia [6, 15, 16].

Several small studies have examined long-term outcomes after intrauterine transfusion for parvovirus B19 infection during pregnancy. These studies, ranging from two to 28 patients, found rates of minor neurodevelopmental impairment from 0 to 18.8% and rates of major neurodevelopmental impairment from 0 to 12.5%. Neurological abnormalities included mild developmental delay and more severe abnormalities such as ataxia and hypertonia. The causes for increased rates of cerebral injury and adverse neurodevelopmental outcomes in antenatal parvovirus B19 are poorly understood. Possible mechanisms include compromised fetal status due to severe anemia and hydrops or adverse reaction related to the virus itself. It is clear that further long-term studies are needed on children who have previously undergone intrauterine fetal transfusion for hydrops related to parvovirus [17–22]. Given this data, patients should be counseled thoroughly on the risks and benefits of intrauterine transfusion for the "cure" of the effects of parvovirus in the fetus, as well as possible long-term sequelae. This should be a shared decision making process with the patient and the physician.

This case, as well as others in the literature, emphasizes parvovirus in the differential of an elevated fetal NT. Parvovirus is the only infectious cause of an increased fetal NT and should be a consideration in these patients along with chromosomal and cardiac abnormalities. Early recognition provides the opportunity for early management of fetal hydrops and increased fetal survival rates. However, long-term sequelae of antenatal parvovirus and intrauterine transfusions on the infant, including neurodevelopmental impairment, are poorly understood and require further study. The case described, as well as others, provides information relevant for patient counseling and shared decision-making.

3. Conclusion

It is our recommendation that parvovirus should be considered in the differential of an increased NT in first trimester. Maternal serology with IgM and IgG specific antibody titers should be performed. A patient's history should be elicited, but this may be noncontributory based on the fact that the majority of parvovirus infections in pregnancy are asymptomatic.

References

[1] G. R. Marhenson and M. K. Yancey, "Parvovirus B19 infections in pregnancy," *Seminars in Perinatology*, vol. 22, no. 4, pp. 309–317, 1998.

[2] J. Crane, "Parvovirus B19 infection in pregnancy," *Journal of Obstetrics and Gynaecology Canada*, vol. 24, no. 9, pp. 744-745, 2002.

[3] K. N. Desai and L. E. Brustman, "Parvovirus in pregnancy," *Postgraduate Obstetrics & Gynecology*, vol. 34, no. 8, pp. 1–5, 2014.

[4] A. Riipinen, E. Väisänen, M. Nuutila et al., "Parvovirus B19 infection in fetal deaths," *Clinical Infectious Diseases*, vol. 47, no. 12, pp. 1519–1525, 2008.

[5] J. Lassen, A. K. Jensen, P. Bager et al., "Parvovirus B19 infection in the first trimester of pregnancy and risk of fetal loss: a population-based case-control study," *American Journal of Epidemiology*, vol. 176, no. 9, pp. 803–807, 2012.

[6] R. L. Schild, R. Bald, H. Plath, A. M. Eis-Hübinger, G. Enders, and M. Hansmann, "Intrauterine management of fetal parvovirus B19 infection," *Ultrasound in Obstetrics & Gynecology*, vol. 13, no. 3, pp. 161–166, 1999.

[7] A. Kempe, B. Rösing, C. Berg et al., "First-trimester treatment of fetal anemia secondary to parvovirus B19 infection," *Ultrasound in Obstetrics & Gynecology*, vol. 29, no. 2, pp. 226–228, 2007.

[8] T. J. Boley and E. J. Popek, "Parvovirus infection in pregnancy," *Semin Perinatolgy*, vol. 17, p. 410, 1993.

[9] F. Forestier, J. Tissot, Y. Vial, F. Daffos, and P. Hohlfeld, "Haematological parameters of parvovirus B19 infection in 13 fetuses with hydrops foetalis," *British Journal of Haematology*, vol. 104, no. 4, pp. 925–927, 1999.

[10] H. J. Porter, A. M. Quantrill, and K. A. Fleming, "B19 parvovirus infection of myocardial cells," *The Lancet*, vol. 1, no. 8584, pp. 535-536, 1988.

[11] A. L. Morey, U. Nicolini, C. R. Welch, D. Economides, P. F. Chamberlain, and B. J. Cohen, "Parvovirus B19 infection and transient fetal hydrops," *The Lancet*, vol. 337, no. 8739, p. 496, 1991.

[12] T. Carraca, A. Matias, O. Brandão, and N. Montenegro, "Early signs of cardiac failure: A clue for parvovirus infection screening in the first trimester?" *Fetal Diagnosis and Therapy*, vol. 30, no. 2, pp. 150–152, 2011.

[13] J. C. Smulian, J. F. X. Egan, and J. F. Rodis, "Fetal hydrops in the first trimester associated with maternal parvovirus infection," *Journal of Clinical Ultrasound*, vol. 26, no. 6, pp. 314–316, 1998.

[14] G. Markenson, L. A. Correia, G. Cohn, L. Bayer, and C. Kanaan, "Parvoviral infection associated with increased nuchal translucency: A case report," *Journal of Perinatology*, vol. 20, no. 2, pp. 129–131, 2000.

[15] T. Imbar, A. Lev-Sagie, S. Cohen, N. Yanai, and S. Yagel, "Diagnosis, surveillance, and treatment of the anemic fetus using middle cerebral artery peak systolic velocity measurement," *Prenatal Diagnosis*, vol. 26, no. 1, pp. 45–51, 2006.

[16] E. Cosmi, G. Mari, L. D. Chiaie et al., "Noninvasive diagnosis by Doppler ultrasonography of fetal anemia resulting from parvovirus infection," *American Journal of Obstetrics & Gynecology*, vol. 187, no. 5, pp. 1290–1293, 2002.

[17] C. H. Rodeck, C. A. Holman, J. Karnicki, J. R. Kemp, D. N. Whitmore, and M. A. Austin, "Direct intravascular fetal blood transfusion by fetoscopy in severe rhesus isoimmunisation," *The Lancet*, vol. 317, no. 8221, pp. 625–627, 1981.

[18] E. Miller, C. K. Fairley, B. J. Cohen, and C. Seng, "Immediate and long term outcome of human parvovirus B19 infection in pregnancy," *British Journal of Obstetrics and Gynaecology*, vol. 105, no. 2, pp. 174–178, 1998.

[19] H. T. Nagel, T. R. de Haan, F. P. Vandenbussche, D. Oepkes, and F. J. Walther, "Long-term outcome after fetal transfusion for hydrops associated with parvovirus B19 infection," *Obstetrics & Gynecology*, vol. 109, no. 1, pp. 42–47, 2007.

[20] J. Dembinski, F. Haverkamp, H. Maara, M. Hansmann, A. M. Eis-Hübinger, and P. Bartmann, "Neurodevelopmental outcome after intrauterine red cell transfusion for Parvovirus B19-induced fetal hydrops," *BJOG: An International Journal of Obstetrics & Gynaecology*, vol. 109, no. 11, pp. 1232–1234, 2002.

[21] E. P. De Jong, I. T. Lindenburg, J. M. van Klink et al., "Intrauterine transfusion for parvovirus B19 infection: long-term neurodevelopmental outcome," *American Journal of Obstetrics & Gynecology*, vol. 206, no. 3, pp. 204.e1–204.e5, 2012.

[22] I. T. M. Lindenburg, J. M. van Klink, V. E. H. J. Smits-Wintjens, I. L. van Kamp, D. Oepkes, and E. Lopriore, "Long-term neurodevelopmental and cardiovascular outcome after intrauterine transfusions for fetal anaemia: A review," *Prenatal Diagnosis*, vol. 33, no. 9, pp. 815–822, 2013.

41

A Case of Preeclampsia with Uterine Necrosis after Uterine Artery Embolization for Postpartum Hemorrhage

Midori Yoshikawa,[1] Takahiro Seyama,[1] Takayuki Iriyama,[1] Seisuke Sayama,[1] Tatsuya Fujii,[1] Masatake Toshimitsu,[1] Moto Nakaya,[2] Ryo Kurokawa,[2] Eisuke Shibata,[2] Takeyuki Watadani,[2] Keiichi Kumasawa,[1] Takeshi Nagamatsu,[1] Kaori Koga,[1] and Yutaka Osuga[1]

[1]*Department of Obstetrics and Gynecology, Faculty of Medicine, The University of Tokyo, 7-3-1 Hongo, Bunkyo-ku, Tokyo 113-8655, Japan*
[2]*Department of Radiology, Faculty of Medicine, The University of Tokyo, 7-3-1 Hongo, Bunkyo-ku, Tokyo 113-8655, Japan*

Correspondence should be addressed to Takahiro Seyama; tseyama123@gmail.com

Academic Editor: John P. Geisler

Uterine necrosis is a rare complication in uterine artery embolization (UAE) for postpartum hemorrhage (PPH). Preeclampsia (PE) is a condition characterized with systemic endothelial damage and intravascular volume depletion. Whether a patient with PE is at high risk for uterine necrosis after UAE for PPH has been unknown. A 30-year-old primipara woman was diagnosed with PE based on hypertension and proteinuria during delivery. UAE was performed for PPH after forceps delivery. After UAE, the patient presented with pleural effusion and massive ascites as well as persistent fever unresponsive to antibiotics. Ultrasonography and contrast-enhanced magnetic resonance imaging (MRI) led to the diagnosis of uterine necrosis, for which we performed total laparoscopic hysterectomy. It should be kept in mind that patients with PE associated with massive ascites may be at high risk for uterine necrosis after UAE due to decreased uterine perfusion. Therefore, it is important to pay attention to persistent symptoms such as fever and abdominal pain after UAE to diagnose uterine necrosis.

1. Introduction

Uterine artery embolization (UAE) is an effective hemostatic treatment for postpartum hemorrhage (PPH) to avoid hysterectomy. Although hemostasis is achieved in over 90% of the cases, uterine necrosis occurs in 1.4% to 2.7% of the patients after UAE [1–3], and hysterectomy is required in nearly all the cases with necrosis [4].

Previous studies have reported that the size and type of embolic agents as well as maternal conditions, such as obesity, caesarean section, and placental abruption, are related to uterine necrosis after UAE [4, 5]. Preeclampsia (PE) is characterized by systemic vascular endothelial dysfunction that leads to enhanced vascular permeability, resulting in intravascular volume depletion and ascites. Ascites is independently associated with adverse maternal outcomes in patients with PE [6]. Patients with PE often present with disseminated intravascular coagulation (DIC) after delivery that can result in PPH [7]. However, the association between uterine necrosis after UAE and PE is not clarified [5]. Here, we report a case of uterine necrosis after UAE for PPH in a patient with PE associated with massive ascites.

2. Case Report

The patient was a 30-year-old, G1P0 woman. The body mass index (BMI) was 18.6 before conception. Her pregnant course was uneventful after natural conception. At 38 weeks and 4 days of gestation, she was hospitalized due to premature rupture of the membrane (PROM). After admission, she was diagnosed with PE since her blood pressure was 146/105 mmHg and urine protein-to-creatinine ratio was

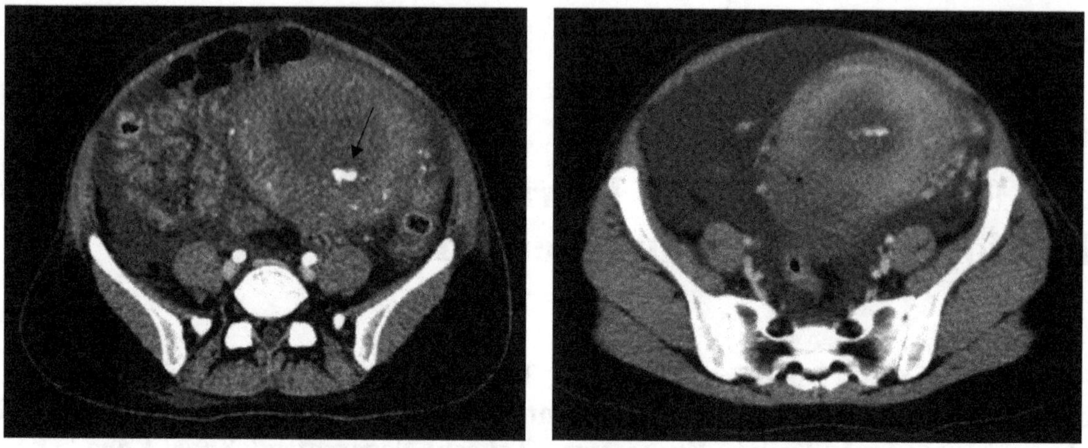

(a) (b)

Figure 1: (a) Contrast-enhanced computed tomography images at the time of massive postpartum hemorrhage: extravasation from the uterine cavity (→). (b) massive ascites.

629 mg/gCr. There was no cardiomegaly or pleural effusion in chest radiograph.

After her cervix was dilated with a metreurynter balloon, labor was induced with oxytocin. However, the labor did not progress on the day of admission or the following day. Labor induction with oxytocin was continued for 2 days after PROM while the patient's blood pressure was maintained around 140/90 mmHg with continuous drip infusion of nicardipine. The labor progressed after onset, and the trans-abdominal ultrasonography showed small volume of ascites. After 3 hours of the second stage of labor, the baby was delivered with forceps due to nonreassuring fetal status. The neonate weighed 2466 g with an Apgar score of 8/9, and umbilical artery pH was 7.159.

The total blood loss was 800 g within 2 hours after delivery, but the hemorrhage increased to a total of 1,500 g 3 hours after delivery. Her heart rate was 100–110 beats per minute, and blood pressure was 110–120/60–80 mmHg. Her hemoglobin decreased to 6.0 g/dl, and fibrinogen was 199 mg/dl. We continuously administered oxytocin, inserted an intrauterine balloon inflated with 200 ml of distilled water, and administered blood transfusion: 2 units of mannitol-adenine-phosphate (MAP), 2 units of fresh frozen plasma (FFP), and 12 units of cryoprecipitate. Her blood pressure persisted over 110/60, and the shock index did not exceed 1 despite the hemorrhage. Contrast-enhanced computed tomography (CT) showed extravasation within the uterus, along with massive ascites (Figure 1). We decided to perform UAE for the hemostasis, and the extravasation from the left uterine artery was confirmed during the procedure. Using 1–2 mm gelatin sponge, we embolized bilateral uterine arteries. The flow from bilateral uterine arteries to the uterus was preserved after the embolization (Figure 2). The vital sign had been stable, and the shock index was constantly below 1 during UAE. The total blood loss was 2,070 g to the end of artery embolization, and the total amount of blood transfusion was 10 units of MAP, 8 units of FFP, and 12 units of cryoprecipitate.

Although UAE enabled hemostasis, ascites resulted in abdominal distention, and pulmonary edema deteriorated (Figure 3). Continuous oxygen supplementation had been continued. Echocardiography did not demonstrate any abnormality, and the B-type natriuretic peptide (BNP) level was within normal. The continuous nicardipine drip also had been restarted after the procedure to control the blood pressure under 140/90. The blood oxygen saturation (SpO_2) had been kept over 95%. On postpartum day 2, she was given oral antihypertensives to replace continuous nicardipine drip. We removed 2,000 ml of ascites by paracentesis and administered albumin 75 g/day because oral intake was difficult and marked respiratory distress occurred. Just after ascites removal, the patient did not demonstrate any drop in blood pressure or tachycardia. We initiated continuous administration of loop diuretics 84 mg/day until postpartum day 4 while tapering the amount due to oliguria. We paid attention to inferior vena cava diameter during diuretic administration, but it never showed any collapse. Hematocrit level, urea nitrogen/creatinine ratio, and electrolyte levels were steady. Her blood pressure and SpO_2 had been stable after the ascites removal. The oliguria was improved from postpartum day 3. On postpartum day 6, oxygen administration and the continuous nicardipine drip were stopped. Pleural effusion and ascites ameliorated on postpartum day 7, and she did not need any diuretics. The proteinuria improved from postpartum day 10.

However, tachycardia, elevated inflammatory response, and spike fever over 38 degrees had continued since postpartum day 2, and *Escherichia coli* was detected from lochia culture. Although the antibiotic was changed from clindamycin to tazobactam and piperacillin on postpartum day 6, then switched to meropenem on day 19, the patient's spike fever persisted. On postpartum day 24, we performed abdominal ultrasonography, using 3D convex probe (Voluson E10 BT19; GE Healthcare, Tokyo, Japan). The power Doppler sonography with slow flow mode, which can depict slow blood flow and microvascular blood flow with high sensitivity, detected no blood flow in the internal myometrium of the uterus. Magnetic resonance imaging (MRI) demonstrated a heterogeneous high-intensity area in the internal myometrium on T2-weighted images without contrast

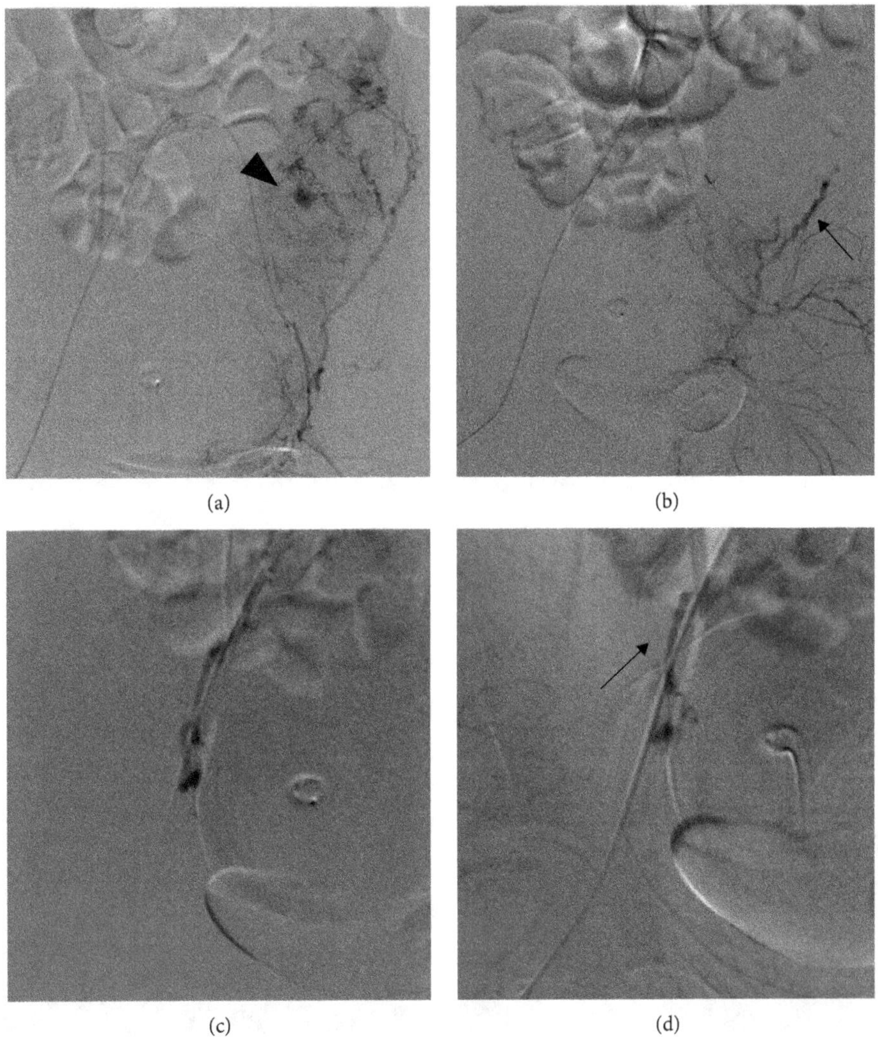

FIGURE 2: (a, b) The images of the left uterine artery before and after embolization. The extravasation (►) is no longer seen after embolization. The flow in the left uterine artery is preserved after embolization (→). (c, d) The images of the right uterine artery before and after embolization. The extravasation is not detected in the right uterine artery. The flow in the right uterine artery is also preserved after embolization (→).

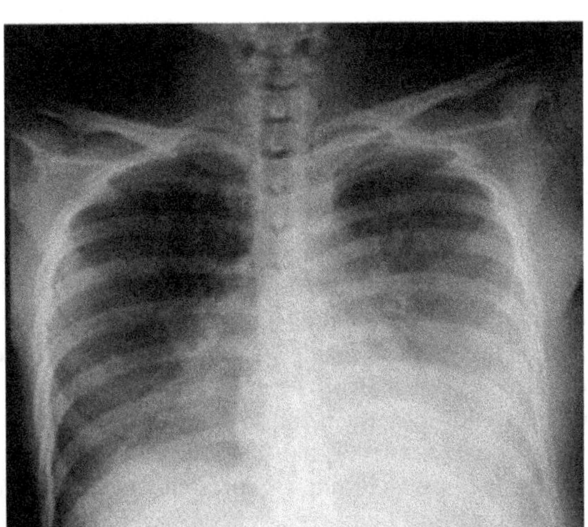

FIGURE 3: Chest radiograph at postpartum day 2 shows bilateral pleural effusion.

enhancement on postcontrast T1-weighted images (Figure 4). We diagnosed the patient with uterine necrosis, and we performed laparoscopic hysterectomy.

Although the surface of the uterus appeared to be normal, the resected internal myometrium was reddish-black and malodorous (Figure 5). Pathology confirmed myometrial necrosis with infiltration of massive inflammatory cells, such as neutrophils, lymphocytes, and plasma cells. The postoperative course was uneventful. She stopped oral antihypertensives on postpartum day 24. She was discharged on postoperative day 6 (postpartum day 30).

3. Discussion

Complications of UAE for obstetric hemorrhage such as intrauterine infection or pelvic abscess are reported to occur in 6%–7% of cases [1]. Uterine necrosis has been reported to occur in 1.4% to 2.7% following UAE [2, 3]. Factors that may associate with uterine necrosis include the size and type of

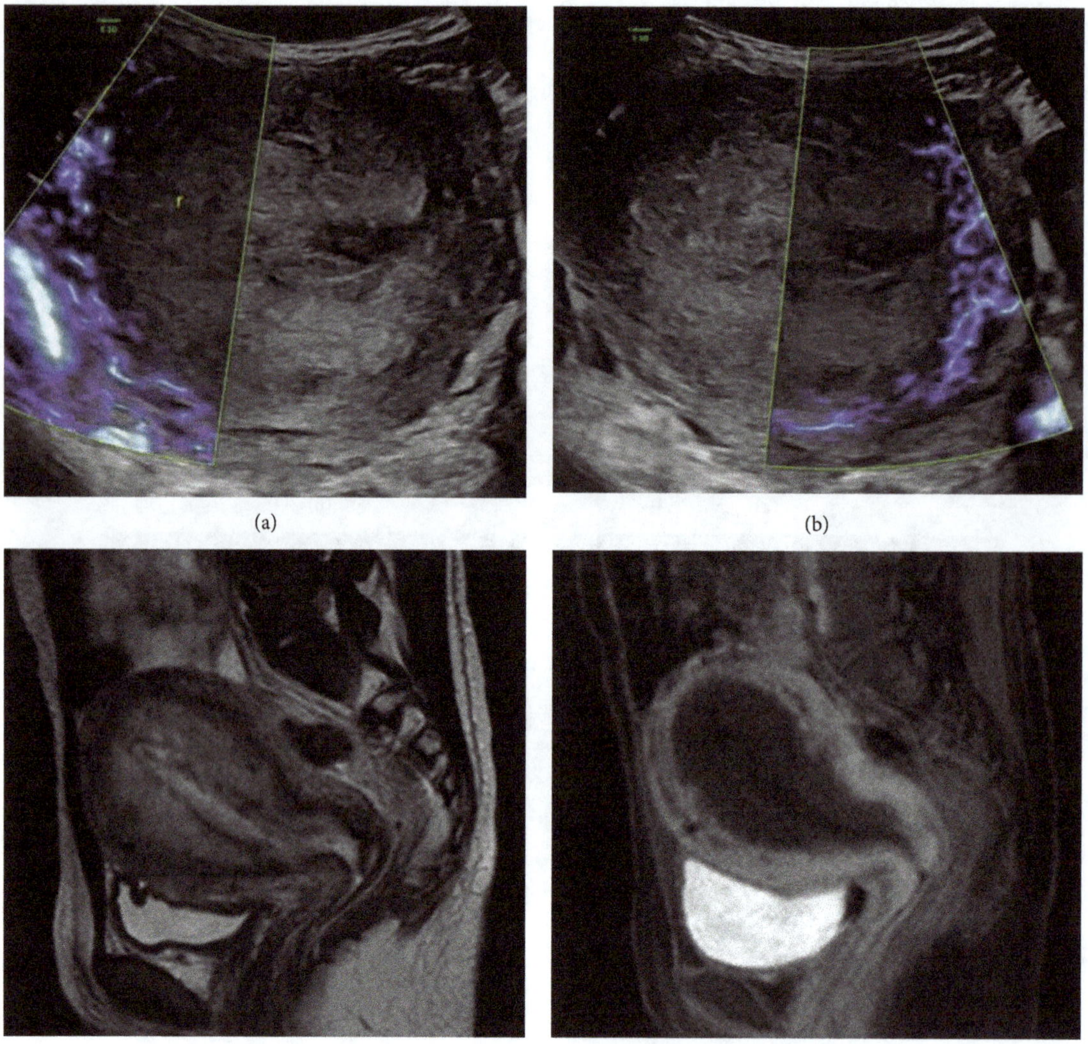

(a) (b) (c) (d)

FIGURE 4: (a, b) Cross section of the internal myometrium in abdominal ultrasonography on postpartum day 24. Abdominal ultrasonography does not show blood flow in the internal myometrium by abdominal ultrasound. (c, d) MRI shows heterogeneous high intensity in internal myometrium on sagittal T2-weighted images (c) without contrast enhancement on sagittal postcontrast T1-weighted images (d), indicating necrosis.

the embolic agent in UAE [4]. Temporary embolic agents < 500 μm cause narrow vessels to be embolized, which may lead to organ necrosis [1, 4]. We used 1–2 mm gelatin sponge, a temporary embolic agent, which is presumed to have little association with uterine necrosis.

The present case developed uterine necrosis after UAE for PPH and required hysterectomy. There is only one case report of uterine necrosis after UAE in a patient with PE by Hirashima et al. [8]. Pleural effusion, proteinuria, and atonic bleeding were observed in our case as well as the case reported by Hirashima et al. In addition, our case showed massive ascites. In PE, systemic vascular endothelial dysfunction is known to trigger various organ damage. Ascites in PE is mainly caused by hypoproteinemia and enhanced vascular permeability [6, 9]. Although transabdominal ultrasonography prior to labor showed a small volume of ascites, it suddenly increased after delivery. It suggests that severe vascular endothelial dysfunction occurred and caused systemic hypoperfusion associated with local circulatory failure in the organs, the mechanism by which the uterus may have become more vulnerable to necrosis. PE with ascites should be considered as a risky condition for uterine necrosis after UAE.

To inspect the pathophysiology mentioned above, we reviewed the past cases in our institution. We experienced 45 postpartum hemorrhage cases which required UAE for hemostasis in the past decade from January 2011 to December 2020. The present case was the first case of uterine necrosis after UAE for PPH. Among 45 cases, 10 cases were complicated with PE. We compared the present case with other PE cases ($n = 9$) (Table 1). Pulmonary edema was observed in 5 cases including the present case. The circulatory disturbance and hemorrhagic shock were confirmed in other cases, but not in this case. Diuretics were used in other PE cases. However, massive ascites was confirmed only in this case. These results support the suggestion that PE with

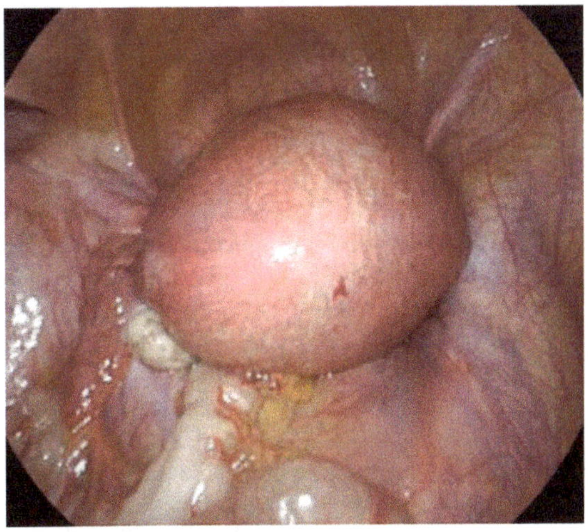

(a)

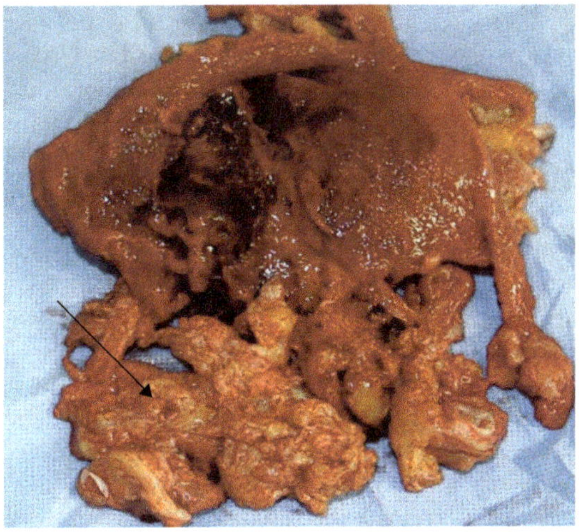

(b)

FIGURE 5: (a) Laparoscopic images of the uterine surface during surgery. The uterine surface appeared normal. (b) Macroscopic finding of the resected uterus shows the inner myometrium of the uterus is necrotized (→).

TABLE 1: The characteristics of PE cases which required uterine artery embolization after delivery in our hospital from January 2011 to December 2020. Massive ascites before delivery is confirmed only in the present case (No. 1). Gelatin sponge is used as embolic agent in all patients except for No. 10.

	Ascites	Pulmonary edema	Diuretics	Embolic agent	Embolization of uterine arteries	Shock index > 1	Transfusion
No. 1	++	+	+	Gelatin sponge	Bilateral	—	+
2	—	—	—	Gelatin sponge	Bilateral	—	+
3	—	—	—	Gelatin sponge	Bilateral	+	+
4	—	+	+	Gelatin sponge	Bilateral	+	+
5	—	+	—	Gelatin sponge	Bilateral	+	+
6	—	+	—	Gelatin sponge	Bilateral	+	+
7	—	+	+	Gelatin sponge	Unilateral	+	+
8	—	—	—	Gelatin sponge	Unilateral	+	+
9	—	+	—	Gelatin sponge	Bilateral	—	+
10	—	+	+	NBCA*	Unilateral	+	+

*NBCA: n-butyl-2-cyanoacrylate.

massive ascites may be at high risk for uterine necrosis after UAE. This study design has been approved by our institutional ethics committee.

In addition, hemorrhagic shock and sepsis have been indicated as risk factors for uterine necrosis after UAE [4]. This patient had complicated premature rupture of membranes before birth comparing other PE cases which needed UAE. This patient also took more than 2 days until delivery and had fever prior to labor with an elevation of inflammatory response, all of which indicating a latent infection localized in the uterus. The association of uterine necrosis with these events, which have potentially exacerbated localized circulatory disturbance, cannot be ruled out.

On the other hand, we performed paracentesis and administered diuretics to control the massive ascites. Furosemide, a loop diuretic, activates the renin-angiotensin system, the vasopressin system, catecholamine, and others, potentially triggering electrolyte imbalances and renal dysfunction; therefore, it should be administered with caution in patients with PE [10, 11]. However, we consider that systemic circulatory disturbance was unlikely to be elicited by these procedures. This is because we kept monitoring the inferior vena cava diameter using ultrasonography while simultaneously administering albumin. The patient did not demonstrate inferior vena cava collapse, renal dysfunction, or any other signs of intravascular volume depletion. And there were three other cases of PE which needed diuretics after UAE without uterine necrosis in our cases.

The characteristic symptoms of uterine necrosis are fever, abdominal pain, pelvic pain, sepsis, metrorrhagia, and vaginal discharge [4]. In our patient, only fever persisted despite the use of multiple antimicrobial agents. Blood flow was confirmed only in the external layer in the uterine myometrium, and no blood flow in the internal layer was observed by ultrasonography. Contrast-enhanced MRI showed loss of contrast enhancement in the internal myometrium, leading us to diagnose uterine necrosis. These imaging findings are characteristic for uterine necrosis [8,

12]. In the event of fever of unknown origin or other persistent symptoms indicative of uterine necrosis after UAE, observing the state of the endometrium with abdominal ultrasonography is important for diagnosis. When hypoperfusion in the internal myometrium is observed by ultrasonography, contrast-enhanced MRI should be considered for definitive diagnosis of uterine necrosis.

In conclusion, patients with PE with massive ascites may possess a greater risk of UAE-induced uterine necrosis due to uterine local circulatory failure associated with intravascular volume depletion. In UAE for patients with PE, care should be taken in the selection of embolic materials and the management of other risk factors such as infection or hypovolemic status for uterine necrosis. After UAE, it is important to pay attention to the symptoms suspecting uterine necrosis, as well as evaluate the vascularity of the uterine with ultrasonography and MRI to achieve timely diagnosis of uterine necrosis.

Consent

Informed patient consent has been obtained.

References

[1] M. Sone, Y. Nakajima, R. Woodhams et al., "Interventional radiology for critical hemorrhage in obstetrics: Japanese Society of Interventional Radiology (JSIR) procedural guidelines," *Japanese Journal of Radiology*, vol. 33, no. 4, pp. 233–240, 2015.

[2] J. Y. Cheong, T. W. Kong, J. H. Son, J. H. Won, J. I. Yang, and H. S. Kim, "Outcome of pelvic arterial embolization for postpartum hemorrhage: a retrospective review of 117 cases," *Obstetrics & Gynecology Science*, vol. 57, no. 1, pp. 17–27, 2014.

[3] S. Inoue, H. Masuyama, Y. Hiramatsu, and Multi-Institutional Study Group of Transarterial Embolization for Massive Obstetric Haemorrhage in Chugoku & Shikoku Area Society of Obstetrics and Gynecology, "Efficacy of transarterial embolisation in the management of post-partum haemorrhage and its impact on subsequent pregnancies," *The Australian & New Zealand Journal of Obstetrics & Gynaecology*, vol. 54, no. 6, pp. 541–545, 2014.

[4] O. Poujade, P. F. Ceccaldi, C. Davitian et al., "Uterine necrosis following pelvic arterial embolization for post-partum hemorrhage: review of the literature," *European Journal of Obstetrics, Gynecology, and Reproductive Biology*, vol. 170, no. 2, pp. 309–314, 2013.

[5] M. J. Kim, I. J. Kim, S. Kim, and I. Y. Park, "Postpartum hemorrhage with uterine artery embolization: the risk of complications of uterine artery embolization," *Minimally Invasive Therapy & Allied Technologies*, vol. 31, no. 2, pp. 276–283, 2022.

[6] J. Y. Suriya, A. Keepanasseril, K. Manikandan, D. K. Maurya, P. Veena, and S. Soundara Raghavan, "Maternal ascites an independent prognostic factor in severe preeclampsia: a matched cohort study," *Archives of Gynecology and Obstetrics*, vol. 296, pp. 63–68, 2017.

[7] A. Sjaus, D. M. McKeen, and R. B. George, "Hypertensive disorders of pregnancy," *Canadian Journal of Anesthesia*, vol. 63, no. 9, pp. 1075–1097, 2016.

[8] H. Hirashima, K. Kaminaga, Y. Koyashiki, K. Tabata, R. Usui, and A. Ohkuchi, "Uterine necrosis following uterine artery embolism due to postpartum hemorrhage: a case report and review," *Hypertension Research in Pregnancy*, vol. 9, no. 1, pp. 11–16, 2021.

[9] S. B. Koseoglu, R. Deveer, A. Camuzcuoglu, B. Kasap, and H. Camuzcuoglu, "Massive ascites and pleural effusion in preeclampsia," *Journal of Clinical and Diagnostic Research: JCDR*, vol. 11, pp. QD08–QD09, 2017.

[10] G. Laffi, G. La Villa, V. Carloni et al., "Loop diuretic therapy in liver cirrhosis with acites," *Journal of Cardiovascular Pharmacology*, vol. 22, pp. s51–s58, 1993.

[11] L. C. Costello-Boerrigter, W. B. Smith, G. Boerrigter et al., "Vasopressin-2-receptor antagonism augments water excretion without changes in renal hemodynamics or sodium and potassium excretion in human heart failure," *American Journal of Physiology. Renal Physiology*, vol. 290, no. 2, pp. F273–F278, 2006.

[12] J. P. Rodenas, L. G. Martínez-Acacio, M. A. Collantes, M. V. García, J. P. G. de la Torre, and A. N. A. Recover, "Uterine necrosis. A rare complication of embolisation due to postpartum haemorrhage," *Journal of Gynecology Obstetrics and Human Reproduction*, vol. 50, no. 2, article 101773, 2021.

42

Preeclampsia, HELLP Syndrome and Postpartum Renal Failure with Thin Basement Membrane Nephropathy: Case Report and a Brief Review of Postpartum Renal Failure

K. C. Janga, Pavani Chitamanni, Shraddha Raghavan, Kamlesh Kumar, Sheldon Greenberg, and Kundan Jana

Maimonides Medical Center, Brooklyn, NY 11219, USA

Correspondence should be addressed to K. C. Janga; kjanga@maimonidesmed.org

Academic Editor: Irene Hoesli

A 36-year-old primigravida female from a birthing center was referred for elevated blood pressure to the hospital two days after normal spontaneous vaginal delivery with nausea, vomiting, and diarrhea. During this two-day period, she was experiencing persistent vaginal bleeding and lower abdominal pains for which she took six doses of 600 mg ibuprofen. Further laboratory evaluation reflected leukocytosis, anemia, thrombocytopenia, elevation of liver enzymes, and renal failure with hyperkalemia requiring emergent hemodialysis once in the Medical Intensive Care Unit (MICU). She was diagnosed with HELLP syndrome with underlying preeclampsia. A week later, due to hypertension controlled with medications and nonoliguric renal failure with no active urine sediments, a renal biopsy was indicated to direct management. The renal biopsy supported the diagnosis of diffuse severe acute tubulointerstitial nephritis with hypereosinophilia and thin basement membrane nephropathy (see figures). She was subsequently treated with high-dose steroids which resulted in the normalization of blood pressures and renal function returning to baseline. We report the first case of acute tubulointerstitial nephritis in an individual with thin basement membrane nephropathy secondary to postpartum complications.

1. Case Summary

1.1. History of Presenting Illness. Our patient is a 36-year-old female primigravida who presented with two-day history of persistent postpartum vaginal bleeding, pelvic pain, nausea, vomiting, diarrhea, and poor oral fluid intake. Patient had received prenatal care limited to vitamins and genetic counselling and went into labor at 41-week-and-4-day gestation at a midwife-assisted birthing center. Castor oil, herbal tea techniques, acupuncture, and various massage maneuvers were used to induce and aid the progression of labor. The patient delivered 11 hours after an artificial rupture of membranes performed by the midwife. Due to a second-degree vaginal tear and postpartum hemorrhage of unknown etiology and duration, oral misoprostol and intramuscular oxytocin were administered, and the patient returned home. Over the next day, she had poor oral intake, pelvic pain, and low urine output. Due to continuing weakness, difficulty walking, and high blood pressure, she was referred to our medical facility. The patient's past medical history includes easy bruising, nosebleeds, and bleeding gums since childhood. Additionally, she used combined hormonal contraceptives for three years prior to her current gestation.

1.2. Hospital Course. In the MICU, the patient was in severe renal failure with metabolic acidosis; azotemia; persistent hyperkalemia even after administration of calcium gluconate, insulin dextrose, bicarbonate pushes, and 2 doses of Kayexalate; hyponatremia unresponsive to fluids; and hypoglycemia. Laboratory findings also included elevated liver enzymes, anemia, thrombocytopenia, leukocytosis, hyperuricemia, subnephrotic-range proteinuria with a urine protein to creatinine ratio of 0.77 (770 mg/dl) and high LDH levels suggestive of HELLP syndrome with preeclampsia. The patient was subsequently started on a nicardipine drip for elevated blood pressures. Although presenting with no neurologic signs, she was started on seizure prophylaxis for eclampsia with levetiracetam. The patient was also placed on broad-spectrum antibiotics for possible intra-abdominal infection. Though the patient was afebrile, her abdominal pain with leukocytosis and history of postpartum hemorrhage prompted initiation of prophylactic treatment for puerperal sepsis. Differential diagnoses at that time included preeclampsia/-HELLP syndrome, acute fatty liver of pregnancy (AFLP), hemolytic uremic syndrome (HUS), thrombotic thrombocytopenic purpura (TTP), and puerperal sepsis.

Due to persistently elevated creatinine and refractory hyperkalemia of 6.3 mg/dl not responding to medical therapy, the patient underwent one cycle of emergent hemodialysis in the Medical Intensive Care Unit. Though her liver function tests, platelets, hematocrit, and electrolytes began to slowly normalize over the next two days, her creatinine remained elevated. She was diagnosed with nonoliguric renal failure of uncertain etiology requiring a kidney biopsy.

By hospital day 5, the patient's electrolytes, leukocytosis, thrombocytopenia, and hemolysis parameters normalized (Table 1). Seizure and antibiotic prophylaxes were discontinued at that time. Her blood pressure remained elevated, and the patient was deescalated to oral labetalol and amlodipine. ADAMTS13 activity levels, ordered on admission, showed a low value of 36.8% (normal 66.8%). However, TTP was ruled out as ADAMTS13 levels should be under 10% for this diagnosis. Rare schistocytes were seen on daily peripheral blood smears; thus, the patient still partially met criteria for atypical HUS. Immunologic workup and viral panels for hepatitis and HIV were unremarkable, with the exception of Epstein-Barr virus immunoglobulin titers evident for chronic infection.

On hospital day 6, the patient regained normal appetite and she was participating in breastfeeding and out-of-bed exercises conducted in the medical ward. Renal biopsy results demonstrated acute tubulointerstitial nephritis with eosinophils and thin glomerular basement membrane (Figures 1–3). Thus, the patient was started on high-dose steroids with a rapid taper over 2 weeks. The management we provided resulted in normalization of renal function.

2. Renal Biopsy Results

3. Discussion

The syndrome of postpartum renal failure has been recognized since 1968 as an idiopathic condition characterized by renal failure in association with microangiopathic hemolytic anemia and thrombocytopenia occurring within a week of apparently normal delivery [1, 2] Postpartum renal failure is associated with high mortality and morbidity primarily from bleeding diathesis and renal failure. Beyond supportive care and hemodialysis, there is no conclusive evidence that specific therapy is effective in mitigating the hemolytic abnormality or reducing the severity of renal failure. Postpartum renal failure can be categorized based on etiologies similar to the nonpregnant population (Table 2).

4. Thin Basement Membrane Nephropathy and Pregnancy

Thin basement membrane nephropathy (TBMN) is characterized by persistent hematuria and thinning of glomerular basement membrane. This disease is clinically defined as isolated glomerular hematuria, minimal proteinuria, normal renal function, and a first-degree relative with hematuria. It is histologically defined by uniform basement membrane thinning (on electron microscopic examination) in the absence of glomerular or interstitial abnormality (on light microscopic or immunological examination). Additionally, WHO criteria for defining TBMN is a basement membrane dimension between 250 and 264 nm [3]. Causes of TBMN include focal segmental glomerulosclerosis (FSGS) and IgA glomerulosclerosis; however, many patients have incidental biopsy findings as with our patient.

Clinical complications of TBMN include hematuria, hypertension, proteinuria, and renal failure [4]. Out of these, hypertension and hematuria are the most common complications. However, hypertension in TBMN is not known to be causal or coincidental. Renal failure is a rare complication of TBMN and is usually known to be precipitated when associated with proteinuria, hypertension, and a coexistent tubulointerstitial or glomerular lesion as seen in our patient [5]. Renal impairment in TBMN is explained by progression of the disease itself or more commonly, predisposition to glomerular or tubulointerstitial lesion [6, 7]. In a study of 16 biopsy-proven TBMN patients with acute renal failure, 15 of them had coexisting glomerular or tubulointerstitial lesions suggesting the prominent role they play in leading to renal failure [5]. Whereas lesions like acute tubulointerstitial nephritis, as seen in our patient, are more likely to be coincidental, lesions like IgA glomerulonephritis need further investigation to understand their association.

Although the disease affects >1% of the population, the effects of TBMN have not been extensively studied in pregnancy. In a study from 2005, records of parous women with a diagnosis of TBMN over 13 years were reviewed. Majority of the patients (89.6%) had no complications with an overall fetal outcome of 95% live births and 4.4% fetal loss in <12 weeks. Particularly, 3 percent of them developed renal impairment, 48 percent developed hypertension, and 53 percent developed proteinuria. Renal impairment was reversible in 100 percent of cases [3].

Our patient presented with nonoliguric acute renal failure with hyperkalemia postpartum warranting a session of emergent hemodialysis. Renal biopsy showed ultrastructural diffuse glomerular basement membrane thinning (mean 215.06 nm; range 135-287 nm) consistent with thin glomerular basement membrane nephropathy. Although patients with thin basement membrane nephropathy are known to have an overall benign course, patients developing proteinuria or hypertension tend to have a higher risk of renal failure [8]. Proteinuria and hypertension in our patient were also associated with elevated liver enzymes and thrombocytopenia suggestive of a broad differential including preeclampsia, HELLP syndrome, acute fatty liver of pregnancy, and atypical hemolytic uremic syndrome.

TABLE 1: Laboratory values of the patient over the course of her hospitalization.

	Day 1	Day 3	Day 5	Day 7	Discharge	3-week follow-up
Glucose	40	147	73	109	96	83
Hemoglobin	8.9	8.5	7.9	7.4	7.0	11.4
WBC count	23.7	16.6	9.1	8.0	8.6	6.4
Eosinophils (%)	0.0	0.0	1.1	1.6	0.0	
Platelet count	57000	115000	144000	183000	253000	211000
Creatinine	5.3	4.7	5.6	5.3	2.1	1.0
BUN	57	45	61	66	53	17
AST	650	166	45	32	18	13
ALT	1308	708	313	184	91	15
ALP	143	142	119	111	102	69
Sodium	113	126	123	132	142	140
Potassium	6.6	4.4	4.2	4.6	4.8	4.0
Bicarbonate	17	20	19	19	21	30
Bilirubin	0.8	0.5	0.4	0.4	0.4	0.4
PT	10.2	11.2		11		
PTT	26.5			30.3		
INR	0.9	0.9		0.9		
LDH	448	360		278	224	

WBC: white blood cell; BUN: blood urea nitrogen; AST: aspartate transaminase; ALT: alanine transaminase; ALP: alkaline phosphatase; PT: prothrombin time; PTT: activated partial thromboplastin time; INR: international normalized ratio; LDH: lactate dehydrogenase.

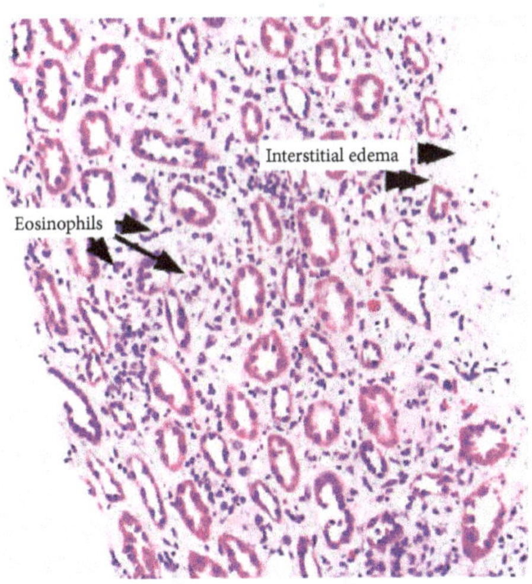

FIGURE 1: Light microscopy findings indicative of diffuse severe acute tubulointerstitial nephritis with eosinophils.

In addition, biopsy finding of acute tubulointerstitial nephritis with hypereosinophilia also suggested acute interstitial nephritis (AIN). Overall, the etiology of acute interstitial nephritis can be grouped into five general categories: drug-induced, infectious, autoimmune, malignant, and idiopathic. Out of these, drug-induced AIN accounts for over two-thirds of all cases and, although many drugs have been implicated, nonsteroidal anti-inflammatory drugs (NSAIDs) and antimicrobial agents have been seen to cause the majority of these cases. It is understood that the pathogenesis of AIN is an immunologic reaction via endogenous nephritogenic or exogenous antigens that are presented by tubular cells to T cells, activating a cascade of effector cells and cytokines eventually leading to interstitial infiltrates [9]. Either patchy or diffuse infiltrates of lymphocytes, macrophages, and plasma cells are commonly seen on renal biopsy, such as in our patient, along with nonsuppurative fluid within the interstitium and/or tubules. The laboratory findings, showing impairment in kidney function, can vary from selective abnormalities of tubular function to acute renal failure with or without oliguria. Historically, BUN and creatinine will increase after tubular dysfunction is detectable, with or without oliguria. The presence of a history consistent with AIN and laboratory findings of acute kidney injury are sufficient to diagnose this condition, although definitive diagnosis is through renal biopsy. Reversal of kidney injury is the rule in 60-65% of cases after the removal of offending agents. The use of steroids in AIN remains controversial but deserves consideration, as it has been shown to have better outcomes for patients when started early in the disease course [9, 10]. The etiology of AIN in our patient was likely the recent use of NSAIDs prior to delivery.

5. Differential Diagnoses

At presentation, the patient met the criteria for preeclampsia with hypertension, proteinuria with urine protein to creatinine ratio of 0.77, elevated creatinine and transaminases, and thrombocytopenia suggestive of end-organ damage (Table 3). Currently, preeclampsia is one of the most prevalent medical complications of acute kidney injury in women and the most reported complication in those women requiring dialysis in the postpartum period [11].

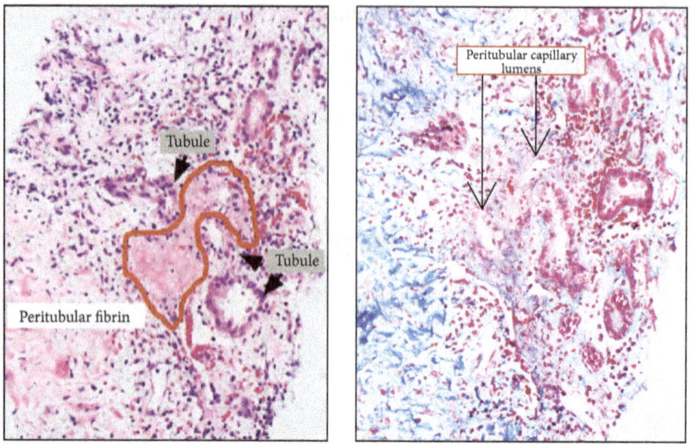

FIGURE 2: (a, b) Light microscopy shows fibrinoid necrosis of the peritubular areas suggestive of microangiopathy.

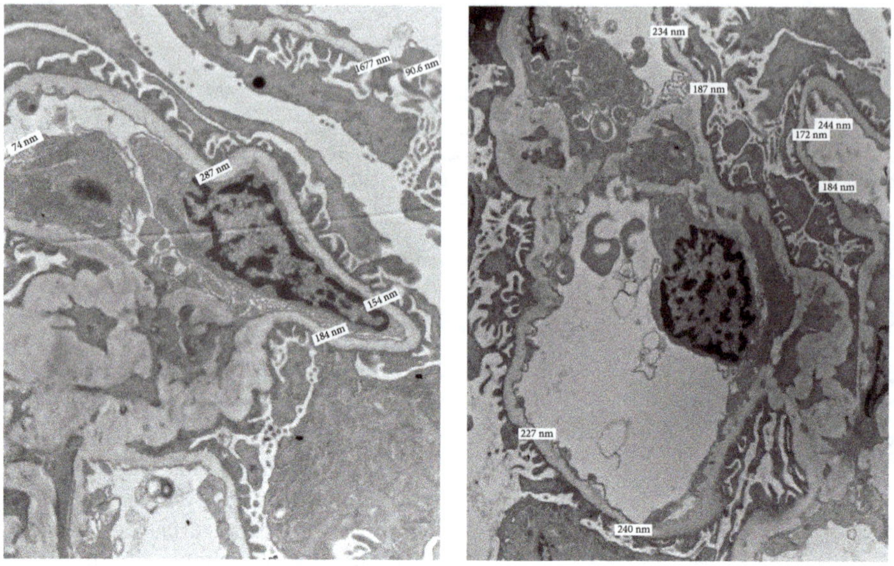

FIGURE 3: (a, b) Electron microscopy demonstrates diffuse glomerular basement thinning with arithmetic mean 215.06 nm (range 135-287 nm with 100% of 41 measures less than 300 nm and 63% less than 215 nm).

The pathogenesis of preeclampsia occurs in several ways. It involves defects in placentation mediated by placental-derived angiogenic factors, such as placental growth factor or soluble endoglin. Along with dysfunction of the complement system, errors in placentation can cause severe kidney injury. Without maternal susceptibility, the complement system is activated in normal pregnancy. However, it is exaggerated in preeclampsia and studies have found this exacerbation cytotoxic to cells [12]. It has also been found that preeclampsia has a direct effect via endothelial injury, vasoconstriction, inflammation, and the overactivation of the coagulation cascade. These mechanisms are sufficient enough to cause catastrophic organ complications and are responsible for high admission rates to the intensive care unit.

HELLP syndrome was also part of the differential as the patient had evidence of hemolysis with elevated liver enzymes and low platelet count (Table 4). This syndrome can present up to 7-day postpartum and is a milder form of microangiopathic hemolytic anemia due to a dysregulation of the complement pathway. Postpartum complications involve bleeding requiring transfusions, DIC, pulmonary edema, and renal failure in 10% of recorded cases. Management is usually supported including magnesium sulfate, antihypertensive medications, and blood transfusions for Hb < 7, and platelet transfusions for <30K. This syndrome is self-limiting in the postpartum phase, and trending the platelet counts is used as a prognostic indicator [13, 14].

Though acute fatty liver of pregnancy (AFLP) is known to typically present between the 30th and 38th week of pregnancy, few cases have been reported to occur postpartum [15]. General clinical symptoms that can be present at the time of diagnosis are nausea, vomiting, abdominal pain,

Table 2: Causes of renal failure in pregnant and nonpregnant patients.

Etiologies of renal failure	Conditions related to pregnancy	Conditions unrelated to pregnancy
Prerenal	Hyperemesis gravidarum, vomiting due to preeclampsia, HELLP/AFLP, hemorrhage (missed abortion, septic abortion, placental abruption, placenta previa, uterine previa, bleeding during surgery, uterine laceration, uterine perforation)	Vomiting due to infections, gastroenteritis, pyelonephritis, malnutrition Others (like diuretics, CHF)
Intrinsic renal	ATN/ACN: preeclampsia, HELLP, AFLP, amniotic fluid embolism, pulmonary embolism TMA: HUS, preeclampsia, HELLP, AFLP, DIC, underlying glomerular diseases	ATN, de novo glomerular disease, AIN
Postrenal	Bilateral hydronephrosis Trauma to the ureters and bladder during surgery	Bilateral ureteral obstruction stone/tumor Tubular obstruction (meds/calcium/uric acid) Obstruction at bladder outlet
Renal allograft related	Similar to nonpregnant conditions	Acute rejection ATN Acute interstitial nephritis, calcineurin inhibitor toxicity, CMV/BK virus nephropathy, postinfectious glomerulonephropathy

HELLP: hemolysis, elevated liver enzymes, low platelet count; AFLP: acute fatty liver of pregnancy; CHF: congestive heart failure; ATN: acute tubular necrosis; ACN: acute cortical necrosis; AIN: acute interstitial nephritis; TMA: thrombotic microangiopathies; HUS: hemolytic uremic syndrome; DIC: disseminated intravascular coagulation; CMV: cytomegalovirus.

Table 3: Diagnostic criteria for preeclampsia fulfilled by our patient.

	Preeclampsia criteria	Our patient's laboratory results on admission	Met or unmet
Blood pressure	New-onset hypertension after 20 weeks of gestation (>140/>90 on 2 occasions at least 4 h apart or >160/>110 within short minutes)	Postpartum blood pressure of 140/60 mmHg, with continuous elevated readings during hospitalization	Met
Proteinuria	Hypertension plus >300 mg/24 h urine collection, protein/creatinine ratio of >0.3, or urine dipstick reading of 1+	Protein/creatinine ratio of 0.7	Met
End-organ damage	Blood pressure criteria plus evidence of thrombocytopenia (platelet < 100K), renal insufficiency (creatinine > 1.1 or doubling), impaired liver function (transaminases twice the normal), pulmonary edema, cerebral or visual symptoms	Platelets: 68,000/μl Creatinine: 5.3 mg/dl AST/ALT: 650/1308	Met

AST: aspartate transaminase; ALT: alanine transaminase.

Table 4: Diagnostic criteria for HELLP syndrome fulfilled by our patient.

Definition	Laboratory range	Met or unmet
Hemolysis	Peripheral smear: schistocytes and burr cells (>5/HPF)	Yes
	Serum bilirubin: >1.2 mg/dl	No
	Haptoglobin: <25 mg/dl	Yes
	LDH > 2x the upper limit of normal	Yes
	Anemia: Hgb < 7 and not related to blood loss	Yes
Elevated liver function tests	AST/ALT > 2x the upper limit of normal	Yes
Low platelets	<100,000 cells/μl	Yes

AST: aspartate transaminase; ALT: alanine transaminase.

and jaundice. The pathogenesis of this disease involves maternal and fetal mutations in the enzyme long-chain 3-hydroxyacyl-CoA dehydrogenase, which processes long-chain fatty acids (LCFA). With dysfunction of this enzyme, LCFAs accumulate and cause hepatotoxicity. Thus, although biopsy is not usually performed, it would demonstrate microvesicular fatty infiltration of hepatocytes [12]. Pregnancy-related acute kidney injury is present in over half the cases of AFLP, as these LCFAs can deposit in the renal tubular epithelium. Our patient similarly reported nausea and vomiting in the postpartum period. A large degree of clinical overlap is very often seen between AFLP, HELLP, and preeclampsia [16]. With elevated transaminases, hypoglycemia, lactic acidosis, and thrombocytopenia, she fell into the spectrum of this disease, although her hypertension also placed her diagnosis in the realm of preeclampsia/HELLP syndrome. Since distinguishing between AFLP and preeclampsia/HELLP can be difficult due to similar parameters of disease, many patients, about 20-40% with AFLP, have a simultaneous diagnosis of preeclampsia/HELLP [12].

Thrombotic microangiopathies were also considered an important differential as the patient had hemolytic anemia, acute kidney injury (AKI), and thrombocytopenia. However, thrombotic thrombocytopenic purpura was ruled out as ADAMTS13 levels were >10%. Atypical hemolytic uremic syndrome (HUS) was still a possibility with marked effect on renal function requiring renal replacement therapy. In the postpartum period, loss of placental protective barrier mechanisms, inflammation, infection, wounded uterus, and influx on fetal cells can trigger systemic activation of alternative complement cascade. Genetic mutations in the regulatory proteins (factor-H, I, CD-46) or complement activators (C3, factor-B) of the alternative complement pathway are found in 50% of the cases [13, 17, 18].

Preeclampsia, AFLP, and HELLP syndrome are commonly associated with cortical or acute tubular necrosis on renal biopsy [19] whereas atypical HUS shows fibrinoid necrosis of arterioles and thrombus in the lumen extending to the glomerular capillary tufts [18]. However, renal biopsy in our patient showed acute tubulointerstitial nephritis with hypereosinophilia and thinning of the basement membrane suggestive of acute interstitial nephritis with thin basement membrane nephropathy. A rare focus of microscopic peritubular fibrin and necrosis was also present (Figure 2(a)) suggestive of a microangiopathy; however, other features of thrombotic microangiopathy (e.g., arterial, arteriolar, or glomerular angiopathy/ultrastructural endotheliosis) were not identified.

In conclusion, we present a case of renal failure in the postpartum period in which an array of factors were considered. Predisposing risk factors for postpartum renal failure include nephrotoxic medications, infections, proteinuria, cystic diseases, chronic kidney disease, transplant, and glomerular diseases. As outlined by our review article, a few of these causes include medication use like NSAIDS in the peripartum period and gestational disease including preeclampsia and HELLP syndrome, as well puerperal sepsis in the postpartum obstetrical infections. Our patient was successfully treated with prompt supportive therapy and a short course of high-dose steroids with normalization of renal indices and urine proteinuria. In such cases of renal failure specifically in the postpartum period, the etiologies contributing are overlapping each other leading to a complex presentation which requires a multidisciplinary approach in the treatment geared towards addressing each of the specific causes [20].

References

[1] L. Neave and M. Scully, "Microangiopathic hemolytic anemia in pregnancy," *Transfusion Medicine Reviews*, vol. 32, no. 4, pp. 230–236, 2018.

[2] M. Salhab, A. Hsu, E. Ryer, J. Appiah, and B. Switzer, "Microangiopathic hemolytic anemia in pregnancy," *Transfusion and Apheresis Science*, vol. 56, no. 3, pp. 354–356, 2017.

[3] D. Packham, "Thin basement membrane nephropathy in pregnancy," *Seminars in Nephrology*, vol. 25, no. 3, pp. 180–183, 2005.

[4] J. E. Collar, S. Ladva, T. D. H. Cairns, and V. Cattell, "Red cell traverse through thin glomerular basement membranes," *Kidney International*, vol. 59, no. 6, pp. 2069–2072, 2001.

[5] S. Tonna, Y. Y. Wang, D. MacGregor et al., "The risks of thin basement membrane nephropathy," *Seminars in Nephrology*, vol. 25, no. 3, pp. 171–175, 2005.

[6] F. G. Cosio, M. E. Falkenhain, and D. D. Sedmak, "Association of thin glomerular basement membrane with other glomerulopathies," *Kidney International*, vol. 46, no. 2, pp. 471–474, 1994.

[7] Y. M. Sue, J. J. Huang, R. Y. Hsieh, and F. F. Chen, "Clinical features of thin basement membrane disease and associated glomerulopathies," *Nephrology (Carlton, Vic.)*, vol. 9, no. 1, pp. 14–18, 2004.

[8] C. M. G. Nieuwhof, F. de Heer, P. de Leeuw, and P. J. C. van Breda Vriesman, "Thin GBM nephropathy: premature glomerular obsolescence is associated with hypertension and late onset renal failure," *Kidney International*, vol. 51, no. 5, pp. 1596–1601, 1997.

[9] R. Raghavan and G. Eknoyan, "Acute interstitial nephritis - a reappraisal and update," *Clinical Nephrology*, vol. 82, no. 9, pp. 149–162, 2014.

[10] M. Praga and E. Gonzalez, "Acute interstitial nephritis," *Kidney International*, vol. 77, no. 11, pp. 956–961, 2010.

[11] A. M. Hildebrand, K. Liu, S. Z. Shariff et al., "Characteristics and outcomes of AKI treated with dialysis during pregnancy and the postpartum period," *Journal of the American Society of Nephrology*, vol. 26, no. 12, pp. 3085–3091, 2015.

[12] S. Rao and B. Jim, "Acute kidney injury in pregnancy: the changing landscape for the 21st century," *Kidney International Reports*, vol. 3, no. 2, pp. 247–257, 2018.

[13] J. P. Hayslett, "Current concepts. Postpartum renal failure," *The New England Journal of Medicine*, vol. 312, no. 24, pp. 1556–1559, 1985.

[14] A. Mancini, G. Ardissino, P. Angelini et al., "HELLP syndrome and hemolytic uremic syndrome during pregnancy: two disease entities, same causation. Case report and literature review," *Giornale Italiano di Nefrologia: Organo Ufficiale Della Società Italiana di Nefrologia*, vol. 36, no. 2, 2019.

[15] M. Knight, C. Nelson-Piercy, J. J. Kurinczuk, P. Spark, P. Brocklehurst, and on behalf of UK Obstetric Surveillance System (UKOSS), "A prospective national study of acute fatty liver of pregnancy in the UK," *Gut*, vol. 57, no. 7, pp. 951–956, 2008.

[16] H. Minakami, M. Morikawa, T. Yamada, T. Yamada, R. Akaishi, and R. Nishida, "Differentiation of acute fatty liver of pregnancy from syndrome of hemolysis, elevated liver enzymes and low platelet counts," *The Journal of Obstetrics and Gynaecology Research*, vol. 40, no. 3, pp. 641–649, 2014.

[17] A. Acharya, J. Santos, B. Linde, and K. Anis, "Acute kidney injury in pregnancy-current status," *Advances in Chronic Kidney Disease*, vol. 20, no. 3, pp. 215–222, 2013.

[18] F. Meibody, M. Jamme, V. Tsatsaris et al., "Post-partum acute kidney injury: sorting placental and non-placental thrombotic microangiopathies using the trajectory of biomarkers," *Nephrology, Dialysis, Transplantation*, vol. 35, no. 9, pp. 1538–1546, 2020.

[19] C. J. Saphier and J. T. Repke, "Hemolysis, elevated liver

enzymes, and low platelets (HELLP) syndrome: a review of diagnosis and management," *Seminars in Perinatology*, vol. 22, no. 2, pp. 118–133, 1998.

[20] M. Jonard, A. S. Ducloy-Bouthors, E. Boyle et al., "Postpartum acute renal failure: a multicenter study of risk factors in patients admitted to ICU," *Annals of Intensive Care*, vol. 4, no. 1, p. 36, 2014.

43

Uterocutaneous Fistula after a C-Section in a Patient with Second Trimester Fetal Demise and Chorioamnionitis

Déborah Wernly,[1] **Valérie Besse**,[2] **and Daniela Huber**[1,3]

[1]*Department of Obstetrics and Gynecology, Sion's Hospital, Valais, Switzerland*
[2]*Department of Radiology, Sion's Hospital, Valais, Switzerland*
[3]*Department of Pediatrics, Obstetrics and Gynecology, Geneva University Hospitals, Switzerland*

Correspondence should be addressed to Déborah Wernly; deborah.wernly@chuv.ch

Academic Editor: Kyousuke Takeuchi

Uterocutaneous fistulae are very rare entities with only about 120 cases reported in the literature. They are mostly described after a C-section or other pelvic surgery. We hereby describe a uterocutaneous fistula in a 41-year-old patient 5 months after a C-section because of a chorioamnionitis and a 22-week fetal demise. One month after the C-section, she underwent a diagnostic hysteroscopy to exclude postoperative intrauterine adhesions. Afterwards, she complained of pelvic pain, persistent metrorrhagia, and significant weight loss during 2 months. She consulted the emergency unit several times, and lastly endometritis was diagnosed. She was treated with antibiotic therapy for 7 days, without significant clinical improvement. She presented at our institution 48 hours after a carbuncle had appeared in her right iliac fossa. A uterocutaneous fistula was diagnosed on the CT scan. The patient received IV antibiotic therapy and underwent a total hysterectomy with bilateral salpingectomy by laparotomy, as she did not want a conservative surgery. The clinical postoperative evolution was favorable. Symptoms of UCF can be very unspecific. To avoid medical wandering and improve the patient's care, UCF should be in the differential diagnostic of abdominal pain after a pelvic surgery. Moreover, in patients with previous C-section and infectious perioperative status, the risk of PID or pelvic abscess must be careful evaluated before intrauterine diagnostic or therapeutic procedures.

1. Introduction

Uterocutaneous fistulae (UCF) are abnormal communications between the endometrium and the skin. Around 20 cases were reported in the literature in the last 10 years [1]. The majority of these cases are complications of a C-section, although some are the result of uterine perforation after curettage for a septic abortion [2–4]. Rarely, UCFs are caused by other surgeries such as polymyomectomy by laparotomy [5] or by other mechanisms such as necrobiosis of an intramural fibroid following a C-section [6]. UCF can also appear after a hysteroscopy, performed after a septic event.

The only pathognomonic symptom is the menstrual bleeding through the abdominal scar. Other symptoms are often atypical and may lead to diagnostic delay. An early diagnostic allows a conservative management of the fistulae: medical treatment with antibiotics and hormonal therapy or conservative surgery with the excision of the fistulous tract. As the majority of UCF appear after a C-section, young patients are concerned. Conservative management is therefore crucial if family planning is incomplete.

2. Case Presentation

In September 2019, a 41-year-old nulliparous patient had undergone a C-section by midline laparotomy with a corporeal hysterotomy at 22 weeks, in the context of fetal demise and chorioamnionitis. She underwent oral antibiotic therapy with metronidazole for 7 days postoperatively. In October 2019, a diagnostic hysteroscopy was conducted and revealed a posterior uterine myoma and no intrauterine adhesions.

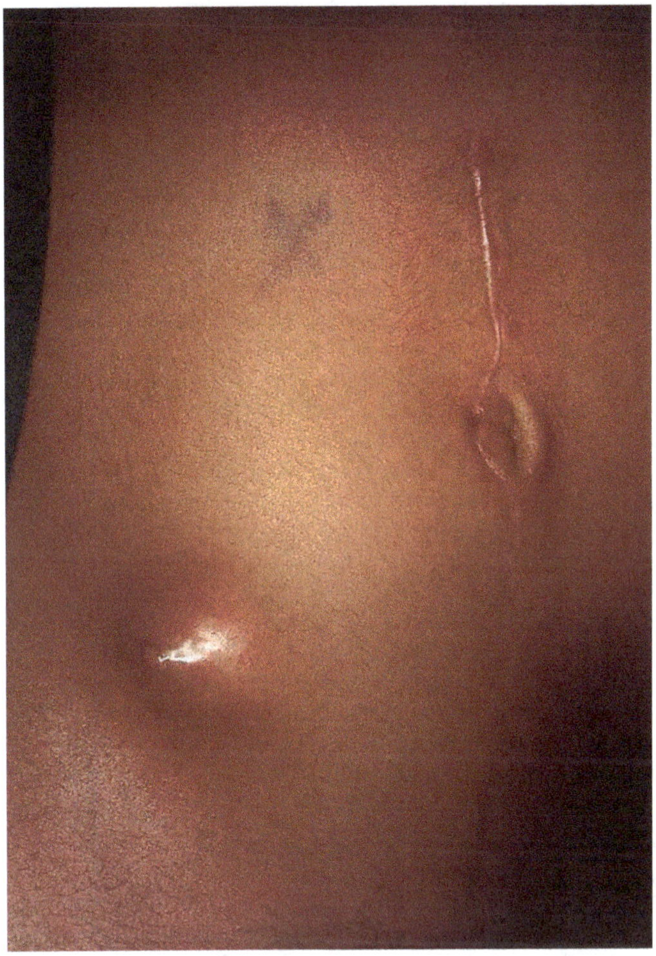

FIGURE 1: Carbuncle in the right iliac fossa.

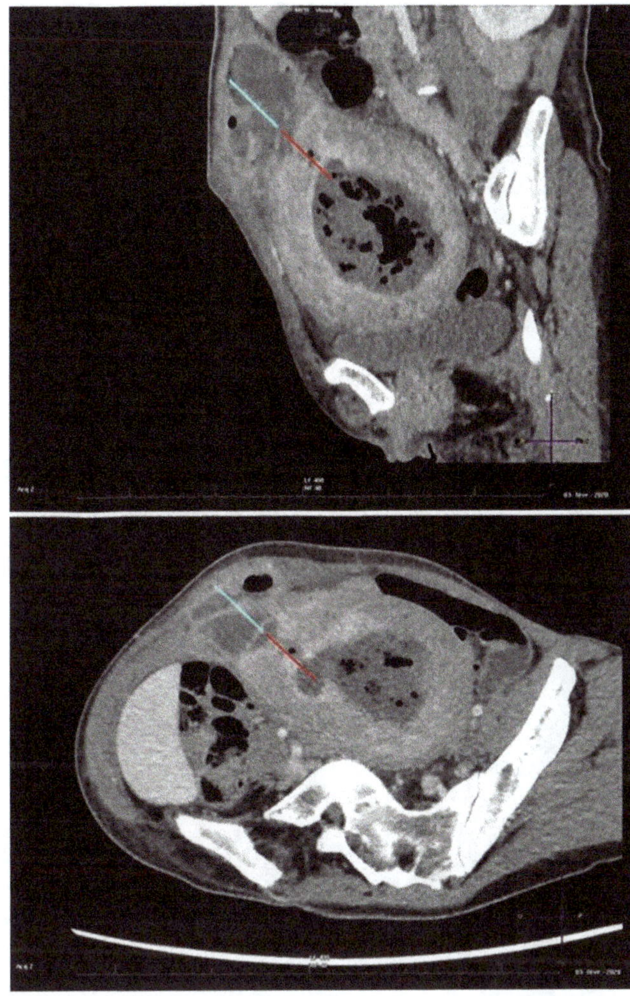

FIGURE 2: Sagittal and axial MPR reconstruction. Portal phase after iodine contrast injection. The blue arrow shows UCF. The red arrow shows uterine wall defect.

Subsequently, the patient complained of abdominal pain, which led to multiple gynecological consultations. In December 2019, she underwent oral antibiotic therapy with metronidazole and co-amoxicillin for 7 days for suspicion of endometritis. The patient felt no clinical improvement and consulted twice again for abdominal pain and metrorrhagia.

In early February 2020, after 4 months of persistent abdominal pain, she presented in our institution because a carbuncle in her right iliac fossa had appeared (Figure 1). She also reported an increased abdominal pain, metrorrhagia, and purulent vaginal discharge. She complained of inappetence and an involuntary 8 kg weight loss during the last 2 months.

She was hemodynamically stable and had no fever. Laboratory findings showed leukocytosis (13.7 G/L), elevated c-reactive protein (244 mg/L), and anemia (hemoglobin 87 g/L). An abdominal CT scan identified a uterocutaneous fistula with a 7.5 × 7.5 × 11 cm intrauterine collection draining from the right antero-lateral uterine fundus to the abdominal wall (Figure 2).

The patient received IV antibiotic therapy. As she was in favor of a radical treatment, a total hysterectomy with bilateral salpingectomy by midline laparotomy was performed. Figure 3 shows the excision of the fistula tract right before the hysterectomy. The bacteriological analyses identified an *Enterococcus faecalis* strain that was sensitive to co-amoxicillin. The antibiotic therapy was pursued for a total of 14 days with a favorable clinical evolution.

The patient was discharged 9 days after surgery. Two months after, she was treated conservatively for bartholinitis. In May 2020, she was evaluated by our general surgeon for a possible right abdominal wall reinforcement. The results of a CT scan showed no need of further surgery.

3. Discussion

UCFs are very rare fistulae with only 120 cases described in the literature over the past 200 years [7]. Complications of a C-section or curettage for septic abortion associated with uterine perforation account for most cases [2, 3]. In 2018, Hardy and Leung described a fistula as the primary presentation of a high-grade endometrioid adenocarcinoma [8]. Risk factors include multiple abdominal surgeries, corporeal hysterotomy, and presence of a foreign body (18), use of drains, or incomplete closure of a uterine wound following a C-section.

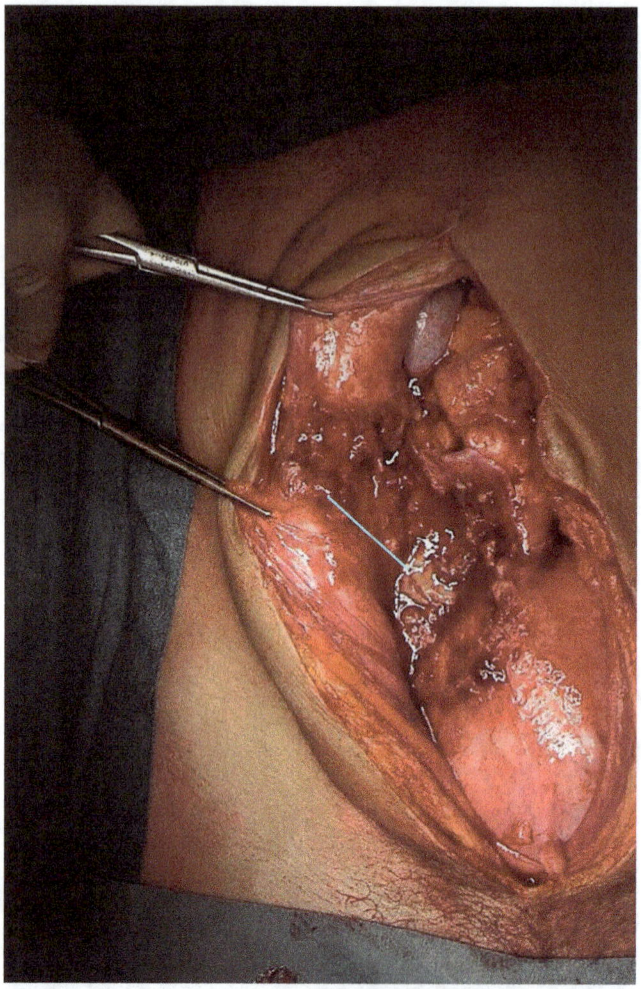

FIGURE 3: The blue arrow shows fistulae's tract (from the right uterine fundus to the skin) after its excision, before hysterectomy. The green star shows the uterus.

The diagnosis of UCF can be challenging. The time between surgery and the diagnosis of UCF ranges from 15 days to 11 years [1]. Whereas a number of reported cases describe bleeding through the C-section scar as a pathognomonic symptom, others mention menstrual blood loss through the fistula, abdominal wall discharge, or undefined abdominal pain [1]. The differential diagnosis includes intra-abdominal infections or tumors. Persistent abdominal pain and significant weight loss should lead to imaging to rule out pelvic tumors, an intra-abdominal abscess, or a fistula. Multiple diagnostic imaging techniques are available: ultrasonography, tomography, or MRI. Others described diagnosis tools including hysterosalpingography and hysteroscopy [1].

The prevalence of infection after hysteroscopy varies between 0.18 and 1.5% [9]. Currently, guidelines do not recommend the use of prophylactic antibiotics for hysteroscopy [10, 11]. Yet limited scientific evidence supports this recommendation. A meta-analysis of 5 studies [12] shows that antibiotics do not reduce the rate of fever, endometritis, or PID after hysteroscopy [12]. However, this study has some limitations. A hysteroscopy performed after chorioamnionitis or PID is likely associated with a greater infectious risk than a hysteroscopy in a patient with no infection history. The risk of infection is also higher after a prolonged operative hysteroscopy, especially after repeated insertion and removal of the hysteroscope through the cervix [13]. Comorbidities such as immunosuppression, connective tissue disorders, heart disease, mitral valve prolapse, history of PID or pelvic abscess, tubal dilation, and endometriosis were reported as risk factors [12, 14, 15]. Screening with a vaginal swab culture and/or prophylactic antibiotics should be considered for high-risk patients, as hysteroscopy can lead to serious complications such as UCF.

The treatment of UCF includes hormonal therapy and surgical excision of the fistulous tract with or without hysterectomy. Surgery is frequently the primary treatment. Medical treatment using the GnRH agonist for 6 months has been described in two cases [16, 17]. For young patients with incomplete family planning, conservative treatment, including resection of the fistula tract and closure of the uterus, should be considered with a risk of recurrence after conservative treatment [18]. A successful pregnancy and delivery were described in 2019 after the excision of a postmyomectomy uterocutaneous fistula tract [19]. After explaining the different available treatments, the patient refused the conservative treatment. After months of persistent symptoms and medical wandering, the patient was adamant for a hysterectomy.

4. Conclusion

Although UCFs are rare conditions, they should be included in the differential diagnosis of persisting symptoms such as metrorrhagia, purulent vaginal discharge, pelvic pain, and significant weight loss in patients with a history of uterine procedures such as C-section, curettage, hysteroscopy, or myomectomy followed or preceded by genital infections as PID or chorioamnionitis. Imaging by a CT scan is an important diagnostic tool in these clinical situations. A fast diagnostic will improve the patient's care and enable a conservative treatment in most cases. As a preventive care, screening with a vaginal swab culture and/or prophylactic antibiotics should be considered when performing a hysteroscopy in patients with recent pelvic or genital infections.

Consent

The patient gave written consent for the case report and images to be published.

Authors' Contributions

Wernly D, the first author, led the writing of the manuscript and compiled the initial literature sources, wrote up the patient's course, asked the patient for her consent for the report to be published, and prepared the manuscript for submission. Besse V. aided in interpreting and creating the CT reconstructions. Huber D, the senior author, assisted in the literature review, supervised the project, and reviewed the manuscript.

References

[1] C. Chattot, P. Aristizabal, S. Bendifallah, and E. Daraï, "Uteroabdominal Wall fistula after cesarean section in a patient with prior colorectal resection for endometriosis: a case report and systematic review," *Journal of Minimally Invasive Gynecology*, vol. 24, no. 7, pp. 1234–1238, 2017.

[2] S. K. Gupta, V. K. Shukla, D. N. Varma, and S. K. Roy, "Uterocutaneous fistula," *Postgraduate Medical Journal*, vol. 69, no. 816, pp. 822-823, 1993.

[3] S. Pratibha and B. Rajni, "Uterocutaneous fistula following septic abortion: can it heal without major surgical intervention?," *Journal of Obstetrics and Gynaecology*, vol. 35, no. 6, pp. 651-652, 2015.

[4] M. Sönmezer, Ö. Şahincioğlu, E. Çetinkaya, and F. Yazıcı, "Uterocutaneous fistula after surgical treatment of an incomplete abortion: methylene blue test to verify the diagnosis," *Archives of Gynecology and Obstetrics*, vol. 279, no. 2, pp. 225–227, 2009.

[5] M. O. Akkurt, A. Yavuz, B. Tatar, M. O. Ozkaya, and E. I. Ekici, "Utero-cutaneous fistula after multiple abdominal myomectomies: a case report," *Balkan Medical Journal*, vol. 32, no. 4, pp. 426–428, 2015.

[6] P. S. Lim, M. N. Shafiee, S. Ahmad, and M. Hashim Omar, "Utero-cutaneous fistula after caesarean section secondary to red degeneration of intramural fibroid," *Sexual and Reproductive Healthcare*, vol. 3, no. 2, pp. 95-96, 2012.

[7] G. Eldem, B. Turkbey, S. Balas, and E. Akpinar, "MDCT diagnosis of uterocutaneous fistula," *European Journal of Radiology*, vol. 67, no. 3, pp. e129–e130, 2008.

[8] L. E. Hardy and Y. Leung, "Uterocutaneous fistula as the primary presentation of a gynaecological malignancy," *BMJ Case Reports*, vol. 18, 2018.

[9] A. Agostini, L. Cravello, R. Shojai, I. Ronda, V. Roger, and B. Blanc, "Postoperative infection and surgical hysteroscopy," *Fertility and Sterility*, vol. 77, no. 4, pp. 766–768, 2002.

[10] ACOG Committee on Practice Bulletins, "ACOG Practice Bulletin No. 74: antibiotic prophylaxis for gynecologic procedures," *Obstetrics & Gynecology*, vol. 108, no. 1, pp. 225–234, 2006.

[11] Collège National Des Gynecologues Et Obstetriciens Francaistional, *Recommandations pour la pratique clinique: prévention des complications de l'hystéroscopie*, Recomm. Pour Prat. Clin, Paris, 2013.

[12] L. Muzii, V. D. Donato, C. D. Tucci et al., "Efficacy of antibiotic prophylaxis for hysteroscopy: a meta-analysis of randomized trials," *Journal of Minimally Invasive Gynecology*, vol. 27, no. 1, pp. 29–37, 2020.

[13] E. J. Bieber, *Hysteroscopy, Resectoscopy and Endometrial Ablation*, CRC Press, 1st edition, 2003.

[14] Y.-H. Lin, J. L. Hwang, K. M. Seow, K. M. Chong, and L. W. Huang, "Tubo-ovarian abscess with septic shock in a case of endometrioma following diagnostic hysteroscopy," *Taiwanese Journal of Obstetrics & Gynecology*, vol. 49, no. 3, pp. 359-360, 2010.

[15] N. Pereira, A. P. Hutchinson, J. P. Lekovich, E. Hobeika, and R. T. Elias, "Antibiotic prophylaxis for gynecologic procedures prior to and during the utilization of assisted reproductive technologies: a systematic review," *Journal of Pathogens*, vol. 2016, Article ID 4698314, 8 pages, 2016.

[16] P. Yadav, S. Gupta, P. Singh, and S. Tripathi, "Successful medical management of uterocutaneous fistula," *International Journal of Gynecology & Obstetrics*, vol. 124, no. 3, pp. 263-264, 2014.

[17] A. Seyhan, B. Ata, B. Sidal, and B. Urman, "Medical treatment of uterocutaneous fistula with gonadotropin-releasing hormone agonist administration," *Obstetrics & Gynecology*, vol. 111, no. 2, pp. 526–528, 2008.

[18] J. A. Kirkland, "Abdominal menstrual fistula: Report of a case and review of the literature," *American Journal of Obstetrics and Gynecology*, vol. 78, no. 6, pp. 1292–1297, 1959.

[19] M. Yesiladali, E. Saridogan, and E. Saridogan, "Successful pregnancy and delivery following surgical treatment of postmyomectomy uterocutaneous fistula," *BML Case Reports*, vol. 12, no. 12, article e231594, 2019.

44

Perinatal Catatonia in a Patient with a Twin Pregnancy of Unknown Chorionicity and Gestational Age Presenting in Spontaneous Preterm Labor

Ryan Farias and Janice Hartnett

University of Connecticut Obstetrics and Gynecology, USA

Correspondence should be addressed to Ryan Farias; farias@uchc.edu

Academic Editor: Seung-Yup Ku

Catatonia during pregnancy is rare and presents unique challenges due to the potential ramifications to mom and baby of the overall disease state and of potential treatment options. The purpose of this case report is to highlight the complexities in the workup and management of a catatonic patient with concurrent acute obstetric concerns requiring urgent intervention. We report a case of acute catatonia due to underlying major depressive disorder in a patient who presented in spontaneous preterm labor, with a twin pregnancy of unknown chorionicity with no known prenatal care. She underwent an extensive workup with no significant findings on lumbar puncture, brain MRI, metabolic labs, and EEG. After exclusion of several acute underlying conditions, a presumptive diagnosis of catatonia secondary to exacerbation of underlying major depressive disorder was made. She was transferred to an inpatient psychiatric facility postdelivery and treated with a course of lorazepam, aripiprazole, and escitalopram with good effect.

1. Introduction

Catatonia is a neuropsychiatric behavioral syndrome characterized by an inability to move normally, abnormal behaviors, and withdrawal. Clinical manifestations encompass a heterogeneous group of signs/symptoms including mutism, stupor, atypical posturing, waxy flexibility, and staring. There are a wide variety of potential underlying etiologies, including bipolar disorder, major depressive disorder, schizophrenia, meningitis, autoimmune encephalitis, neoplasm, or various other infectious, metabolic, neurologic, and rheumatologic disorders, which can make diagnosis and management difficult. During pregnancy, catatonia is more commonly due to an underlying organic process such as neuroleptic malignant syndrome, paraneoplastic encephalitis, atypical posterior reversible encephalopathy, eclampsia, and cerebrovascular disease. Catatonia during pregnancy is rare and presents unique challenges due to the potential ramifications to mom and baby of the overall disease state and of potential treatment options. We report a case of catatonia due to underlying major depressive disorder in a pregnant patient who presented to labor and delivery with a spontaneous twin pregnancy of unknown chorionicity, with no prenatal care, at an unknown gestational age.

2. Case

A 36-year-old G6P5005 with no prenatal care and a spontaneous twin pregnancy of unknown chorionicity presented with altered mental status. She was accompanied by her partner, and he reported that she was "two days past her due date" and was becoming "more unresponsive." The patient was not able to speak any words and would respond to questions only with simple noises. She was able to point to the words "yes" and "no" written on paper to answer certain questions and was able to express that she felt safe with her partner and did not feel as if she was in any danger. The majority of the patient history was obtained from the patient's partner, who denied any history of psychiatric illness or hospitalization. Limited bedside growth scan was consistent with approximately 36-week gestational age, and both babies were in breech presentation. The psychiatry team was consulted, and, on their evaluation, they noted that she required multiple verbal prompts to follow simple commands and demonstrated reduced response to stimulation over time with progressive difficulty moving her fingers to point to "yes/no" written on paper. On mental status exam, she was noted to have poor eye contact, psychomotor slowing, and flat affect and appeared to be internally occupied. She pointed to "yes" when asked about hearing voices. Given the constellation of mutism, difficulty moving, waxy flexibility on prompting, fluctuating alertness, and internal preoccupation, a diagnosis of hypoactive catatonia was made. She was started on lorazepam 1 mg every two hours.

From an obstetric standpoint, she was also noted to have an irritable contraction pattern on tocometry and, after consenting to a cervical exam, was found to be 4 cm dilated/50% effaced/-3 station. Fetal cardiotocography from time of admission is shown in Figure 1. She became very combative during attempts at IV placement and was unable to be put in wrist restraints to safely obtain IV access. The case was discussed with the hospital Risk Management team and Maternal-Fetal Medicine. Per Risk Management, the team should care for the patient as medically necessary, including the use of medical sedation and physical restraints, if needed. She was given 5 mg intramuscular haloperidol and 2 mg intramuscular lorazepam for sedation which allowed for safe placement of an IV. She continued to regularly contract and on repeat exam was found to be 5-6 cm dilated/75% effaced/-2 station with breech-breech presentation reconfirmed on ultrasound. Per prior psychiatry evaluation, the patient did not have capacity to give informed consent and would be unable to consent for primary cesarean section for spontaneous preterm labor with fetal malpresentation. She was able to respond "okay" when informed of need to proceed with surgery but was unable to sign consent. She underwent an uncomplicated primary cesarean section under general anesthesia.

The Psychiatry team continued to follow postoperatively, and she was transitioned to Lorazepam 2 mg every six hours, which slowly began to produce a clinical response. On postop day 0, she was noted to be intermittently verbal with more purposeful movements and was able to answer questions at times. On postop day 1, she was able to ambulate with supervision, eat and use the bathroom on her own, and visit her babies in the NICU. However, her overall mental status would wax and wane throughout the day, and she continued to have nonverbal periods with psychomotor slowing. It was determined that she met criteria for inpatient psychiatric hospitalization given her grave disability secondary to her catatonic state. She was transitioned to lorazepam 2 mg every 8 hours and underwent lumbar puncture to rule out autoimmune encephalitis prior to being discharged to the nearby psychiatric hospital on postop day 3. Her workup prior to discharge to the psychiatric hospital included normal LP, metabolic labs, and no evidence of seizure on EEG. Brain MRI showed artifact versus reduced diffusivity within the caudate nuclei bilaterally and the cerebral cortex bilaterally, which can frequently be seen in acute catatonia. The diagnostic findings from the case are summarized in Table 1. Prior to her discharge, records from a hospital in a different state were obtained which showed a long-standing history of major depressive disorder with catatonic features, for which she had previously been prescribed lorazepam 1 mg three times daily. During her psychiatric admission, lorazepam was uptitrated to 3 mg three times daily due to continued persistent catatonia and frequent relapses. The lorazepam treatment had a waxing and waning effect on her catatonic features, showing baseline functionality after her dosages that regressed back to catatonic before the next dose was due. She was also started on aripiprazole due to possible psychosis with reported auditory hallucinations, as well as escitalopram due to depressed mood and a previous diagnosis of major depressive disorder. ECT was offered several times during the patient's admission, but each time, the patient declined. She was eventually discharged to the care of her father after a 33-day stay with improved mood and a Bush-Francis score of 0 with continued lorazepam treatment. She was discharged on lorazepam, aripiprazole, and escitalopram, with plan for close outpatient follow-up.

3. Discussion

Catatonia generally occurs in patients with an underlying psychiatric or general medical disorder such as bipolar disorder, major depressive disorder, schizophrenia, meningitis, autoimmune encephalitis, neoplasm, or various other infectious, metabolic, neurologic, and rheumatologic disorders. There are three main subtypes of catatonia, hypoactive, excited, and malignant. Hypoactive, which is what our patient displayed, is characterized by mutism, inhibited movement, negativism, and staring. Patients with excited catatonia exhibit excessive and purposeless motor activity in their extremities with restlessness, impulsivity, and combativeness. Finally, malignant catatonia is a life-threatening state that is accompanied by fever, autonomic instability, delirium, and rigidity. These subtypes exist on a spectrum, and patients may transition back-and-forth at any given time. The most widely used scoring system in the evaluation and tracking of treatment over time in catatonic patients is the Bush-Francis Catatonia Rating Scale, which is a 23-item rating scale with good interrater reliability.

Overall, catatonia is rare in the peripartum period. A search of the National Library of Medicine database by Gonzales et al. discovered 16 reported cases of catatonia occurring during pregnancy or in the immediate postpartum period [1]. Many of these cases were due to organic medical conditions including NMS, paraneoplastic encephalitis, atypical posterior reversible encephalopathy, eclampsia, and cerebrovascular disease. Thus, when any pregnant patient presents with catatonic features, it is important to keep a broad differential and rule out underlying medical conditions that could potentially be fatal to mom and/or baby. The first-line treatment of catatonia is high-dose benzodiazepines, which also aids in making the diagnosis. The lorazepam challenge involves administering an IV bolus of 1 to 2 mg and closely observing for improvement in symptoms. Partial relief of signs/symptoms 5 to 10 minutes after

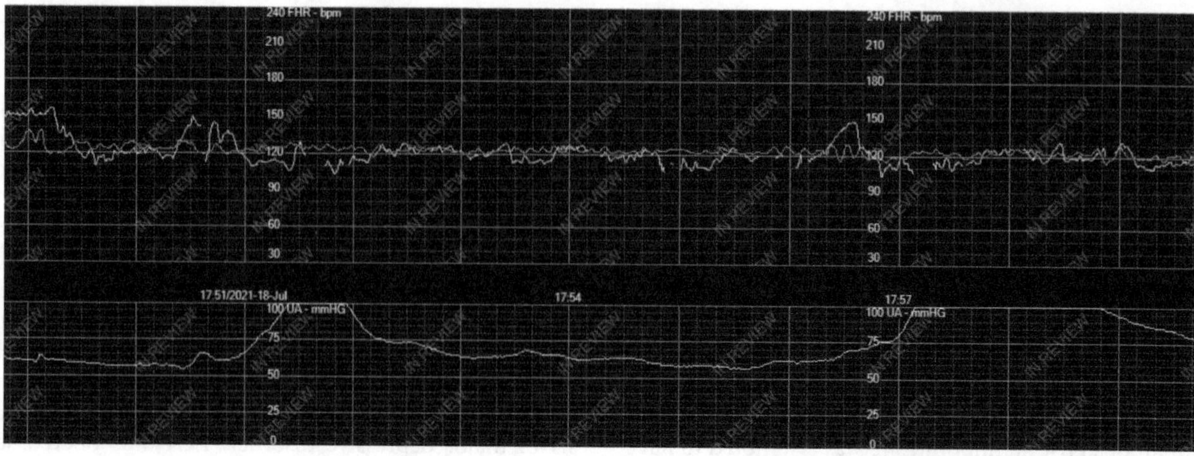

Figure 1: Fetal cardiotocography tracing on admission to labor and delivery.

Table 1: Summary of diagnostic findings.

MRI brain	"Artifact versus reduced diffusivity within the caudate nuclei bilaterally and the cerebral cortex bilaterally that can be correlated with underlying encephalitis, hypoxic ischemic changes, and/or toxic/metabolic derangements"
EEG	"Essentially normal natural sleep inpatient bedside routine EEG for age during awake and drowsy. Excessive diffuse beta activity was noted likely due to benzodiazepine use"
Lumbar puncture	Negative paraneoplastic autoantibody evaluation
Vitamin D	10 ng/mL (NL = 30-100 ng/mL)
Vitamin B12	165 pg/mL (NL = 243-894 pg/mL)
Folate	4.2 ng/mL (NL ≥ 7.2 ng/mL)
Complete blood count	Unremarkable
Complete metabolic panel	Unremarkable
Ammonia level	14 mmol/L (NL = 11-51 mmol/L)
Thyroid stimulating hormone level	1.62 mIU/L (NL = 0.27-4.20 mIU/L)
Urine toxicology screen	Negative

administration is consistent with a diagnosis of catatonia [2, 3]. Treatment then involves a continued regimen of high-dose benzodiazepines, frequently followed by electroconvulsive therapy. Multiple prospective open-label studies, cases series, and retrospective studies suggest that benzodiazepines alone, ECT alone, or benzodiazepines followed by ECT lead to recovery in approximately 60 to 80 percent of patients [4]. Treatment guidelines from the American Psychiatric Association recommend treating catatonia with either a benzodiazepine or ECT, depending upon the clinical scenario [5].

The case presented demonstrates several of the unique challenges of catatonia during pregnancy. The immobility, mutism, and withdrawal of hypoactive catatonia, especially when combined with other socioeconomic factors, can make it very difficult for patients to receive adequate prenatal care. Our patient presented to the hospital with no available records, with a twin pregnancy of unknown chorionicity, at an unknown gestational age. Her partner was also unable to provide any reliable collateral information, which raised concern for domestic violence, unstable housing, and/or sex trafficking. Furthermore, she presented in spontaneous labor with a twin pregnancy with breech-breech presentation necessitating cesarean delivery. The patient's presentation made this case unique from prior reported cases of catatonia during pregnancy, as our patient presented both with acute catatonia and an acute obstetric concern necessitating delivery. It also presented a very ethically challenging situation as her partner was unavailable, and she was deemed to not have capacity to make medical decisions or provide informed consent. In this scenario, there is an ethical obligation to determine an alternative decision maker, which is ideally someone chosen by the patient in advance in the form of a spouse, child, sibling, or other close relative. Our patient had no immediately available alternative decision maker, and a prompt decision was needed given the acute change in clinical status and need for cesarean section.

An additional challenge of catatonia during pregnancy is the potential effects of the standard treatment options on the pregnancy. A 2011 meta-analysis of nine studies with more than one million pregnancies found that in general, benzodiazepines did not appear to increase teratogenic risk [6]. However, retrospective case-control studies suggest that fetal exposure to benzodiazepines may increase the risk of oral cleft from the general population base rate of 6 in 10,000 births to 11 in 10,000 births [7]. Furthermore, benzodiazepine use in the third trimester can lead to neonatal abstinence syndrome, temperature dysregulation, hypotonia, and poor feeding at birth [8]. Antenatal benzodiazepine use may also be associated with preterm birth and low birth weight [8]. In our case, benzodiazepine therapy was started very shortly prior to delivery, likely negating any possible negative effects. Postdelivery in breastfeeding moms, lorazepam has low levels in breastmilk and does not cause any adverse effects in breastfed infants [9]. The other mainstay of treatment of catatonia, electroconvulsive therapy, is largely considered to be safe at any stage of pregnancy. However, there have been case reports of placental abruption, preterm labor, miscarriage, and fetal heart rate decelerations associated with ECT [10]. Although not an issue in this case, as our patient had an urgent obstetric indication for delivery, the decision of when to deliver and route of delivery can be very difficult in catatonic patients. In general, decision making will depend on gestational age, severity of disease, other underlying medical conditions, and a risk-benefit analysis of intrapartum treatment vs. delay until after delivery.

This case also demonstrates the importance of a complete workup to determine the underlying cause of catatonia. Our patient underwent bloodwork to assess for any metabolic derangements, evaluation for preeclampsia, brain MRI to assess for structural abnormality, EEG to assess for seizures, and a lumbar puncture to assess for autoimmune encephalitis. With continued work to obtain further collateral information, we were able to attain records that endorsed a history of catatonia secondary to major depressive disorder, which aided in evaluation and allowed for a more definitive diagnosis. This case also highlights the benefits of having a multidisciplinary care team, which included general Obstetrics and Gynecology, Maternal-Fetal Medicine, Psychiatry, Neurology, Social Work, and Risk Management.

References

[1] N. Gonzales, D. K. Quinn, and W. Rayburn, "Perinatal catatonia: a case report and literature review," *Psychosomatics*, vol. 55, no. 6, pp. 708–714, 2014.

[2] M. Fink and M. A. Taylor, *Catatonia: A Clinician's Guide to Diagnosis and Treatment*, Cambridge University Press, Cambridge, UK, 2009.

[3] M. Fink and M. A. Taylor, "The many varieties of catatonia," *European Archives of Psychiatry and Clinical Neuroscience*, vol. 251, Suppl 1, pp. I8–13, 2001, PMID: 11776271.

[4] J. Coffey, P. Roy-Byrne, S. Marder, and D. Solomon, *Catatonia: treatment and prognosis. UpToDate*, 2021, https://www.uptodate.com/contents/catatonia-treatment-and-prognosis?search=catatonia%20treatment&source=search_result&selectedTitle=1~92&usage_type=default&display_rank=1.

[5] A. J. Gelenberg, M. P. Freeman, J. C. Markowitz et al., "American Psychiatric Association practice guidelines for the treatment of patients with major depressive disorder," *American Journal of Psychiatry*, vol. 167, Suppl 10, pp. 9–118, 2010.

[6] E. Enato, M. Moretti, and G. Koren, "Motherisk rounds: the fetal safety of benzodiazepines: an updated meta- analysis," *Journal of Obstetrics and Gynaecology Canada*, vol. 33, no. 1, pp. 46–48, 2011.

[7] K. A. Yonkers, K. L. Wisner, Z. Stowe et al., "Management of bipolar disorder during pregnancy and the postpartum period," *The American Journal of Psychiatry*, vol. 161, no. 4, pp. 608–620, 2004.

[8] B. N. Wikner, C. O. Stiller, U. Bergman, C. Asker, and B. Källén, "Use of benzodiazepines and benzodiazepine receptor agonists during pregnancy: neonatal outcome and congenital malformations," *Pharmacoepidemiology and Drug Safety*, vol. 16, no. 11, pp. 1203–1210, 2007.

[9] Drugs and Lactation Database (LactMed), *Lorazepam*, National Library of Medicine (US), Bethesda (MD), 2006, https://www.ncbi.nlm.nih.gov/books/NBK501231/.

[10] O. Saatcioglu and N. B. Tomruk, "The use of electroconvulsive therapy in pregnancy: a review," *The Israel Journal of Psychiatry and Related Sciences*, vol. 48, no. 1, pp. 6–11, 2011.

Subcutaneous Extended-Release Buprenorphine use in Pregnancy

Craig V. Towers and Heather Deisher

Obstetrics and Gynecology, Maternal-Fetal Medicine, High Risk Obstetrical Consultants, Knoxville, Tennessee 37920, USA

Correspondence should be addressed to Craig V. Towers; ctowers@utmck.edu

Academic Editor: Seung-Yup Ku

Background. Opioid use disorder (OUD) in pregnancy is managed by medication-assisted treatment. Sublingual buprenorphine is one option, but subcutaneous extended-release buprenorphine (Sublocade®) is an alternate form administered in monthly injections. Through an extensive literature search, we did not find any prior publication on the use of Sublocade in pregnancy. *Case.* Two patients with OUD switched from sublingual buprenorphine to Sublocade. One patient received a total of eight injections and then discovered she was pregnant. Based on ultrasound dating, the last 5 administrations occurred during her pregnancy. The second patient received 6 injections with the last occurring at the time of her last menstrual period. Both declined further injections, as well as oral buprenorphine. Serial urine drug screens remained positive for buprenorphine through delivery in both cases. Neither the mothers nor the neonates experienced withdrawal symptoms or adverse outcomes. No birth anomalies were found. *Discussion.* Though further research is needed regarding the use of Sublocade in pregnancy, it is likely that other pregnancies will occur during this treatment modality. If this long-acting form of buprenorphine medication is found to be safe, it might play a role in managing some pregnant patients with OUD.

1. Background

Opioid use disorder (OUD) in pregnancy is a rising epidemic, especially in the United States. The Centers for Disease Control and Prevention reported that the prevalence of OUD more than quadrupled in the United States from 1999 to 2014 (from 1.5/1000 deliveries to 6.5/1000) [1]. The mainstay of medical management is to place these patients on medications for opioid use disorder (MOUD) that use longer-acting opioid drugs such as methadone or buprenorphine [2–6]. These two medications are administered in daily oral/sublingual dosages. Buprenorphine is also available in a subcutaneous extended-release form called Sublocade® [7]. Through a literature search of PubMed, Embase, Cochrane, Google Scholar, and Scopus, we did not find any prior publication on the use of Sublocade in pregnancy.

The objective of this report is to describe the pregnancy and delivery outcome of two patients who were receiving monthly Sublocade injections and then became pregnant.

2. Case Presentation

Patient number one had an 8-year history of opioid use disorder. She was being managed with sublingual buprenorphine and then chose to transition to monthly Sublocade injections; the first of which was administered about 3 months prior to her last menstrual period. The first two injections were 300 mg doses followed by monthly 100 mg doses. The last injection occurred at a gestational age of $17^{4/7}$ weeks. A total of 8 injections had been given (2-300 mg and 6-100 mg). At $18^{3/7}$ weeks' gestation, the patient discovered she was pregnant (unplanned) and declined any further injections. Oral buprenorphine was offered for continued MOUD during her pregnancy, but she wanted to be opioid-free at delivery and again declined.

Patient number two had a 6-year history of opioid use disorder. She was also being managed with sublingual buprenorphine but was transitioned to monthly Sublocade injections. She received a total of 6 injections (2-300 mg and 4-100 mg). The last injection occurred at the time of her last menstrual period. Oral buprenorphine was again offered for continued MOUD during her pregnancy, but she also declined. The prenatal care of both patients included an intensive behavioral health component.

Urine drug screens were performed throughout both pregnancies, and the buprenorphine and norbuprenorphine levels are seen in Table 1 for patient one and in Table 2 for patient two. Liver enzymes were checked and were normal in both cases. Urine drug screens were negative for any other drugs except buprenorphine. For both patients, subcutaneous nodules were palpable across the upper abdomen area (the location of the injection sites). These disappeared at around 34 weeks' gestation for patient number one and at 22 weeks' gestation for patient number two. Both patients delivered vaginally at term without complications. Both newborns had normal Apgar scores and were discharged with their mothers. No birth anomalies were identified. Both mothers required only acetaminophen and ibuprofen during the postpartum period for pain control.

Neither patient experienced any symptoms of opioid withdrawal. Both infants were monitored closely for 5 days postdelivery for signs of neonatal abstinence syndrome (NAS). NAS did not develop in either case. Patient number one was seen 8 weeks postdelivery, and her urine drug screen was still positive for buprenorphine and norbuprenorphine but at very low levels. She was doing well with no signs of opioid withdrawal. Patient number two was seen 6 weeks postdelivery, and her urine drug screen was negative. Both patients were continuing in intensive behavioral health, and the plan was to continue this for a minimum of 12 months postpartum. Both declined restarting any form of MOUD. Both newborns at follow-up (8 months for newborn one and 2 months for newborn two) were evaluated and had normal examinations and were progressing with normal milestones.

Table 1: Urine buprenorphine and norbuprenorphine levels for patient one obtained through gestation, at delivery, and 8 weeks postdelivery—the last administration of subcutaneous extended-release buprenorphine was at $17^{4/7}$ weeks' gestation.

Gestational age (weeks)	Buprenorphine level (ng/mg creatinine)	Norbuprenorphine level (ng/mg creatinine)
$22^{4/7}$	111	313
$25^{5/7}$	85	156
$28^{6/7}$	90	155
$32^{6/7}$	64	88
$35^{5/7}$	67	101
$37^{5/7}$	59	104
Delivery $39^{3/7}$	43	87
8 weeks postdelivery	11	24

Table 2: Urine buprenorphine and norbuprenorphine levels for patient two obtained through gestation, at delivery, and 6 weeks postdelivery—the last administration of subcutaneous extended-release buprenorphine was at the time of her last menstrual period.

Gestational age (weeks)	Buprenorphine level (ng/mg creatinine)	Norbuprenorphine level (ng/mg creatinine)
$9^{3/7}$	73	46
$14^{2/7}$	54	33
$18^{2/7}$	19	19
$25^{2/7}$	8	11
$28^{2/7}$	3	6
$30^{2/7}$	4	0
$33^{2/7}$	5	0
Delivery $37^{4/7}$	1	0
6 weeks postdelivery	0	0

3. Discussion

The primary recommended treatment approach in managing opioid addiction is MOUD. A recurring problem in treating the OUD patient population is noncompliance with therapy leading to relapse or continued use of illicit opioid drugs, as well as drug diversion. This long-lasting injectable form of buprenorphine needs to be further studied to see if it has the potential benefit of preventing or limiting noncompliance as well as drug diversion.

Through our literature search, Sublocade use in pregnancy has not been previously reported. In these 2 cases, both women were receiving outpatient treatment for OUD with Sublocade injections. However, their outpatient management did not include contraception counseling despite being sexually active females of reproductive age. Both had unplanned pregnancies, desired to discontinue their Sublocade injections, and declined oral buprenorphine treatment. Urine drug levels for buprenorphine and the primary metabolite norbuprenorphine were serially monitored and consistently stayed positive for up to 30 weeks after the last injection for patient one and for 37 weeks in patient two. These also remained positive after the palpable subcutaneous injection site nodules resolved (13 weeks for patient one and 15 weeks for patient two). Both patients never experienced any symptoms of withdrawal, and both had uncomplicated pregnancies and deliveries. Neither newborn developed signs of NAS, and no anomalies were found.

Though this report only discusses two patients, the lack of withdrawal symptoms needs further discussion. These patients' urine drug levels slowly tapered over time to very low levels. This raises further questions and potential concerns. Are these lower levels still effective in preventing cravings and possible relapse or do they increase the possibility of relapse? This potential risk needs to be closely monitored in anyone who discontinues using the injectable form of buprenorphine and does not supplement their MOUD with another form of therapy. Additionally, many urine drug screens for buprenorphine have lower limits of detection and the levels for patient two could report out negative starting at 25 weeks' gestation and beyond, even though she was still positive.

Subcutaneous buprenorphine (Sublocade) was FDA approved in 2017 for the treatment of OUD. It is a monthly injection that can be used in place of daily oral buprenorphine [7]. Sublocade is designed to release a controlled rate of buprenorphine over the span of one month. It is dosed every four weeks so that a steady serum level can be maintained [7]. Sublocade has not been recommended for use in pregnancy due to a lack of safety studies. Buprenorphine is recommended for use in pregnancy, and therefore, the concern with using Sublocade is primarily the delivery system (Atrigel®) that for Sublocade is a 50:50 mixture of poly (D, L-lactate-co-glycolide) and N-methyl-2-pyrrolidone [7]. Poly (D, L-lactate-co-glycolide) has a molecular weight of 66,000 to 107,000 g/mol and is unlikely to cross the human placenta. N-Methyl-2-pyrrolidone (NMP) has a molecular weight of 99 g/mol and more than likely would cross the placenta.

Human studies on NMP use in pregnancy are lacking. In pregnant rats, NMP exposure by inhalation at doses equivalent to that delivered by Sublocade resulted in an increase in preimplantation losses, reduced fetal body weight, and delayed ossification [8]. At doses 3 times the maximum human daily dose based on body surface area, an increase in malformations and resorptions was seen [9]. However, studies that evaluate the effect of a drug and/or chemical used during pregnancy in animals versus humans do not often correlate.

A limitation in this case report is that both patients were not continuously observed to verify that oral buprenorphine was not taken by either patient (illicitly) after their last injection. However, urine buprenorphine and norbuprenorphine levels were always low; no other drugs were ever found in the random urine toxicology screens; both were actively involved in intensive behavioral health; and both desired to be drug-free at delivery. Therefore, it is unlikely any other additional buprenorphine was consumed by either patient.

In conclusion, subcutaneous extended-release buprenorphine will more than likely increase in use in the treatment of patients with OUD. With the large number of women of childbearing age suffering from this disease, most likely, there will be an increase in the number of pregnancies seen in women receiving this form of MOUD. Therefore, management of this specific population should include contraceptive counseling. In addition, further reports on the use of subcutaneous buprenorphine in pregnancy are also needed to better evaluate safety. If no adverse events are found, using subcutaneous buprenorphine may become an additional form of MOUD in pregnancy.

Authors' Contributions

Dr. Towers conceptualized and codesigned the study, coordinated and supervised the maternal and neonatal data collection, carried out the initial analyses, and finalized and approved the manuscript as submitted. Dr. Deisher codesigned the study, coordinated and supervised the maternal and neonatal data collection, drafted the initial manuscript, and approved the final manuscript as submitted.

References

[1] S. C. Haight, J. Y. Ko, V. T. Tong, M. K. Bohm, and W. M. Callaghan, "Opioid use disorder documented at delivery hospitalization – United States, 1999-2014," *Morbidity and Mortality Weekly Report*, vol. 67, no. 31, pp. 845–849, 2018.

[2] S. Abuse and M. H. S. Administration, *Clinical guidance for treating pregnant women and parenting women with opioid use disorder and their infants. HHS Publication No. (SMA) 18-5054*, Substance Abuse and Mental Health Services Administration, Rockville, MD, 2018.

[3] Committee on Obstetric Practice American Society of Addiction Medicine, "Committee Opinion No. 711: Opioid Use and Opioid Use Disorder in Pregnancy," *Obstetrics & Gynecology*, vol. 130, no. 2, pp. e81–e94, 2017.

[4] U. M. Reddy, J. M. Davis, Z. Ren, M. F. Greene, and for the Opioid Use in Pregnancy, Neonatal Abstinence Syndrome, and Childhood Outcomes Workshop Invited Speakers, "Opioid use in pregnancy, neonatal abstinence syndrome, and childhood outcomes: executive summary of a joint workshop by the Eunice Kennedy Shriver National Institute of Child Health and Human Development, American College of Obstetricians and Gynecologists, American Academy of Pediatrics, Society for Maternal-Fetal Medicine, Centers for Disease Control and Prevention, and the March of Dimes Foundation," *Obstetrics and Gynecology*, vol. 130, no. 1, pp. 10–28, 2017.

[5] A. Ordean, S. Wong, and L. Graves, "No. 349-Substance Use in Pregnancy," *Journal of Obstetrics and Gynaecology Canada*, vol. 39, no. 10, pp. 922–937.e2, 2017.

[6] L. P. McLafferty, M. Becker, N. Dresner et al., "Guidelines for the management of pregnant women with substance use disorders," *Psychosomatics*, vol. 57, no. 2, pp. 115–130, 2016.

[7] Product Information, *Sublocade. Indivior Pharmaceuticals*, 2017, July 2019, http://www.accessdata.fda.gov/drugsatfda_docs/label/2017/209819s000lbl.pdf.

[8] A. M. Saillenfait, F. Gallissot, and G. Morel, "Developmental toxicity of N-methyl-2-pyrrolidone in rats following inhalation exposure," *Food and Chemical Toxicology*, vol. 41, no. 4, pp. 583–588, 2003.

[9] A. M. Saillenfait, F. Gallissot, I. Langonne, and J. P. Sabate, "Developmental toxicity of N-methyl-2-pyrrolidone administered orally to rats," *Food and Chemical Toxicology*, vol. 40, no. 11, pp. 1705–1712, 2002.

Early Fetal Growth Restriction of Both Twins in a Transgender Man

Alicia Martínez-Varea,[1] **Clara Martínez-Sáez**,[1] **María Patrocinio Tarrazó-Millet**,[2] **and Vicente Diago-Almela**[1]

[1]*Department of Obstetrics and Gynaecology, La Fe University and Polytechnic Hospital, Avenida Fernando Abril Martorell 106, 46026 Valencia, Spain*
[2]*Department of Obstetrics and Gynaecology, Dr. Peset University Hospital, Avenida de Gaspar Aguilar 90, 46017 Valencia, Spain*

Correspondence should be addressed to Alicia Martínez-Varea; martinez.alicia.v@gmail.com

Academic Editor: Maria Grazia Porpora

Gender dysphoria affects 0.5% of people worldwide. Transgender men display a divergence between the female genetic sex and the gender male identity. To the best of our knowledge, we describe the first case report with regard to a transgender man with a dichorionic diamniotic twin pregnancy obtained by artificial insemination using donor sperm as a monoparental family, presenting early fetal growth restriction of both twins. The patient is a 35-year-old transgender man who had previously received gender-affirming hormone therapy based on testosterone for five years and had a prior bilateral mastectomy as gender-affirming surgery. Whether assisted reproductive techniques have any influence on obstetrical outcomes among these patients and whether prior long-term intake of gender-affirming hormone therapy has an impact on pregnancy and obstetrical outcomes remain to be elucidated.

1. Introduction

Gender dysphoria, a disparity between genetically determined sex and gender identity, affects roughly 0.5% of people worldwide [1]. Transgender men display a divergence between the female genetic sex and the gender male identity [1]. The gender-affirming process often includes gender-affirming hormone therapy (GAHT) [1, 2] as well as gender-affirming surgery (GAS) [1, 3]. GAHT is based on the use of testosterone and its derivatives to provide transgender men the longing masculine appearance [1, 2]. GAS may include mastectomy, genital reconstruction, and hysterectomy with or without salpingo-oophorectomy [1, 3, 4]. Interestingly, it has been described that the vast majority of transgender men retain their female reproductive organs and, hence, their potential ability to become pregnant [4, 5].

The precise prevalence of pregnancy among transgender men is unknown [5]. Nonetheless, expert opinion suggests that the number of pregnant transgender men is increasing [4, 5]. The impact on fertility and pregnancy outcomes of long-term testosterone treatment among transgender men is unknown. Additionally, data regarding pregnancy in transgender pregnant men are still limited. To the best of our knowledge, we describe the first case report with regard to a transgender man with a dichorionic diamniotic twin pregnancy obtained by artificial insemination presenting early fetal growth restriction of both twins.

2. Case Report

The patient is a 35-year-old transgender man with a dichorionic diamniotic twin pregnancy obtained by the second artificial insemination using donor sperm as a monoparental family. Previous medical background includes a childhood history of asthma without the requirement of current treatment. He had previously received GAHT based on testosterone (intramuscular testosterone cypionate 250 mg/mL every

18 days) for 5 years. This therapy was ceased 3 months prior to initiating the fertility treatment. Prior surgical history includes gastric bypass surgery, abdominoplasty, and bilateral mastectomy as GAS.

The patient weight at the beginning of pregnancy was 70 kilograms, and the height was 164 centimeters, resulting in a body mass index mass of 26. He smoked 20 cigarettes per day, which was reduced to 2-3 cigarettes daily after becoming pregnant. During pregnancy, the transgender man received daily pregnancy vitamins which included 400 micrograms of folic acid and 150 milligrams of acetylsalicylic acid to prevent early preeclampsia.

The dichorionic diamniotic twin pregnancy was confirmed by ultrasound at 10 weeks gestation. The risk for trisomy 21, 13, and 18 was low at the combined screening performed at 12 weeks gestation. The morphological fetal ultrasound performed at 20 weeks gestation was within normal limits. The pregnancy was uneventful until 29^{+0} weeks gestation, when selective fetal growth restriction of the first twin was diagnosed. Thus, the patient underwent weekly monitoring. At 31^{+5} weeks gestation, early fetal growth restriction of both twins was detected. Ultrasound study revealed biometry of biparietal diameter (BPD) 75.3, head circumference (HC) 266.0, abdominal circumference (AC) 206.0, femur length (FL) 55.2, with an estimated fetal weight of 1046 grams (<percentile 1 for gestational age, Hadlock) of the first twin, which was in cephalic presentation and presented normal amniotic fluid (maximum vertical pocket of 3.0 cm). The second twin was also in cephalic presentation and displayed biometry of BPD 69.5, HC 283.7, AC 242.4, and FL 55.3, with an estimated fetal weight of 1300 grams (percentile 1 for gestational age, Hadlock), as well as normal amniotic fluid (maximum vertical pocket of 4.8 cm). The color Doppler study showed an intermittent absent end-diastolic flow of the umbilical artery of both twins. The pulsatility index of the middle cerebral artery of both twins was within normal limits (1.62 and 2.13, respectively). The blood flow of the ductus venosus was normal in both twins, as well as the mean pulsatility index of the uterine arteries (0.46). Cardiotocography disclosed a stable baseline of approximately 130 beats per minute and a reassuring variability of both twins. Due to the early fetal growth restriction with the intermittent absent end-diastolic flow of the umbilical artery of both twins, the patient was admitted into the hospital in order to initiate fetal lung maturation with betamethasone 2 mL/24 h, 2 doses, and to monitor daily both fetuses with cardiotocography and ultrasound. During the hospital admission, the patient showed a blood pressure within normal limits, being the blood and urine tests nonremarkable. The soluble fms-like tyrosine kinase-1/placental growth factor (sFlt-1/PlGF) ratio was 12 at 31^{+5} weeks gestation.

At 32^{+2} weeks gestation the fetal color Doppler study revealed a persistent absent end-diastolic flow of the umbilical artery in both fetuses with growth restriction. Given that the American College of Obstetricians and Gynecologists suggest delivery between 32^{+0} and 37^{+6} weeks gestation in growth-restricted fetuses with additional risk factors for adverse outcomes, such as abnormal umbilical artery Doppler [6], the risk of emergent cesarean section at labor exceeds 50% in fetuses with growth restriction and absent end-diastolic flow of the umbilical artery [7], and the unknown effects of long-term GAHT on myometrium and placenta, an elective cesarean delivery was performed as individualized management. The patient agreed and signed the informed consent. The first newborn was a male of 1250 grams, who displayed an Apgar score of 10/10/10, an arterial pH of 7.39, and a venous pH of 7.39. The second newborn was a female of 1390 grams, who showed an Apgar score of 10/10/10, an arterial pH of 7.30, and a venous pH of 7.36. The transgender man underwent an uneventful postpartum recovery and was discharged 48 hours after the cesarean section. Both newborns were discharged four weeks after birth and have not presented major morbidity.

3. Discussion

Transgender men have previously received scarce attention with respect to reproductive health and obstetrical care. Although the number of transgender individuals is rising [8], there is a lack of information regarding fertility, pregnancy, and neonatal outcomes among transgender people. Additionally, the impact of GAHT on fertility and pregnancy outcomes is unknown. This case report presents a dichorionic diamniotic twin pregnancy obtained by artificial insemination in a transgender man with early fetal growth restriction and absent end-diastolic flow of the umbilical artery of both twins. We hypothesize that the history of long-term use of testosterone as GAHT may have a potential impact on myometrium and on the subsequent placental development and function, as well as on fetal growth.

It has been described that GAHT in transgender men entails breast atrophy without an associated increased risk of breast cancer [2]. Moreover, the androgen treatment in transgender men induces ovarian effects after 6 months of therapy that consists of modifications of ovarian morphology that simulate the ovarian appearance seen in women with polycystic ovary syndrome but without a variation on antral follicle count [2]. Long-term androgen therapy in transgender men induces a similar metabolic profile to cisgender men with regard to lipid profile, insulin resistance, and mortality [2]. Although data regarding cardiometabolic risk is reassuring, some authors have reported conflicting results [2]. Actually, given that GAHT increases leukocyte-endothelium interactions and proinflammatory cytokines, it has been suggested that cardiovascular risk should be monitored in transgender men [9]. Concerning pregnancy in transgender men, a cross-sectional study based on a web-based survey has reported that pregnancy, delivery, and neonatal outcomes do not differ according to prior testosterone use as GAHT. A total of 36 out of 41 patients (88%) used their own oocytes, the mean gestational age at delivery was 38+6 weeks gestation, and 29 out of 41 patients (71%) underwent vaginal delivery [10]. Although patients with previous use of GAHT underwent more cesarean deliveries compared to those without the prior intake of GAHT (36% [9/25] versus 19% [3/16], respectively), the difference was not statistically significant [10]. A subsequent cross-sectional study based on a quantitative survey is in line with the finding that only a minority (23%) of transgender individuals deliver by cesarean section, although prior GAHT is not taken into account [11]. Both studies lack the comparison of pregnancy outcomes between singleton and multiple pregnancies, as well as between spontaneously conceived gestations and those obtained through assisted reproductive techniques. Ultimately, the impact of prior GAHT on labor and obstetrical outcomes is largely unknown [5, 11].

Regarding psychological aspects of pregnancy in transgender men, it is noteworthy that the interruption of GAHT before pregnancy accompanied by the increase of female hormones due to pregnancy status may increase gender dysphoria [4, 5, 12]. Moreover, it is crucial to closely monitor transgender men during postpartum in order to rule out postpartum depression, given that baseline depression among transgender individuals is higher compared to adult average and a number of these patients experience a lack of social support as well as individual loneliness during pregnancy and parenting [4, 12, 13].

Transgender men have to decide whether to reinitiate testosterone during the postpartum period [4]. For those who have not undergone a mastectomy as GAS and desire to breastfeed, it has been shown that 100 mg subcutaneous testosterone pellet is not associated with a marked increase of milk testosterone levels [14]. Although subcutaneous testosterone cypionate increases milk testosterone levels, testosterone displays low oral bioavailability due to its extensive first-pass metabolism, and apparently, it does not increase serum testosterone levels in breastfed infants [14]. Breastfed infants appear not to be adversely affected by transgender paternal GAHT [14]. High doses of testosterone are able to suppress lactation [4, 14]. On the other hand, for transgender men who do not seek to breastfeed, data to guide the new beginning of GAHT after delivery is limited [5]. It has been suggested to wait between 4 and 6 weeks after delivery [5].

It is essential to address postpartum contraception with transgender men [5, 13], given that ovulation and pregnancy may still occur while amenorrheic with GAHT [15] and testosterone induces virilization during embryogenesis [5]. All contraceptive options may be offered to transgender men because testosterone is not a contraindication to any form of contraception [15].

In conclusion, the number of transgender individuals is increasing [8], and data regarding fertility, pregnancy, and neonatal outcomes among transgender people is limited. Notably, the impact of GAHT on labor and obstetrical outcomes is largely unknown [5, 11]. Thus, the need for obstetrician-gynecologists and reproductive specialists to improve care for transgender men should be highlighted. Further prospective studies are needed in order to clarify fertility and pregnancy outcomes among transgender men and the impact, if any, of prior GAHT. It has been presented a dichorionic diamniotic twin pregnancy in a transgender man obtained by artificial insemination with early fetal growth restriction and absent end-diastolic flow of the umbilical artery of both twins. The patient underwent GAHT for 5 years before pregnancy. Whether assisted reproductive techniques have any influence on obstetrical outcomes among these patients and whether prior long-term intake of GAHT has an impact on fertility, pregnancy, and obstetrical outcomes remain to be elucidated.

References

[1] D. de Ziegler and P. de Sutter, "Transgender men: clinical care and implications in reproductive medicine: introduction," *Fertility and Sterility*, vol. 116, no. 4, pp. 919–921, 2021.

[2] P. Pirtea, J. M. Ayoubi, S. Desmedt, and G. T'Sjoen, "Ovarian, breast, and metabolic changes induced by androgen treatment in transgender men," *Fertility and Sterility*, vol. 116, no. 4, pp. 936–942, 2021.

[3] M. Carbonnel, L. Karpel, B. Cordier, P. Pirtea, and J. M. Ayoubi, "The uterus in transgender men," *Fertility and Sterility*, vol. 116, no. 4, pp. 931–935, 2021.

[4] J. Obedin-Maliver and H. J. Makadon, "Transgender men and pregnancy," *Obstetric Medicine*, vol. 9, no. 1, pp. 4–8, 2016.

[5] J. S. Brandt, A. J. Patel, I. Marshall, and G. A. Bachmann, "Transgender men, pregnancy, and the "new" advanced paternal age: a review of the literature," *Maturitas*, vol. 128, pp. 17–21, 2019.

[6] American College of Obstetricians and Gynecologists, "ACOG Practice Bulletin No. 204: fetal growth restriction," *Obstetrics and Gynecology*, vol. 133, no. 2, pp. e97–e109, 2019.

[7] F. Figueras and E. Gratacos, "An integrated approach to fetal growth restriction," *Best Practice & Research. Clinical Obstetrics & Gynaecology*, vol. 38, pp. 48–58, 2017.

[8] E. L. Meerwijk and J. M. Sevelius, "Transgender population size in the United States: a meta-regression of population-based probability samples," *American Journal of Public Health*, vol. 107, no. 2, pp. e1–e8, 2017.

[9] F. Iannantuoni, J. D. Salazar, A. M. de Marañon et al., "Testosterone administration increases leukocyte-endothelium interactions and inflammation in transgender men," *Fertility and Sterility*, vol. 115, no. 2, pp. 483–489, 2021.

[10] A. D. Light, J. Obedin-Maliver, J. M. Sevelius, and J. L. Kerns, "Transgender men who experienced pregnancy after female-to-male gender transitioning," *Obstetrics and Gynecology*, vol. 124, no. 6, pp. 1120–1127, 2014.

[11] H. Moseson, L. Fix, J. Hastings et al., "Pregnancy intentions and outcomes among transgender, nonbinary, and gender-expansive people assigned female or intersex at birth in the United States: results from a national, quantitative survey," *International Journal of Transgender Health*, vol. 22, no. 1-2, pp. 30–41, 2021.

[12] M. Besse, N. M. Lampe, and E. S. Mann, "Experiences with achieving pregnancy and giving birth among transgender men: a narrative literature review," *The Yale Journal of Biology and Medicine*, vol. 93, no. 4, pp. 517–528, 2020.

[13] A. Hoffkling, J. Obedin-Maliver, and J. Sevelius, "From erasure to opportunity: a qualitative study of the experiences of transgender men around pregnancy and recommendations for providers," *BMC Pregnancy and Childbirth*, vol. 17, Supplement 2, p. 332, 2017.

[14] "(US) DaLDLIBMNLoM. Testosterone 2006," 2021, https://www.ncbi.nlm.nih.gov/books/.

[15] C. Krempasky, M. Harris, L. Abern, and F. Grimstad, "Contraception across the transmasculine spectrum," *American Journal of Obstetrics and Gynecology*, vol. 222, no. 2, pp. 134–143, 2020.

Spontaneous Heterotopic Pregnancy: Diagnosis and Management

Katie P. Nguyen,[1] Marlekah Hudspeth,[2] and Honey Milestone[3]

[1]*Department of Family Medicine, Riverside Community Hospital, HCA Healthcare, Riverside, CA, USA*
[2]*University of California Riverside, School of Medicine, Riverside, CA, USA*
[3]*Department of Obstetrics & Gynecology, University of California Riverside, School of Medicine, Riverside Community Hospital, Riverside, CA, USA*

Correspondence should be addressed to Katie P. Nguyen; katie.nguyen2@hcahealthcare.com

Academic Editor: Daniel Martin

Background. Heterotopic pregnancies albeit rare are conceivably life-threatening if missed. With the development of assisted reproductive techniques, the incidence has increased. Confirmation of an intrauterine pregnancy (IUP) should not preclude the existence of a heterotopic pregnancy. *Case.* A healthy 27-year-old patient (gravida 4, term 1, preterm 0, abortion 2, living 1) at approximately 5 weeks gestation through natural conception presented to the emergency room with acute abdominal pain and vaginal bleeding. Pelvic ultrasound showed evidence of an IUP and a right adnexal mass, raising suspicion for a heterotopic pregnancy. The patient underwent an uncomplicated laparoscopic right salpingectomy. An IUP was confirmed on ultrasound postoperatively. The patient had an early pregnancy loss at 8 weeks of gestation. *Conclusion.* With a high index of suspicion from clinical presentation and pelvic imaging, heterotopic pregnancy, while rare, should not be ruled out.

1. Introduction

A heterotopic pregnancy is the presence of an intrauterine pregnancy (IUP) and a concurrent extrauterine pregnancy. It is both rare and life-threatening. The risk of having a heterotopic pregnancy from natural conception is estimated to be from 1 in 4,000 to 1 in 30,000 [1]. With the emergence of assisted reproductive technology, the incidence has been reported to be as high as 1 in 100 [1, 2]. Despite its rarity, the presence of a confirmed IUP should not exclude a concurrent extrauterine pregnancy. Ectopic pregnancies and heterotopic pregnancies are similar in presentation. Obtaining serial human chorionic gonadotropin (hCG) has limited diagnostic value as production is likely from the intrauterine pregnancy. This case report details the diagnosis and management of a naturally conceived heterotopic pregnancy in a healthy patient.

2. Case Presentation

A healthy 27-year-old patient (gravida 4, term 1, preterm 0, abortion 2, living 1) at 5 weeks and 5 days gestation through natural conception presented to the emergency department with acute lower abdominal pain and vaginal bleeding. She had associated nonbilious nonbloody vomiting. Obstetrical history included one spontaneous vaginal delivery and two spontaneous abortions. The medical, surgical, and family histories were noncontributory. On presentation, she was tachycardic at 117 beats per minute. The physical exam was significant for rebound tenderness of the lower abdomen, worse on the right side at McBurney's point. The pelvic exam showed blood in the vaginal vault. Labs were notable for an hCG at 16,108 mIU/mL and leukocytosis. Pelvic ultrasound showed evidence of an IUP measuring 5 weeks and 5 days with a fetal heart rate of 128 bpm (Figure 1). A 2.4 cm hyperechoic structure with a 1.3 cm internal hypoechoic structure was noted in the right adnexa. Weak peripheral vascularity was noted. No fetal pole was identified (Figure 2). There was a weak "ring of fire" sign present with internal septations possibly indicative of a yolk sac (Figure 3). There was a small volume of complex free fluid in the pelvis (Figure 4). Vascular waveforms were seen in both ovaries.

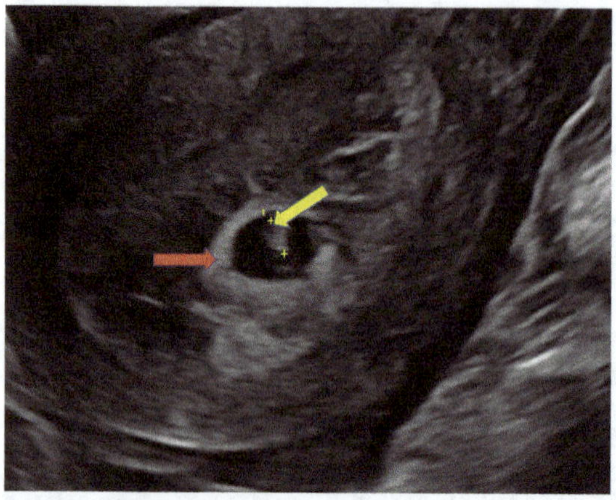

FIGURE 1: Longitudinal transvaginal ultrasound demonstrates an intrauterine gestational sac (red arrow) with a fetal pole (yellow arrow). Crown rump length measures 0.37 cm which correlates to the gestational age of 5 weeks and 5 days. Fetal heart rate was 128 beats per minute.

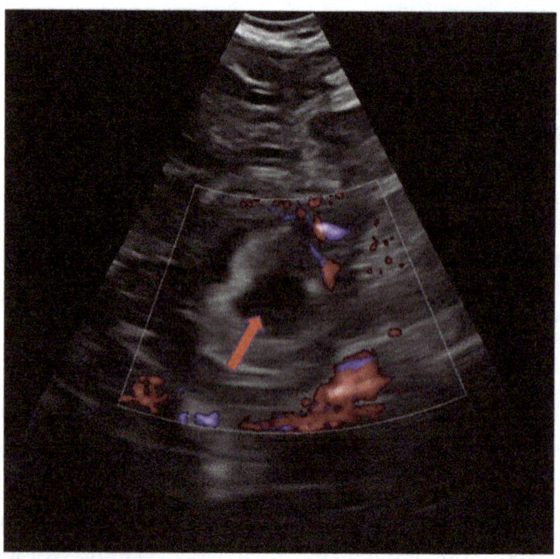

FIGURE 2: Longitudinal transvaginal ultrasound of the right adnexa demonstrates a thick walled hypoechoic cystic structure (red arrow) with weak peripheral vascularity ("ring of fire"). There is no fetal pole present.

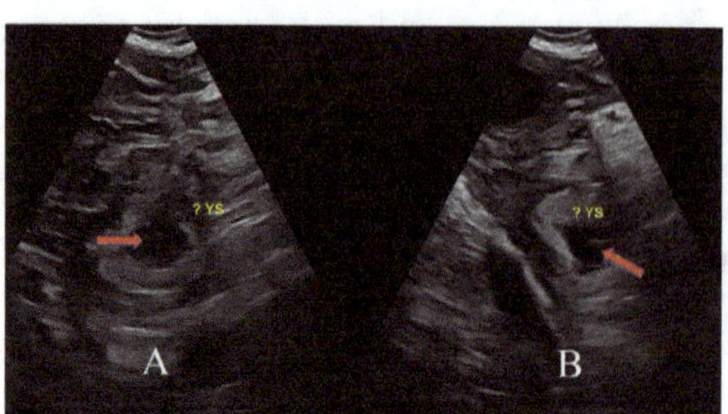

FIGURE 3: Longitudinal (a) and transverse (b) transvaginal ultrasound images of the right adnexa structure demonstrate possible internal echogenicity or septations (red arrow) which may represent a yolk sac or reverberation artifact.

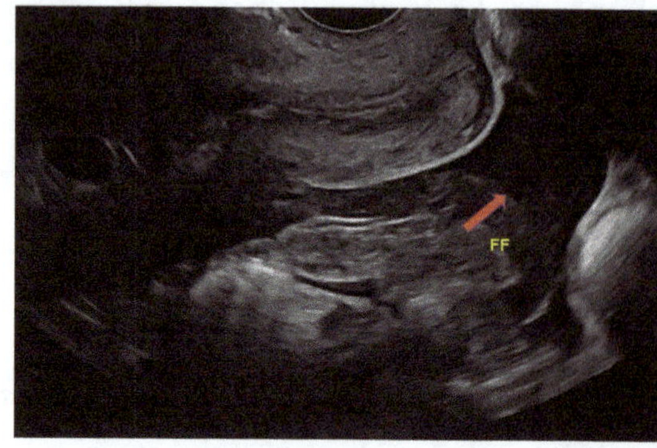

FIGURE 4: Sagittal transvaginal ultrasound image of the cervix with the posterior cul-de-sac with free fluid concerning for hemorrhage (red arrow).

Given findings of an acute abdomen and pelvic ultrasound highly suspicious for an ectopic pregnancy, the patient was consented for laparoscopic evaluation. The patient was counseled on the risk of having an early pregnancy loss with the surgical intervention. General surgery was consulted for possible appendectomy. The patient underwent a laparoscopic right salpingectomy with evacuation of hemoperitoneum. Significant operative findings included an enlarged uterus, an enlarged right fallopian tube with a purple-red hue, and notable rupture with hemoperitoneum (Figures 5, 6, and 7). The estimated blood loss was 500 mL. Bilateral ovaries, left fallopian tube, appendix, and liver were normal in appearance. The pathology results confirmed the presence of the right fallopian tube from the ruptured ectopic gestation. The postoperative course was unremarkable. A postoperative ultrasound confirmed a viable IUP, and the patient was discharged home on postoperative day one. Follow up confirmed an early pregnancy loss at 8 weeks of gestation.

3. Discussion

Heterotopic pregnancies are rare, but could be life-threatening if missed. The presence of a confirmed IUP usually rules out an extrauterine pregnancy if there is no evidence for another concurrent pregnancy located elsewhere. A systematic review of the literature from 2005 to 2010 revealed that as many as 33% of heterotopic cases had prior sonography of a normal IUP which led to false reassurance and misdiagnosis [3]. Studies report a wide variability for hCG concentrations in early pregnancy warranting cautious interpretation of a single hCG value for the diagnosis and management of suspected ectopic and/or heterotopic pregnancies. At around 6 weeks gestation, the hCG range could vary from 105 to 106,520 mIU/mL [4, 5]. A review of the literature shows a wide range of hCG levels for heterotopic pregnancies at similar gestational ages [6, 7]. With in vitro fertilization studies, hCG levels tend to be lower in heterotopic pregnancies compared to intrauterine twin pregnancies, but tend to be higher than intrauterine single pregnancies [8]. Patients who have higher than expected hCG levels especially with known singleton gestations need

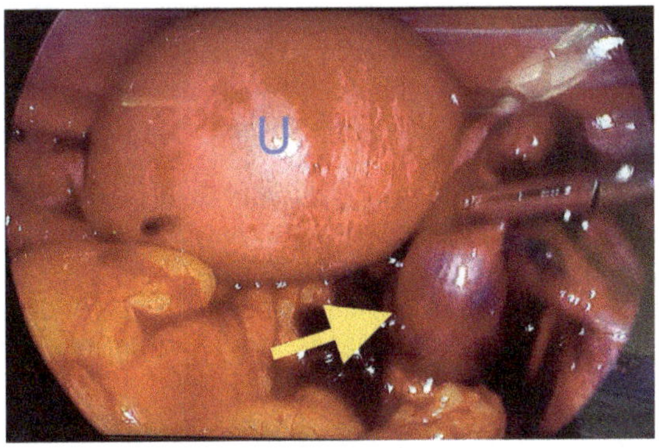

Figure 5: Intraoperative view of an enlarged uterus (U) and enlarged right fallopian tube with a purple-red hue (yellow arrow).

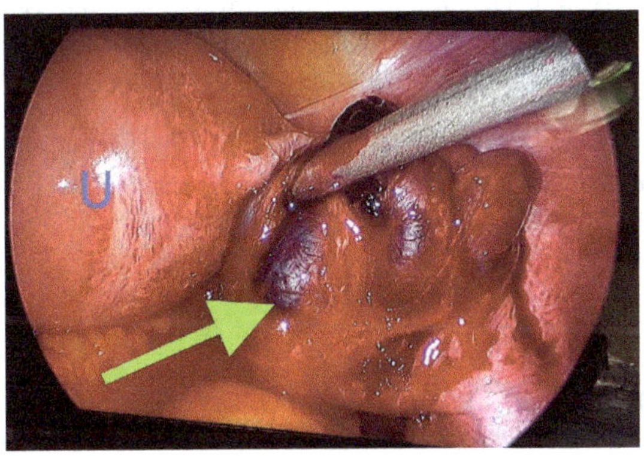

Figure 6: Intraoperative view of an enlarged uterus (U) and enlarged right fallopian tube with hemoperitoneum from the ruptured ectopic gestation (green arrow).

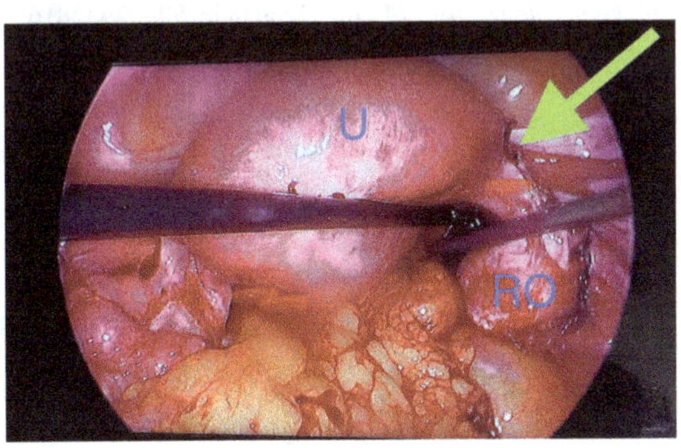

Figure 7: Intraoperative view of an enlarged uterus (U), right ovary (RO), and right salpingectomy (green arrow).

close monitoring with repeat hCG levels and ultrasound to subsequently rule out multiple gestations and heterotopic pregnancies. Prompt and accurate diagnosis remains a challenge. Major risk factors include prior tubal diseases or use of ART. There are also heterotopic pregnancy cases without any risk factors as demonstrated by the patient in this case report. The most common presentation is abdominal pain and vaginal bleeding which should prompt evaluation for an ectopic pregnancy versus a threatened abortion. In fact, a presumptive diagnosis of heterotopic pregnancy can be made if a patient has a combination of abdominal pain, signs of peritonitis, and ultrasound findings showing an adnexal mass with an enlarged uterus. There are also heterotopic pregnancies that are asymptomatic [3].

The diagnosis of heterotopic pregnancy is straightforward with the sonographic visualization of both an IUP; a complex adnexal mass containing either a yolk sac, embryo, or fetal pole; or echogenic fluid in the posterior cul-de-sac [9]. The difficulty lies in differentiating between an adnexal mass with a gestational sac but no embryo present versus a hemorrhagic corpus luteal cyst [10]. Doppler ultrasound allows assessment of the maternal fetal circulation and the uteroplacental blood flow velocity waveform; there is continuous maternal blood flow in the intervillous space, and the fetal blood flow velocity waveform is detectable as early as 5 weeks of gestation [9, 11]. Transvaginal color Doppler ultrasound can detect a high diastolic vascular flow, also known as the "ring of fire" sign, for a gestational sac of abnormal location if the ectopic pregnancy is unruptured [12]. Echogenic free fluid, if present, is suggestive of intraperitoneal hemorrhage from a ruptured ectopic pregnancy as was the case for this patient. If there was prior ovarian hyperstimulation, enlarged ovaries would be present [12].

This patient had evidence of an IUP measuring at 5 weeks with cardiac activity (Figure 1). There was a right adnexal hypoechoic structure with an internal hypoechoic structure. The "ring of fire" sign is indicative of a hypervascular lesion with peripheral vascularity commonly seen in corpus luteal cysts or an ectopic pregnancy. For every IUP, its corpus luteal cyst with the "ring of fire" is located in the ovary and not in the adnexa. The diagnosis was not definitive here because despite its presence in the adnexa, the "ring of fire" was weak and without a fetal pole. The possible internal echogenicity or septations seen may represent a yolk sac or artifact (Figures 2 and 3). With a high index of suspicion from the clinical presentation (pregnant patient with acute abdomen and vaginal bleeding) and concerning pelvic ultrasound (i.e., IUP, free fluid in pelvis, and complex adnexal mass), the possibility for heterotopic pregnancy, albeit rare, cannot be ruled out (Figure 4).

If clinical presentation and/or sonography findings are not definitive as was the case for this patient, a diagnostic laparoscopy or laparotomy (if hemodynamically unstable) would be indicated. This patient's serial abdominal exams worsened which warranted prompt surgical evaluation (Figures 5, 6, and 7). Appropriate management of heterotopic pregnancies requires taking into consideration the following: hemodynamic stability, prognosis or desired outcome for the IUP, site of implantation of the ectopic pregnancy, and the least invasive therapeutic approach. Laparoscopy is preferred over laparotomy if the patient is hemodynamically stable. Patients who are hemodynamically unstable are more likely to require laparotomies to prevent hemoperitoneum and hypovolemic shock from a ruptured ectopic pregnancy. The first line of treatment is a salpingectomy. Extra precautions should be taken to avoid cannulation or excessive manipulation of the uterus in order to preserve the IUP [13]. If the IUP is not desired, patients who are hemodynamically stable with definitive diagnosis on ultrasound are candidates for conservative systemic medical management with methotrexate. If the IUP is desired and the ectopic pregnancy is unruptured, consider transvaginal local injection of feticidal substances such as potassium chloride or hyperosmolar glucose. Both are effective in terminating the ectopic pregnancy, do not affect the fallopian tube, and are tolerated by the IUP [14]. Patients should still be counseled that conservative management could fail and that subsequent salpingectomy may be required. While it is crucial to counsel the patient on the increased risk of the IUP ending in an early pregnancy loss, a review of the literature shows an improvement in the survival rate from between 48% and 51% in 1957 [15] to 69% in 2007 [3].

Having a high index of suspicion for heterotopic pregnancy, despite its rarity, allowed prompt diagnosis and management in this otherwise healthy pregnant patient with natural conception.

Consent

Written informed consent was obtained from the patient for this case report.

Disclosure

The views expressed in this publication represent those of the author(s) and do not necessarily represent the official views of HCA Healthcare or any of its affiliated entities.

Acknowledgments

This research was supported (in whole or in part) by the HCA Healthcare and/or an HCA Healthcare affiliated entity.

References

[1] American College of Obstetricians and Gynecologists, "Tubal ectopic pregnancy. ACOG Practice Bulletin No. 193," *Obstetrics and Gynecology*, vol. 131, no. 3, pp. e91–103, 2018.

[2] A. Maleki, N. Khalid, C. Rajesh Patel, and E. El-Mahdi, "The rising incidence of heterotopic pregnancy: current perspectives and associations with in-vitro fertilization," *European Journal of Obstetrics, Gynecology, and Reproductive Biology*, vol. 266, article S0301211521004863, pp. 138–144, 2021.

[3] K. Talbot, R. Simpson, N. Price, and S. R. Jackson, "Heterotopic pregnancy," *Journal of Obstetrics and Gynaecology*, vol. 31, no. 1, pp. 7–12, 2011.

[4] J. Larsen, P. Buchanan, S. Johnson, S. Godbert, and M. Zinaman, "Human chorionic gonadotropin as a measure of pregnancy duration," *International Journal of Gynaecology and Obstetrics*, vol. 123, no. 3, pp. 189–195, 2013.

[5] C. Gnoth and S. Johnson, "Strips of hope: accuracy of home pregnancy tests and new developments," *Geburtshilfe und Frauenheilkunde*, vol. 74, no. 7, pp. 661–669, 2014.

[6] G. Cucinella, G. Gullo, A. Etrusco, E. Dolce, S. Culmone, and G. Buzzaccarini, "Early diagnosis and surgical management of heterotopic pregnancy allows us to save the intrauterine pregnancy," *Prz Menopauzalny*, vol. 20, no. 4, article 111277, pp. 222–225, 2021.

[7] M. Diakosavvas, N. Blontzos, G. Daskalakis et al., "Vaginal delivery at term in a woman with a spontaneous heterotopic pregnancy treated with laparoscopic salpingectomy," *Case Reports in Obstetrics and Gynecology*, vol. 2020, Article ID 8892273, 5 pages, 2020.

[8] M. Liu, X. Zhang, L. Geng et al., "Risk factors and early predictors for heterotopic pregnancy after in vitro fertilization," *PLoS One*, vol. 10, no. 10, article e0139146, 2015.

[9] E. W. Scibetta and C. S. Han, "Ultrasound in early pregnancy: viability, unknown locations, and ectopic pregnancies," *Obstetrics and Gynecology Clinics of North America*, vol. 46, no. 4, article S0889854519300944, pp. 783–795, 2019.

[10] L. D. Goyal, R. Tondon, P. Goel, and A. Sehgal, "Ovarian ectopic pregnancy: a 10 years' experience and review of literature," *Iranian Journal of Reproductive Medicine*, vol. 12, no. 12, pp. 825–830, 2014.

[11] C. Wen, L. Huang, and H. Jiang, "Diagnosis of interventional transvaginal maternal diseases based on color Doppler ultrasound," *Journal of Healthcare Engineering*, vol. 2021, Article ID 5517785, 10 pages, 2021.

[12] A. Chukus, N. Tirada, R. Restrepo, and N. I. Reddy, "Uncommon implantation sites of ectopic pregnancy: thinking beyond the complex adnexal mass," *Radiographics*, vol. 35, no. 3, pp. 946–959, 2015.

[13] J. B. Li, L. Z. Kong, J. B. Yang et al., "Management of heterotopic pregnancy: experience from 1 tertiary medical center," *Medicine*, vol. 95, no. 5, article e2570, 2016.

[14] J. L. Allison, M. Aubuchon, J. D. Leasure, and D. J. Schust, "Hyperosmolar glucose injection for the treatment of heterotopic ovarian pregnancy," *Obstetrics and Gynecology*, vol. 120, Part 2, pp. 449–452, 2012.

[15] A. E. Winer, W. D. Bergman, and C. Fields, "Combined intra- and extrauterine pregnancy∗," *American Journal of Obstetrics and Gynecology*, vol. 74, no. 1, article S0002937816370181, pp. 170–178, 1957.

48

A Case of Pregnancy Complicated with ATIII Deficiency in a Patient Who Developed Severe Venous Thromboembolism in Her Fourth Pregnancy and Had a Favourable Outcome in Her Subsequent Pregnancy with Careful Management of Anticoagulation Therapy including Edoxaban

Mie Sakai, Jumpei Ogura, Koji Yamanoi, Takahiro Hirayama, Tsutomu Ohara, Haruka Suzuki, Yoshihide Inayama, Koji Yasumoto, and Koh Suginami

Department of Obstetrics and Gynecology, Toyooka Public Hospital, Japan

Correspondence should be addressed to Koji Yamanoi; kojiymni@kuhp.kyoto-u.ac.jp

Academic Editor: Giampiero Capobianco

Congenital ATIII deficiency is one of the congenital thrombophilia diseases that can cause severe venous thromboembolism (VTE) in pregnant patients. A 30-year-old female, 4 gravida and 2 para, came to the emergency department with a complaint of oedema and pain in the left lower leg at 11 weeks of gestation. An inferior vena cava thrombus and pulmonary embolism were found. Because VTE was very severe, artificial abortion was performed, and VTE disappeared rapidly. She maintained oral administration of edoxaban (NOAC) and got pregnant naturally fifty-five weeks later after the abortion. Anticoagulation therapy was changed from NOAC to ATIII formulation and unfractionated heparin at 5 weeks of gestation. The course of pregnancy was good, and a healthy female newborn of 2310 g was delivered vaginally at 37 weeks 6 days of gestation. In puerperium, anticoagulation therapy was changed to warfarin. Currently one and one-half years had passed after delivery and no major adverse events or thrombosis has occurred. This case indicates that severe VTE can develop even in multipara pregnancy and that those who take NOAC may be able to continue pregnancy when they get pregnant.

1. Introduction

Venous thromboembolism (VTE) is quite an important disease because it sometimes directly relates to severe events. It is well known that pregnancy itself is one of the risk factors of VTE and is one of the major reasons of maternal death during pregnancy and postpartum [1–3]. If patients have hereditary thrombophilia disease, risk of VTE during pregnancy rises markedly [4–8].

Congenital ATIII deficiency is one of the autosomal dominant congenital thrombophilia diseases. Mutation of more than 250 ATIII-related genes suppresses transcription and decreases the antigen amount or activity, thereby decreasing the antithrombotic action and frequently causing thrombosis [9, 10]. The mutation was first reported by Warren et al. [11] in 1935, and the incidence rate is said to be approximately 1/2500 [10]. Thrombosis often presents as an initial symptom in young ATIII-deficient patients between the ages of 10 and 35, and it is well known that its frequency increases markedly during pregnancy [12–15]. However, not all ATIII-deficient patients have a family history. Furthermore, because not all ATIII-deficient patients develop VTE during pregnancy, it can happen that VTE does not develop at their first or second pregnancy.

Here, we present the case of a patient who developed severe VTE and was diagnosed as congenital ATIII deficiency in her fourth pregnancy. Although she was forced to undergo an artificial abortion because of the seriousness of VTE, she got pregnant naturally with administration of edoxaban (NOAC). In her fifth pregnancy, we cooperated closely with cardiovascular doctors, performing prophylactic anticoagulant therapy, and she delivered a healthy baby.

2. A Case Report

2.1. Development of Severe VTE and Treatment and Diagnosis of Congenital ATIII Deficiency. The patient was a 30-year-old woman (4 gravida, 2 para, and 1 artificial abortion) who got pregnant naturally and came to our department. She had no family history of VTE. She had no major illness in the past. Her menstrual cycle was approximately 30 days regularly. At 24 years old, she delivered a male baby of 2900 g vaginally at 40 weeks of gestation. In addition, at 27 years old, she delivered a female baby of 2345 g vaginally at 38 weeks of gestation. She is a nonsmoker and nonalcoholic drinker.

At 11 weeks of gestation, she presented to the emergency department of our hospital with a complaint of edema and pain in the left lower leg. Because VTE was strongly suspected, a contrast-enhanced computed tomography (CT) examination was performed with the consent of the patient. Then, a bilateral peripheral pulmonary embolism and venous thromboembolism from the left femoral vein to the inferior vena cava (renal vein level) were detected (Figures 1(a), 1(b), and 1(c)).

The IVC filter was placed emergently, and anticoagulation therapy with continuous heparin infusion started immediately. A blood examination taken at the day of admission revealed a decrease in protein S activity (33%) and ATIII (54%) (Table 1(a)). Those findings strongly suggested the existence of some congenital thrombophilia disease, such as protein S deficiency and ATIII deficiency. Because VTE was very severe, the cardiologists recommended a termination. With consent of the patient and her family, followed by enough discussion with us and the cardiologists, an artificial abortion was performed at 15 weeks of gestation. After surgery, VTE improved dramatically and finally disappeared (Figures 1(d) and 1(e)). The IVC filter was removed, and the anticoagulation therapy was changed to oral administration of NOAC. Then, she was discharged from the hospital.

After discharge, we repeated blood examination and found that the ATIII value maintained at a low level, 33.9% (Table 1(b)). Further detailed examination was performed in another hospital, and congenital ATIII deficiency was diagnosed.

2.2. Management of Antithrombosis Therapy during Subsequent Pregnancy. The patient strongly hoped for pregnancy. Followed by detailed explanation to her and her family, we decided to maintain NOAC treatment and allowed her to become pregnant.

Fifty-five weeks after the abortion, she came to our department with a complaint of 4 weeks of amenorrhea, and a gestational sac was detected by ultrasound examination. At that time, there were no symptoms of thrombosis clinically. We immediately changed anticoagulation treatment from NOAC to a regular administration of ATIII formulation. To keep ATIII value above 70%, we appropriately changed the dose and frequency (Figure 2(a)).

Although no thrombosis was detected by ultrasound examination, we thought it was better to conduct administration of unfractionated heparin (UFH) at the same time. To maintain an APTT value of approximately 50 to 60 seconds, we appropriately changed the dose and frequency (Figure 2(a)). During pregnancy, no symptoms of thrombosis were observed.

The development of the baby was observed carefully by ultrasonic examination. Foetal estimated body weight was from -1.5 to -1.0 SD during pregnancy (Figure 2(b)). No obvious anomaly was detected, and amniotic fluid volume was within normal range. There was no obvious abnormality in the blood flow of the umbilical artery and middle cerebral artery. Foetal heart beat monitoring was observed once a week from 36 weeks of pregnancy, and there were reassuring patterns.

2.3. Management of Delivery. As for delivery, we decided to have a planned vaginal delivery. We discussed with the cardiovascular doctors and paediatricians and planned a delivery as below (also, a flowchart is shown in Figure 2(c)).

At term, UFH was administered at fixed times, 5:00, 13:00, and 21:00. If delivery was expected within 4 hours, UFH would be postponed. The ATIII formulation would be administered on schedule. After delivery, we would resume UFH 4 hours later and return to the scheduled subcutaneous injection.

At the time of admission (37+5 weeks of gestation), internal examination revealed that the cervix opened to 2.5 cm in dilatation. A balloon catheter (120 ml of distilled water) was inserted at noon. An irregular uterine contraction started approximately 14:00. At 21:00, the cervix dilated to 8 cm. We expected that delivery would be within 4 hours, and APTT value at that time was prolonged to 59 seconds. The scheduled administration of UFH was postponed.

The delivery gradually progressed. At 0:58, a baby of 2310 g was delivered vaginally with Apgar score 9/9 and an umbilical artery pH of 7.352. The total blood loss during delivery was 420 ml. At 5:00, we resumed administration of UFH because 4 hours after delivery had passed, and no symptoms of bleeding tendency were observed. The amount of vaginal bleeding did not increase after resuming UFH.

We gradually switched ATIII and UFH to warfarin from the second day of postpartum.

Warfarin was started from 3.0 mg / day and was gradually increased until the PT-INR reached the range of 2.0 to 3.0. At the same time UFH was gradually decreased from 15000 units/day. We changed the dose of reagents very carefully so as not to cause any complications. Since PT-INR was kept within 2.0 to 3.0 by only oral administration of warfarin from the 11th day of postpartum, she was discharged from the hospital on the 14th day of postpartum. Currently about one and one-half years had passed since delivery, and she has maintained warfarin treatment without development of VTE.

Because the baby's weight was less than that of the 10th percentile, we examined the placenta pathologically. The placenta weight was 486 g, which is relatively smaller than that of average. Macroscopically, a circumferential-like

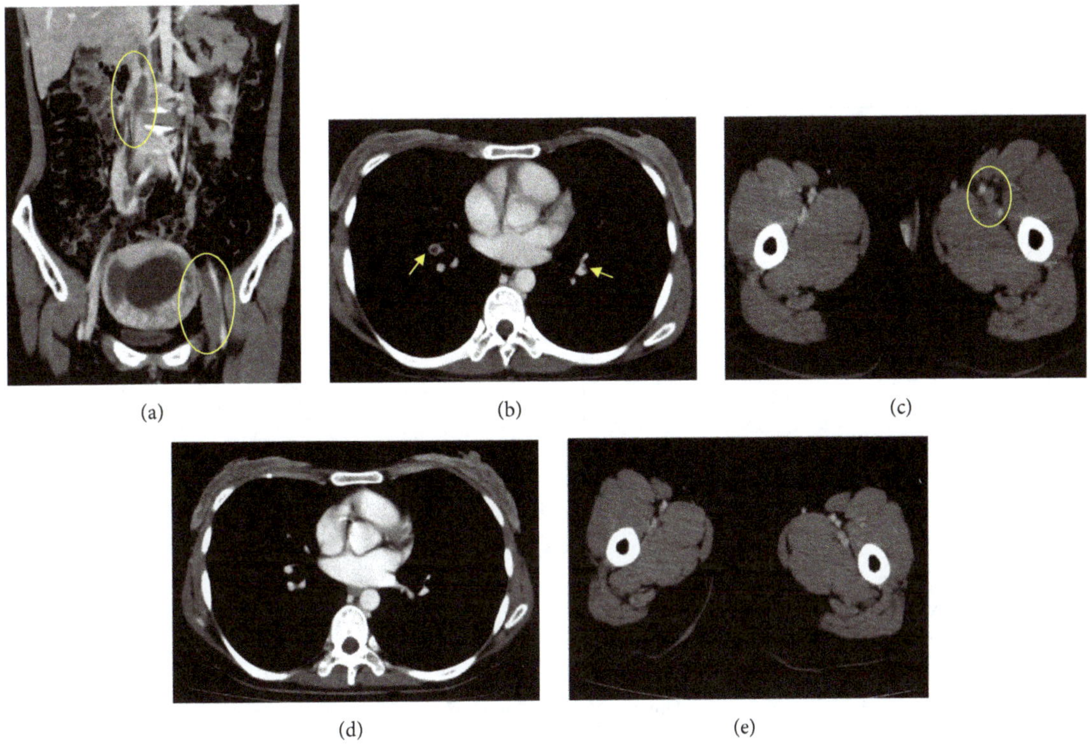

FIGURE 1: Development of severe VTE, and its disappearance after treatment at patient's fourth pregnancy. (a~c) Contrast CT image taken at the admission day. (a) Coronal plane, large thrombosis exists in inferior vena cava and femoral vein. (b) Transverse plane at the level of trunk of pulmonary artery. (c) Transverse plane at the level of femoral vein. Yellow circle and arrow indicate the location of venous thrombosis. (d, e) Contrast CT image taken at the start of oral administration of edoxaban. (d) Transverse plane at the level of trunk of pulmonary artery. (e) Transverse plane at the level of femoral vein.

TABLE 1

(a) Results of blood examination taken at the onset of VTE.

ATIII (%)	54.1
Protein S Activity (%)	33
Protein C Activity (%)	94
Anti-dsANA (titer)	<40
Anti-Cardiolipin (U/ml)	<1.2
MPO-ANCA (titer)	<40

(b) Results of blood examination taken after pregnancy.

	1 day after delivery	91 days after delivery
ATIII (%)	33.9	51.4
Protein S Activity (%)		75

infarction was observed in a portion approximately 4 cm in radius around the umbilical cord (Figure 3(a)). Necrosis of the amniotic membrane and chorion was observed microscopically at that site. In addition, necrosis of villi and fibrin precipitation was observed around that site (Figures 3(b) and 3(c)). These findings are probably due to the influence of congenital ATIII deficiency.

3. Discussion

This time, we experienced a case of congenital ATIII deficiency, which was first diagnosed when development of VTE was observed at her fourth pregnancy.

Congenital ATIII deficiency is one of the hereditary thrombophilia diseases, and it is known that the risk of VTE is very high especially during pregnancy. Charles et al. report that the VTE rate of pregnant women who do not have a history of VTE is 3-7%, while that of pregnant women with congenital ATIII deficiency is 40%, which is 6-13 times higher than that in normal pregnant women [10]. However, in this case, she had no family history or medical history of VTE and developed VTE for the first time during her fourth pregnancy. Although the risk of VTE in congenital ATIII deficiency patients during pregnancy is extremely high, VTE does not develop in all patients. In addition, such as this case, patients do not always have family history or medical history of VTE. When severe VTE is detected during pregnancy, even if she has no family or medical history and is multipara pregnant, the presence of some hereditary thrombosis should be taken into consideration.

There is a domestic guideline for the prevention and treatment of VTE during pregnancy in Japan. For VTE high-risk pregnancies, preventive anticoagulation with UFH is recommended, and in the case of ATIII deficiency, it is

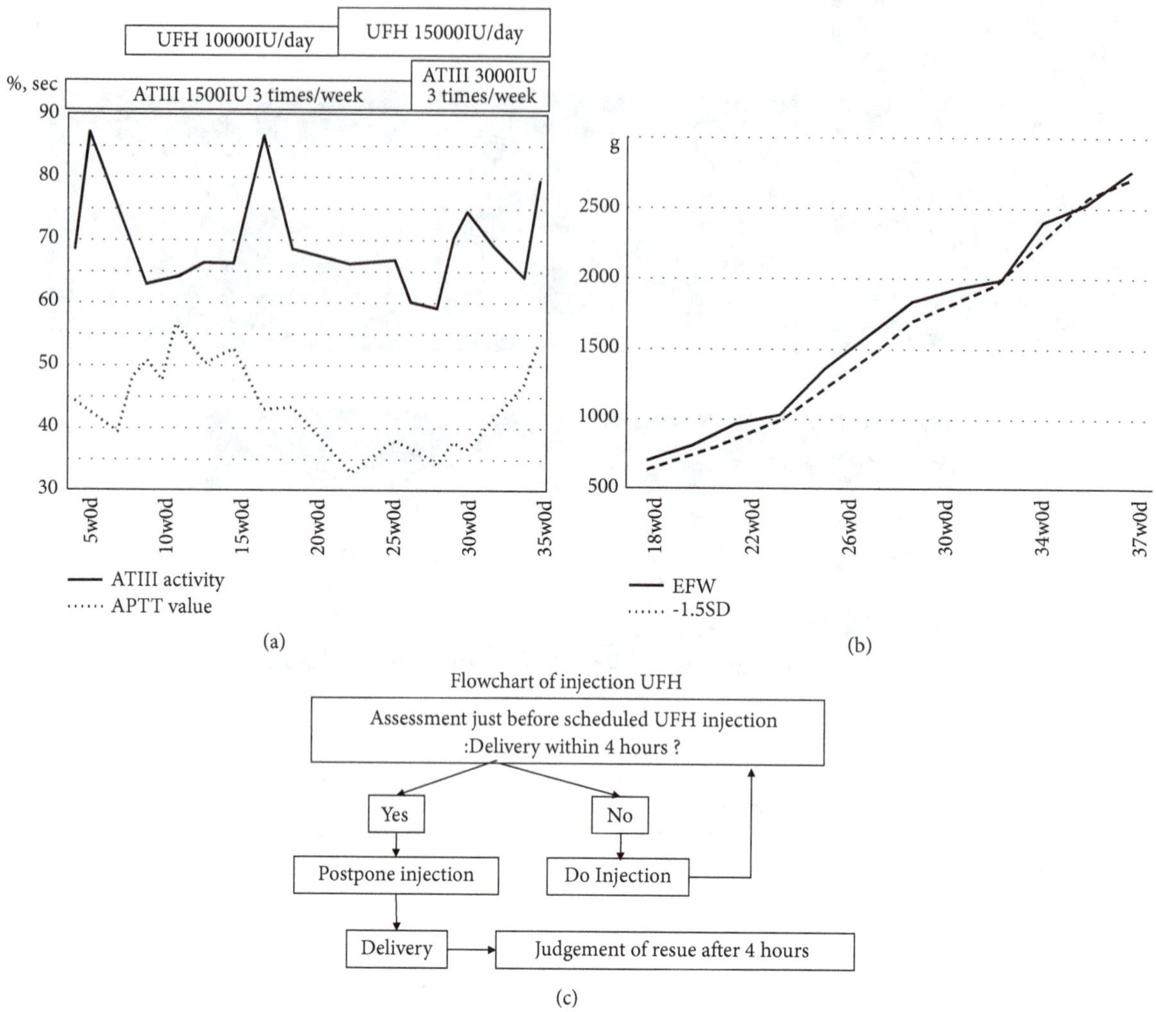

FIGURE 2: Clinical course in patient's fifth pregnancy, and flow chart in delivery. (a) Treatment process and change of ATIII activity and APTT value during pregnancy. Y-axis; % (ATIII) and seconds (sec, APTT). (b) Change of the estimated fetal weight (EFW) of fetus. Dot line indicates the line of -1.5SD. (c) Flowchart that we considered at the delivery.

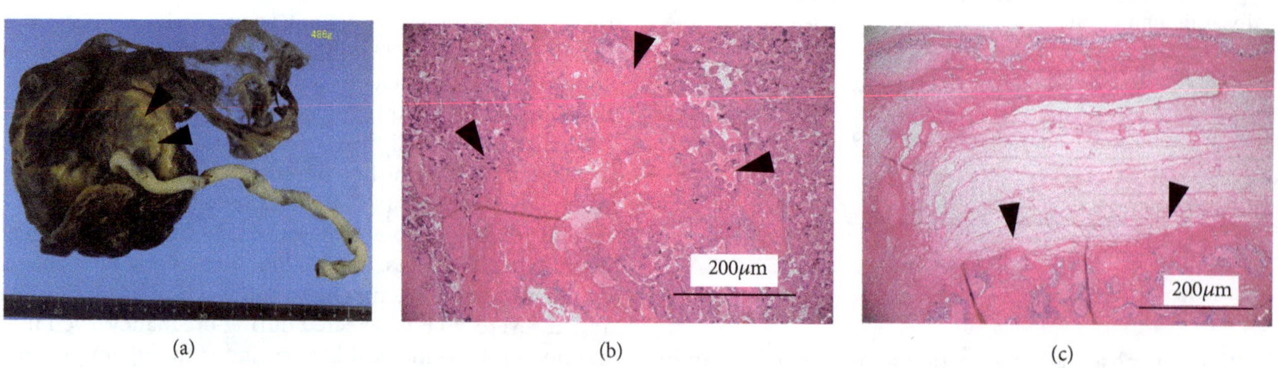

FIGURE 3: Pathological findings of placenta. Macroscopic view and HE staining are shown. Scale is shown in each figure. (a) Macroscopic view; circumferential-like infarction was observed in a portion approximately 4 cm in radius around the umbilical cord. (b) x40 magnification. Necrosis of villi was observed around that site. Black arrows indicate the necrosis of villi. (c) x40 magnification. Necrosis of the amniotic membrane and chorion, and fibrin precipitation was observed. Black arrows indicate the necrosis, and fibrin precipitation.

recommended to add the use of ATIII formulations. In some other countries, we can see more reports using low molecular weight heparin (LMWH) for pregnant women compared to those using UFH. ACCP guidelines mostly recommend LMWH as a first choice for anticoagulation therapy for pregnant women [16]. Some retrospective analyses and systematic reviews show that the risk of bleeding during pregnancy due to LMWH administration is low compared to that due to UFH [17, 18]. In addition, because UFH can maintain the anticoagulant effect for a long time, management of UFH during delivery may be slightly more complicated compared to LMVH. However, in Japan, we are currently not allowed to use LMWH with public insurance. We hope that we can use LMVH for pregnant women in the near future.

At the delivery during antithrombotic therapy, we should pay attention to the adverse effects of both bleeding tendency caused by antithrombotic therapy itself and development of thrombosis caused by interruption of antithrombotic therapy. In this case, we devised a flowchart (Figure 2(c)) to prevent administration of UFH within at least 4 hours before delivery, since UFH was administered every 8 hours. We also had a close meeting with ward staff, midwives, paediatricians, and anaesthesiologists in advance.

Foetal growth restriction (FGR) is frequently observed in the patients with congenital AT III deficiency [19]. In this case, the estimated foetal body weight of her baby was relatively small compared to average, about -1.5 to -1.0 SD, but the amount of amniotic fluid was normal. The baby's birthweight was 2310 g, which was below the 10th percentile and was defined as small for gestational age (SGA). In the pathological examination of the placenta, the infarction existed in a relatively wide range, suggesting a thrombotic tendency due to ATIII deficiency, which might be the reason of SGA.

In this case, the patient got pregnant naturally during the oral administration of NOAC. NOAC is currently preferred to UFH and/or LMWH for nonpregnant patients from the viewpoint of administration route and management. Nonetheless, the influence of NOAC on pregnancy has not been established today. Hence, we should use UFH or LMWH during pregnancy, not NOAC. Burnet et al. have summarized cases taking NOAC in early pregnancy [20]. In their report, among 10 pregnant women who were exposed to NOAC during the first 6 weeks of gestation, 4 were full-term births, 2 were preterm births, 1 was a first-trimester spontaneous abortion, and 3 were elective pregnancy terminations. NOAC animal studies demonstrated no fetal harm. In addition, they say that NOAC is not contraindication to those who are pregnant. In this case, the patient was exposed to NOAC during the first 5 weeks of gestation, and she had a full-term birth without any anomaly in her baby. Evaluating the influence of NOAC on pregnancy is highly recommended in the near future. We hope we will be able to use NOAC even during pregnancy.

In conclusion, we experienced a case of a pregnant patient who had a congenital ATIII deficiency, which developed into severe VTE for the first time in her fourth pregnancy. We should take some heredity diseases into account in the case of severe VTE, even if they are multipara and have no family or medical history. In addition, when those who have hereditary thrombophilia disease with medication of NOAC get pregnant, they may not have to choose an elective pregnancy termination and be able to continue pregnancy.

Disclosure

Present affiliation of Koji Yamanoi is Department of Dermatology, Cutaneous Biology Research Center, Massachusetts General Hospital.

Authors' Contributions

Mie Sakai and Jumpei Ogura equally contributed to this report.

References

[1] J. Hasegawa, A. Sekizawa, H. Tanaka et al., "Current status of pregnancy-related maternal in Japan," *BMJ Open*, vol. 6, no. 3, p. e010304, 2016.

[2] H. S. Wik, A. F. Jacobsen, L. Sandvik, and P. M. Sandset, "Prevalence and predictors for post-thrombotic syndrome 3 to 16years after pregnancy-related venous thrombosis: A population-based, cross-sectional, case-control study," *Journal of Thrombosis and Haemostasis*, vol. 10, no. 5, pp. 840–847, 2012.

[3] F. Melis, J. P. Vandenbrouke, H. R. Büller, L. P. Colly, and K. W. M. Bloemenkamp, "Estimates of risk of venous thrombosis during pregnancy and puerperium are not influenced by diagnostic suspicion and referral basis," *American Journal of Obstetrics & Gynecology*, vol. 191, no. 3, pp. 825–829, 2004.

[4] A. Tosetto, M. Frezzato, and F. Rodeghiero, "Prevalence and risk factors of non-fatal venous thromboembol ism in the active population of the VITA Project," *Journal of Thrombosis and Haemostasis*, vol. 1, no. 8, pp. 1724–1729, 2003.

[5] P. G. Lindqvist, P. J. Svensson, K. Maršál, L. Grennert, M. Luterkort, and B. Dahlbäck, "Activated protein C resistance (FV:Q506) and pregnancy," *Thrombosis and Haemostasis*, vol. 81, no. 4, pp. 532–537, 1999.

[6] L. Robertson, O. Wu, P. Langhorne et al., "Thrombophilia in pregnancy: a systematic review," *British Journal of Haematology*, vol. 132, no. 2, pp. 171–196, 2006.

[7] M. Kovač, Ž. Miković, L. Rakičević et al., "A successful outcome of pregnancy in a patient with congenital antithrombin deficiency," *Vojnosanitetski Pregled*, vol. 68, no. 2, pp. 175–177, 2011.

[8] A. García-Botella, S. Asenjo, M. E. De La Morena-Barrio et al., "First case with antithrombin deficiency, mesenteric vein thrombosis and pregnancy: Multidisciplinary diagnosis and successful management," *Thrombosis Research*, vol. 144, pp. 72–75, 2016.

[9] O. Egeberg, "Inherited antithrombin deficiency causing thrombophilia," *Thrombosis et Diathesis Haemorrhagica*, vol. 13, pp. 516–530, 1965.

[10] L. Charles, W. George, and S. Neil, "Practice Bulletin No. 138: Inherited Thrombophilias in Pregnancy," *Obstetrics & Gynecology*, vol. 122, no. 3, pp. 706–716, 2013.

[11] S. Warren and T. P. Eberhardt, "Mesenteric venos thrombosis," *Surgery Gynecolgy & Obstetrics*, vol. 61, pp. 102–120, 1935.

[12] H. H. Van Boven and D. A. Lane, "Antithrombin and its inherited deficiency states," *Seminars in Hematology*, vol. 34, no. 3, pp. 188–204, 1997.

[13] H. H. Van Boven, J. P. Vandenbroucke, R. G. J. Westendorp, and F. R. Rosendaal, "Mortality and causes of death in inherited antithrombin deficiency," *Thrombosis and Haemostasis*, vol. 77, no. 3, pp. 452–455, 1997.

[14] P. W. Friederich, B.-J. Sanson, P. Simioni et al., "Frequency of pregnancy-related venous thromboembolism in anticoagulant factor-deficient women: Implications for prophylaxis," *Annals of Internal Medicine*, vol. 125, no. 12, pp. 955–960, 1996.

[15] L. Skeith, A. Aw, J. Hews-Girard, and N. Rydz, "A case that illustrates the challenges of managing pregnant patients with antithrombin deficiency: More questions than answers," *Thrombosis Research*, vol. 157, pp. 1–6, 2017.

[16] S. M. Bates, I. A. Greer, S. Middeldorp, D. L. Veenstra, A. Prabulos, and P. O. Vandvik, "VTE, thrombophilia, antithrombotic therapy, and pregnancy," *CHEST*, vol. 141, no. 2, pp. e691S–e736S, 2012.

[17] B.-J. Sanson, A. W. A. Lensing, M. H. Prins et al., "Safety of low-molecular-weight heparin in pregnancy: A systematic review," *Thrombosis and Haemostasis*, vol. 81, no. 5, pp. 668–672, 1999.

[18] I. A. Greer and C. Nelson-Piercy, "Low-molecular-weight heparins for thromboprophylaxis and treatment of venous thromboembolism in pregnancy: A systematic review of safety and efficacy," *Blood*, vol. 106, no. 2, pp. 401–407, 2005.

[19] F. G. Cunningham, K. J. Leveno, S. L. Bloom et al., *Williams Obstetrics*, McGraw Hill, New York, NY, USA, 24th edition, 2014.

[20] A. E. Burnett, C. E. Mahan, S. R. Vazquez, L. B. Oertel, D. A. Garcia, and J. Ansell, "Guidance for the practical management of the direct oral anticoagulants (DOACs) in VTE treatment," *Journal of Thrombosis and Thrombolysis*, vol. 41, no. 1, pp. 206–232, 2016.

49

A Case Report of Overcoming an Obstructive, Pedunculated Cervical Fibroid at the Time of Uterine Evacuation

Jayesh Tigdi[1] **and Cynthia Chan**[2]

[1]*Department of Obstetrics & Gynecology, McMaster University, Hamilton, Ontario, Canada*
[2]*Department of Obstetrics & Gynecology, Western University, London, Ontario, Canada*

Correspondence should be addressed to Jayesh Tigdi; jayesh.tigdi@medportal.ca

Academic Editor: Maria Grazia Porpora

Background. Fibroids, which can impact pregnancies at later gestations, such as obstructing delivery, may also affect the pregnancy termination process. *Case.* We present the case of a 28-year-old G1 at 18 weeks who consented for a genetic pregnancy termination via dilation and evacuation. During the typical preparatory procedure with laminaria, it was noted that a 5-6cm cervical fibroid prolapsed into the vagina obstructing access to the uterine cavity. Through osmotic dilation followed by cervical Foley catheter ripening, a planned myomectomy was possible with minimal blood loss prior to uterine evacuation. *Conclusion.* Through appropriate counselling, planning, and effective cervical dilatation, a planned myomectomy for prolapsing fibroids at the time of termination of pregnancy is possible. This can prevent unnecessary hysterotomy and avoid need for subsequent cesarean section.

1. Introduction

A number of terminations of pregnancy are for prenatally confirmed fetal genetic diagnoses [1]. Due to the timeline of the routine prenatal genetic screening process, the decision to end these pregnancies tends to be taken further along in gestational age. Therefore, complications of later pregnancy can have an impact on the delivery of care in the process of pregnancy termination.

During evacuation of the uterus, cervical dilatation is important as instrumentation is required to allow passage of contents with reduced cervical trauma and to minimize risk of retained tissue [2]. Indeed, fibroids can impede this passage and, at term, delivery sometimes necessitates hysterotomy. An obstructive cervical fibroid is a known indication for operative term delivery via cesarean section [3]. There are case reports of cervical fibroid posing issues in peripartum care at or near term [4, 5]. However, there is little literature on the management of elective termination for pregnancies complicated by cervical fibroid. In this case report, we describe, in accordance with SCARE criteria [6], an unusual technique of dilatation and evacuation through an obstructive fibroid at an academic centre.

2. Case Report

The patient involved was a healthy 28-year-old G1 at 18 weeks of gestation who consented for pregnancy termination via preparatory laminaria dilators and subsequent operative dilatation and evacuation for a confirmed, lethal diagnosis of Trisomy 18. Aside from an ultrasound-diagnosed lower uterine fibroid, her antenatal course was unremarkable and she had had a normal pelvic examination just prior to conceiving.

On preparation of the cervix for dilatation, a speculum exam revealed an obstructing 5-6cm fibroid protruding through the cervix into the vagina. The cervix itself was not visualized due to the size of the fibroid and its protrusion into the vagina. On bimanual exam, the internal os was closed around the fibroid, which appeared to arise from the level of the internal os of the cervix. In order to prepare the cervix for dilation, osmotic dilators were tucked around the fibroid within the cervix. After three hours, the internal os was a finger tip dilated with further ripening required. Rather than a sequential set of dilators which would be challenging to place and maintain around the fibroid due to angulation, a cervical Foley catheter was employed to ripen the cervix

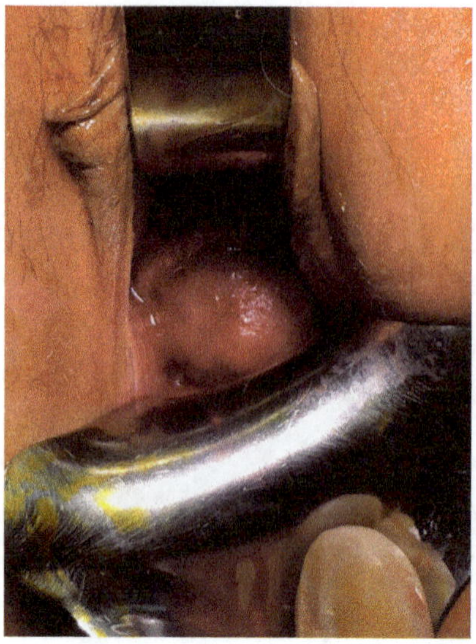

FIGURE 1: Obstructive cervical fibroid prolapsing through into vagina.

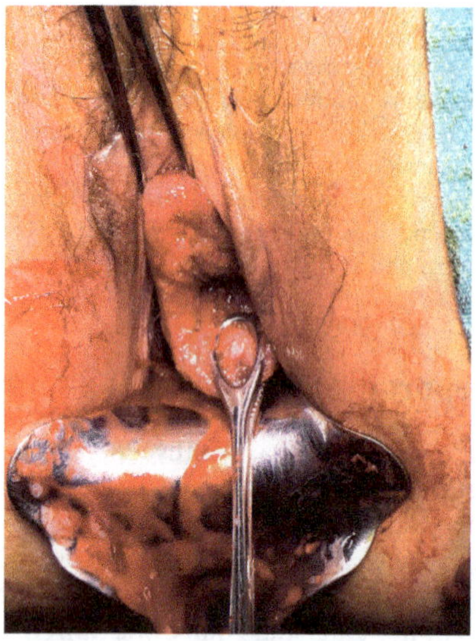

FIGURE 2: Cervix postmyomectomy with cauterized fibroid stalk base. Ring forceps on posterior lip of cervix and single-toothed tenaculum on anterior surface of cervix.

further. The intent was to allow proper placement of a dilator without increasing the risk of false passage creation.

Given the obstructive fibroid, the patient consented for a myomectomy prior to the evacuation, with the added, increased risk of hemorrhage. The possibility of an operative hysteroscopy was explained, as it would allow for removal of the stalk of the fibroid in its entirety, as well as cauterization of the base itself should it be required. Prior ultrasound had indicated that the fibroid was within the lower uterine segment, and the location of the base could not yet be identified.

The following day with the Foley having fallen out and under general anesthetic, examination revealed a sufficiently 3-4cm dilated cervix with the prolapsed fibroid now slightly recessed into the cervix due to the dilatation of the internal os. There was clear visualization of the fibroid stalk originating from within the endocervix (Figure 1). To minimize blood loss intraoperatively, dilute vasopressin (8 units) with 1% lidocaine (20ml) was infiltrated as a paracervical block and at the base of the fibroid. The fibroid was grasped and transected at its base with cautery used to maintain hemostasis. With the obstruction cleared (Figure 2), the remainder of the uterine evacuation was carried forth in the usual manner utilizing a 12mm suction curette. Sharp curettage confirmed that there was no fibroid base remaining. At the conclusion of the case, hemostasis was noted. The patient's postoperative course was uncomplicated.

3. Discussion

To our knowledge, this is the first case report of an obstructive fibroid at the time of performing a uterine evacuation for products of conception. Before pregnancy, the patient's fibroid likely remained intrauterine as she had had a Pap smear just prior to pregnancy with no note of any visible abnormalities. With the growing uterus, through mass effect, the fibroid likely prolapsed through the cervical canal, creating a challenge in dilating the cervix for the required procedure.

Although a reportedly more painful procedure, the cervical Foley catheter can be used for cervical ripening when cervical dilators may prove ineffectual. However, to reduce the risk of spontaneous abortion/preterm labour outside the hospital, this is not routine practice [7]. This patient came from a distance, and when performing serial cervical dilatation, our centre requires that patients remain in town after placement of dilators due to the small risk of labour [8].

The cervical Foley was successful in dilating the cervix, as on returning the next day the cervix was dilated with enough access to the uterine cavity and the base of the fibroid stalk was easily visualized. By securing the vascular supply of the fibroid, we were able to successfully perform the myomectomy; with this removed, we had unobstructed access for evacuation of the uterine contents.

In other cases of obstructing fibroids, often hysterotomy is performed rather than attempting a dilation and evacuation because this would allow definitive removal of tissue, rather than having difficulty accessing the tissue and increasing the risk of retained products. However, a hysterotomy is known to have a higher risk of morbidity than dilation and evacuation, in addition to the risk for later pregnancy. Certainly with term pregnancies, an obstructing fibroid is an indication for a cesarean section as it may prevent descent of the fetus [9].

A controlled clinical setting is required to ensure patient safety when performing a myomectomy in pregnancy, as hemorrhage risk is significant [10]. The combination of appropriate patient counselling, assured cervical dilatation with a cervical Foley catheter, and intraoperative blood loss prophylaxis was key in saving this patient from the morbidity of hysterotomy [11]. Further to the patient's benefit, removal of this fibroid may have prevented a cesarean section and other potential complications in a subsequent pregnancy [12].

References

[1] H. Brandenburg, W. De Koning, M. G. J. Jahoda et al., "Reproductive behaviour and prenatal diagnosis following genetic termination of pregnancy in women of advanced maternal age," *Prenatal Diagnosis*, vol. 12, no. 12, pp. 1031–1035, 1992.

[2] A. M. Autry, E. C. Hayes, G. F. Jacobson, and R. S. Kirby, "A comparison of medical induction and dilation and evacuation for second-trimester abortion," *American Journal of Obstetrics & Gynecology*, vol. 187, no. 2, pp. 393–397, 2002.

[3] D. James, P. J. Steer, C. P. Weiner, and B. Gonik, *High Risk Pregnancy: Management Options*, Cambridge University Press, New York, NY, USA, 5th edition, 2017.

[4] A. Gandhi, H. I. Dugad, and Y. Shah, "A rare presentation of cervical fibroid in pregnancy," *Annals of African Medicine*, vol. 13, no. 2, p. 88, 2014, Academic OneFile, http://link.galegroup.com.libaccess.lib.mcmaster.ca/apps/doc/A364125364/AONE?u=ocul_mcmaster&sid=AONE&xid=5d356a7f.

[5] S. Sengupta, K. Reddy, and M. Pillai, "Prolapsed cervical fibroid in pregnancy: A challenging obstetric dilemma," *Journal of Obstetrics & Gynaecology*, vol. 26, no. 8, pp. 823-824, 2009.

[6] R. Agha, R. A. Agha, A. J. Fowler et al., "The SCARE statement: consensus-based surgical case report guidelines," *International Journal of Surgery*, vol. 34, pp. 180–186, 2016.

[7] G. A. Hackett, P. Reginald, and D. Paintin, "Comparison of the Foley catheter and dinoprostone pessary for cervical preparation before second trimester abortion," *British Journal of Obstetrics & Gynaecology*, vol. 96, pp. 1432–1434, 1989.

[8] A. Edelman, "General obstetrics and gynaecology: Cervical preparation using laminaria with adjunctive buccal misoprostol before second-trimester dilation and evacuation procedures: a randomized control trial," *American Journal of Obstetrics & Gynecology*, vol. 194, no. 2, pp. 425–430, 2006.

[9] D. Abam and T. Kasso, "Uterine fibroids and pregnancy: A review of the challenges," *IntechOpen*, 2007.

[10] D. Brown, H. M. Fletcher, M. O. Myrie, and M. Reid, "Cesarean myomectomy- a safe procedure. a retrospective case controlled study," *Obstetrics & Gynecology*, vol. 19, pp. 139–141, 1999.

[11] J. K. Basu and D. Basu, "The management of failed second-trimester termination of pregnancy," *Contraception*, vol. 80, no. 2, pp. 170–173, 2009.

[12] H. Lee, E. R. Norwitz, and J. Shaw, "Contemporary management of fibroids in pregnancy," *Reviews in Obstetrics Gynecology*, vol. 3, no. 1, pp. 20–27, 2010.

50

Placenta Accreta in a Woman with Childhood Uterine Irradiation: A Case Report and Literature Review

Nanayo Sasagasako, Hirohiko Tani, Yoshitsugu Chigusa, Shingo Io, Haruta Mogami, Junzo Hamanishi, Akihito Horie, Eiji Kondoh, Yukiyasu Sato, and Masaki Mandai

Department of Obstetrics and Gynecology, Kyoto University Hospital, Kyoto, Japan

Correspondence should be addressed to Hirohiko Tani; tanita@kuhp.kyoto-u.ac.jp

Academic Editor: Shawky Z. A. Badawy

The pregnancies of childhood cancer survivors who have received uterine irradiation are associated with a high risk of several obstetrical complications, including placenta accreta. The present case was a 26-year-old pregnant woman with a history of myelodysplastic syndrome treated with umbilical cord blood transplantation following chemotherapy and total body irradiation at the age of 10. Despite every possible measure to prevent preterm labor, uterine contractions became uncontrollable and a female infant weighing 892 g was vaginally delivered at 27^{+4} weeks of gestation. Under the postpartum ultrasonographic diagnosis of placenta accreta, we selected to leave the placenta *in situ*. Although emergency bilateral uterine artery embolization was required, complete resorption of the residual placenta was accomplished on the 115th day postpartum. Our experience highlighted the following points. (1) The expectant management of placenta accreta arising in an irradiated uterus may not only fulfill fertility preservation, but may also reduce possible risks associated with cesarean hysterectomy. (2) Due to extreme thinning of and a poor blood supply to the myometrium, reaching an antepartum diagnosis of placenta accreta in an irradiated uterus is difficult. (3) The recurrence of placenta accreta in subsequent pregnancies needs to be considered after successful preservation of the uterus.

1. Introduction

Due to advances in cancer treatment modalities, including radiotherapy, the number of childhood cancer survivors (CCS) is increasing. As a result, significant numbers of CCS have reached their reproductive ages and wish to have their own children. Nevertheless, most of the CCS who have received irradiation to fields involving the ovary and uterus in their childhood have reduced fertility mainly due to premature ovarian failure [1]. Moreover, even if they become pregnant, their pregnancy courses may be hampered by several complications, such as preterm labor, fetal malposition, and low-birth weight infants [2, 3], which are attributable to myometrial fibrosis causing a reduced uterine volume and distensibility as well as vascular damage resulting in a reduced uterine blood supply [4].

Placenta accreta, which is defined as the myometrial invasion of placental villi without intervening decidual tissue, is one of the major causes of serious postpartum hemorrhage leading to significant maternal mortality. According to the depth of placental invasion, placenta accreta is divided into three types: placenta accreta, in which placental villi attach directly to the myometrium; placenta increta, in which placental villi extend into the myometrium; and placenta percreta, in which the villi penetrate through the myometrium to the uterine serosa and may invade adjacent organs [5]. The underlying etiology of placenta accreta is considered to be a failure in normal decidual formation due to a deficient endometrium. Since uterine irradiation can induce endometrial injury [4], pregnancies after uterine irradiation may be complicated by placenta accreta. Indeed, a history of uterine irradiation is listed as one of the risk factors predisposing women to placenta accreta [5]. However, since there have only been a few cases of placenta accreta reported in women with a history of uterine irradiation, an optimal management strategy has not yet been established.

We herein present a case of placenta accreta that developed in a woman with prior total body irradiation (TBI) during her

TABLE 1: Changes in serum hormone levels after menarche.

Age (years-months)	15-7	16-0	16-8	17-4	17-8	18-3	18-7	20-1	20-7
LH (mIU/ml)	104	2.7	2.2	11.8	2.2	12.8	14.6	14.3	2.8
FSH (mIU/ml)	135.7	8.2	2.6	9.4	7.9	22	9	8	3.9
E2 (pg/ml)	14.2	30.3	69	30	19.2	34.8	45.3	39.6	107.2

childhood. The placenta was left *in situ* after the delivery and expectant management was instituted. Although emergency bilateral uterine artery embolization (UAE) was required to control massive uterine bleeding on the 10th day postpartum, the residual placenta was completely resolved by the 115th day postpartum. We also reviewed the literature describing similar cases to approach an optimal management strategy against this condition.

2. Case

The present case was a 26-year-old para 0, gravida 0, woman with a history of myelodysplastic syndrome (MDS) at the age of 10. She was treated with umbilical cord blood transplantation (CBT) following chemotherapy with cytarabine (3.4 g for 2 days), cyclophosphamide (60 mg/kg/day for 2 days), etoposide (150 mg/m^2/day for 7 days), and mitoxantrone (5 mg/m^2/day for 5 days) as well as 12 Gy of TBI. Complete remission with 100% donor chimerism was confirmed on the 90th day after CBT. Her pubertal development progressed normally, culminating in menarche at the age of 13 and a final height of 162 cm. Although she only had menstrual bleeding a few times every year, exogenous estrogen was not administered because her serum estradiol level remained detectable in periodic blood sampling (Table 1).

At the age of 20, the patient married and visited our fertility clinic. She was oligomenorrheic with hypergonadotropic hypogonadism (serum LH 12.4 mIU/ml, FSH 28.9 mIU/ml, and E_2 12.2 pg/ml). The extremely low level of serum anti-Mullerian hormone (AMH, 0.01 ng/ml) suggested a reduced ovarian reserve due to her history of chemotherapy and TBI. Furthermore, a small uterus measuring only 48.3 mm in length was noted on the ultrasonographic scan. After nearly four years of unsuccessful timed intercourse, which was considered to be mainly attributable to oligo-ovulation, she decided to undergo *in vitro* fertilization (IVF). Since three courses of embryo transfer failed to result in pregnancy, she discontinued fertility treatment at the age of 25.

Two months after the cessation of fertility treatment, when the patient was 26 years old, she naturally conceived and returned to our obstetric clinic at 6^{+2} weeks of gestation. At 13^{+6} weeks of gestation, prophylactic Shirodkar cerclage was performed as the uterine cervix had shortened to 20 mm and oral nifedipine (40 mg/day) was started for tocolysis. Despite these treatments, her cervical length continued to shorten due to frequent uterine contractions. Therefore, continuous intravenous ritodrine hydrochloride was added from 16^{+3} weeks of gestation. At 17^{+3} weeks of gestation, emergency McDonald cerclage was placed at the periphery of the previous Shirodkar suture due to painless prolapse of the amniotic sac. The dose

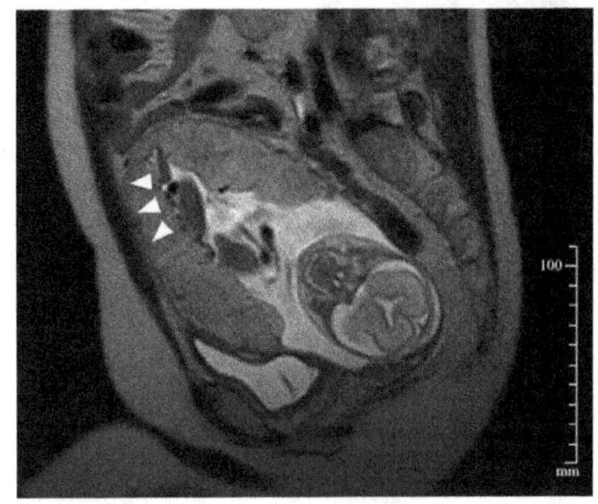

FIGURE 1: Sagittal T2-weighted magnetic resonance image of the uterus at 22^{+4} weeks of gestation. The myometrium is extremely thin throughout the uterus with partial bulging of the anterior uterine wall (arrowheads).

of oral nifedipine was increased to 60 mg/day and continuous intravenous magnesium sulfate was added. At 22^{+4} weeks of gestation, the patient underwent magnetic resonance imaging (MRI) scan to assess precise state of the pregnant uterus, revealing an extremely thin myometrium with only 2 mm in thickness throughout the uterus. Partial bulging of the anterior uterine wall was also noted, implying the presence of placenta accreta (Figure 1). In ultrasonography, however, we could not find any characteristic findings of placenta arcreta such as placental lacunae, loss of hypoechoic space, and abundant vascularity in the myometrium. Fetal well-being and uterine contractions were screened by daily cardiotocography. Fetal growth and amniotic fluid volume were also monitored by ultrasonography twice a week.

At 27^{+1} weeks of gestation, the passage of amniotic fluid through the uterine cervix was noted. Two doses of betamethasone (12 mg) were administered intramuscularly 24 h apart. Intravenous flomoxef (1.0 g) was given every 12 h to prevent intrauterine infection, and the dose of oral nifedipine was increased further to 160 mg/day. At 27^{+4} weeks of gestation, uterine contractions became uncontrollable. After the cerclage was removed, a female infant weighing 892 g (small for gestational age) was vaginally delivered with Apgar scores of 5 and 6 at 1 and 5 min, respectively. Under the suspicion of placenta accreta raised by the MRI finding, spontaneous placenta expulsion was awaited instead of exerting traction on the umbilical cord. The placenta remained *in situ* for more than one hour. An ultrasonographic scan revealed that the placenta was still tightly attached to the uterine wall with significant blood flow from the myometrium into the attached placenta, leading to the diagnosis of placenta accreta. Since uterine bleeding was minimal at that time and the patient expressed

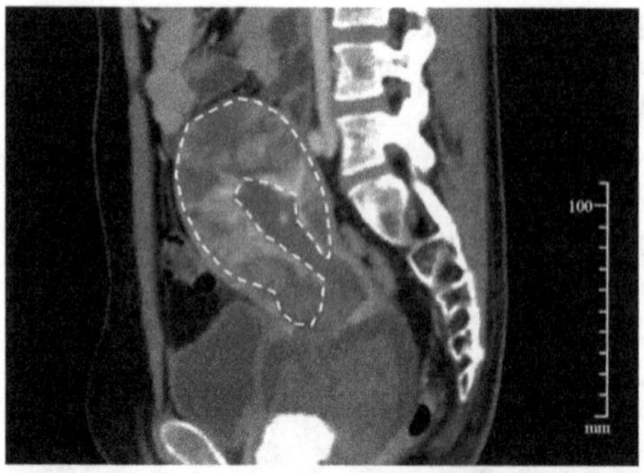

FIGURE 2: Sagittal contrast-enhanced computed tomographic image of the uterus on the 10th postpartum day. The retained placenta is circumscribed by a dashed line. Note that the placenta is enhanced by contrast medium in a patchy manner.

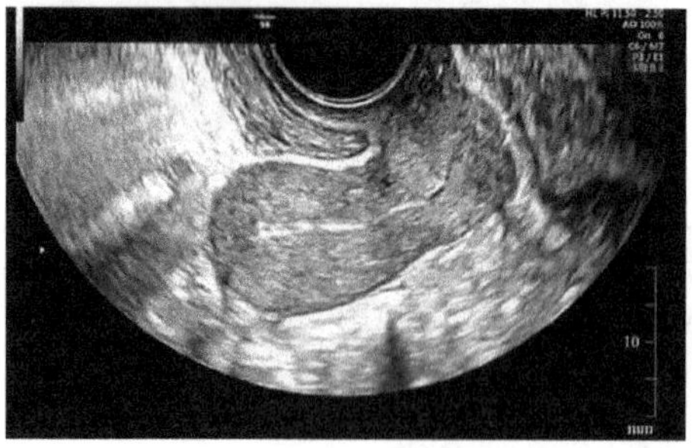

FIGURE 3: Sagittal ultrasound image of the uterus on the 115th postpartum day. The placenta has become undetectable in the uterine cavity. Note that myometrial thickness has returned to normal.

her desire to preserve fertility, we selected to leave the placenta *in situ*.

On the 10th postpartum day, intractable uterine bleeding of more than 300 ml per hour suddenly occurred. Contrast-enhanced computed tomography (CT) revealed the persistence of a significant placental blood supply (Figure 2). Six units of red blood cells were transfused and emergency bilateral uterine artery embolization (UAE) was conducted. Uterine bleeding subsequently subsided and she was discharged from the hospital with the whole placenta left *in situ* on the 28th postpartum day. Her condition was followed up weekly at the outpatient clinic. Her serum hCG levels became lower than the cut-off value on the 87th postpartum day, and complete resorption of the residual placenta was ultrasonographically verified on the 115th day postpartum (Figure 3).

The neonate suffered from respiratory distress syndrome and was given surfactant immediately after the birth. She also had duodenal stenosis with annular pancreas, which required an operation at the age of 8 days. Her postoperative course was uneventful. Respiratory care became unnecessary at the age of 50 days and she was discharged home at the age of 116 days, when her body weight reached 2922 g.

3. Discussion

According to our Pubmed search using "placenta accreta" and "total body irradiation" or "radiotherapy" as key words, only five cases of placenta accreta, including the present case, have been reported in women with a history of radiotherapy involving the uterus [6–9] (Table 2). The degree of uterine damage depends not only on the total irradiation dose, but also on a patient's age at the time of radiotherapy [4]. The irradiation doses in these five cases (8.75–72 Gy) exceeded the threshold value of 4 Gy, below which patients were reported to be free of the risk of subfertility [10]. Notably, radiotherapy was given before menarche in all the five cases except for case 3, which is consistent with the fact that pre-pubertal uterus is more radiosensitive than post-pubertal uterus [4]. In contrast, the risk of early ovarian functional loss becomes greater with increasing age at the time of radiotherapy [11]. In case 3, post-pubertal irradiation deprived the patient of her ovarian function, necessitating oocyte donation to become pregnant, whereas in the other four cases, the patients naturally conceived, indicating that their ovarian function had been preserved post-irradiation. In summary, women whose uteri and ovaries were irradiated during the pre-pubertal period may preserve their potential to conceive naturally; however, their pregnancies are associated with a high risk of developing placenta accreta.

Cesarean hysterectomy is currently the gold standard treatment for placenta accreta, but is associated with high rates (~40%) of maternal complications, such as massive blood loss, bladder injury, thromboembolism, and fistula formation [12, 13]. Since surgeries in previously irradiated fields have an increased risk of postoperative complications mainly due to delayed wound healing [14, 15], complication rates may be even higher if cesarean hysterectomy is performed on an irradiated uterus. Expectant management, i.e., leaving the placenta *in situ* and waiting for its spontaneous resorption, has the potential to reduce the necessity for invasive surgery, and, thus, may be preferable to cesarean hysterectomy as a strategy to manage placenta accreta that develops in women with a history of uterine irradiation. In the present case, since the patient had given birth vaginally and late postpartum hemorrhage was successfully controlled by UAE, we were able to circumvent any type of surgery, including cesarean section. Nevertheless, antenatal care and attempt at vaginal delivery in women with prior uterine irradiation need to be undertaken with great caution because these uteri are liable to rupture, as reported in cases 1 and 2, for which spontaneous uterine rupture occurred at 13 and 17 weeks of gestation, respectively (Table 2).

An antepartum diagnosis of placenta accreta allows for a planned, controlled delivery, which may minimize maternal and fetal risks [16]. Therefore, the diagnosis of placenta accreta needs to be aggressively pursued in any woman with risk factors, including uterine irradiation. In all five cases, including the present case, the diagnosis of placenta accreta was made during laparotomy or after vaginal delivery. The mainstay of an antepartum diagnosis is ultrasonography. Characteristic ultrasonographic findings associated with placenta accreta include the presence of placental lacunae, retroplacental myometrial thinning of less than 1 mm, the loss of a normal hypoechoic retroplacental zone, and hypervascularity at the bladder-myometrium interface [17]. MRI has been used for diagnoses when ultrasonography yielded equivocal results [18]. Characteristic MRI findings associated with placenta accreta include uterine bulging, heterogeneous signal intensity

TABLE 2: Cases of placenta accreta after uterine irradiation.

No.	Type	Primary disease	Age		Gravida and parity	Irradiation		Method of conception	Cerclage	Pregnancy outcome	Treatment	Reference
			Irradiation	Pregnancy		Site	Dose					
1	Percreta	Clear cell sarcoma	7	23	G1P0	Pelvis	70 Gy	Spontaneous	Not described	Uterine rupture abortion (13 weeks)	Hysterectomy	[6]
2	Percreta	Chronic myeloid leukemia	5	23	G1P0	Total body	8.75 Gy	Spontaneous	Not described	Uterine rupture abortion (17 weeks)	Hysterectomy	[7]
3	Accreta	Hodgkin's lymphoma	16	31	G1P0	Right hemipelvis, Mediastinum	36 Gy, 36 Gy	Oocyte donation (twin pregnancy)	Not described	Cesarean section live birth (35 weeks)	Hysterectomy	[8]
4	Accreta	Wilms tumor	4	23	G3P1 spontaneous abortion	Whole abdomen	10.8 Gy	Spontaneous	Performed at 11 weeks' gestation	Cesarean section live birth (37 weeks)	Manual placental removal. Hemostatic sutures	[9]
5	Accreta	Myelo-dysplastic syndrome	10	26	G1P0	Total body	12 Gy	Spontaneous	Performed at 13 and 17 weeks' gestation	Vaginal delivery live birth (27 weeks)	Placenta left *in situ*. Uterine artery embolization	This case

in the placenta, dark intra-placental bands on T2-weighted sequences, focal interruption of the myometrium, and tenting of the bladder, resulting in overall diagnostic accuracy with a sensitivity of 94.4% and specificity of 84.0% [19]. In the present case, even a retrospective review of all ultrasonographic and MRI photos did not clearly reveal any characteristic findings of placenta accreta other than uterine bulging on MRI. This paucity of diagnostic clues may be attributed to the extreme thinning of and a relatively poor blood supply to the myometrium. Therefore, in the case of pregnancy in an irradiated uterus, it is important to note that placenta accreta may be present even without characteristic imaging findings, and, thus, a delivery needs to be scheduled accordingly.

The recurrence of placenta accreta in subsequent pregnancies needs to be considered after the successful preservation of an irradiated uterus. An adequate endometrial thickness in the peri-implantation period may contribute to minimizing this recurrent risk. In women with pre-pubertal uterine irradiation, even high-dose estrogen supplementation failed to increase uterine sizes, uterine artery blood flow, or endometrial thickness [20], indicating that pre-pubertal irradiation deprives all uterine components, i.e., the myometrium, endometrium, and uterine artery, of their estrogen reactivities. This is in contrast to a uterus irradiated post-pubertally, which at least in part preserves estrogen reactivity [21]. Therefore, some measures other than estrogen supplementation were required to recover endometrial thickness in our patient, whose uterus was irradiated pre-pubertally. In 2002, promising findings were reported by Ledee-Bataille et al., who demonstrated that a treatment with the combination of pentoxifylline (800 mg/day) and vitamin E (1,000 IU/day) significantly increased the uterine size, uterine artery blood flow, and endometrial thickness of a pre-pubertally irradiated uterus [22]. This treatment needs to be investigated in the present case in order to establish whether it has the potential to prevent the recurrence of placenta accreta.

In conclusion, our experience of the present case and a literature review of similar cases have highlighted the following three points concerning placenta accreta developing in an irradiated uterus. (1) The expectant management of placenta accreta arising in an irradiated uterus may not only fulfill fertility preservation, but may also reduce the possible risks associated with cesarean hysterectomy against an irradiated uterus. (2) Difficulties are associated with reaching an antepartum diagnosis of placenta accreta in an irradiated uterus because of the extreme thinning of and a poor blood supply to the myometrium. (3) The recurrence of placenta accreta in subsequent pregnancies needs to be considered after the successful preservation of the uterus. Future studies are needed to investigate reliable methodologies for an antepartum diagnosis of placenta accreta in an irradiated uterus. Furthermore, the development of measures to prevent the recurrence of placenta accreta needs to be pursued.

Disclosure

The authors have nothing to disclose. They report no declaration of interest. The authors alone are responsible for the content and writing of the manuscript.

Authors' Contributions

Conception and design of study: N.S., H.T. acquisition of data: Y.C., S.I., J.H. Drafting the manuscript: N.S., H.T., E.K., Y.S. revising the manuscript critically for important intellectual content: H.M., A.H., E.K., Y.S., M.M.

Acknowledgments

The authors are grateful to Dr. Akira Kido for providing informative comments on MRI.

References

[1] W. H. Wallace, A. B. Thomson, and F. Saran, "Predicting age of ovarian failure after radiation to a field that includes the ovaries," *International Journal of Radiation Oncology*Biology*Physics*, vol. 62, no. 3, pp. 738–44, 2005.

[2] D. M. Green, E. M. Peabody, and B. Nan, "Pregnancy outcome after treatment for Wilms tumor: a report from the National Wilms Tumor Study Group," *Journal of Clinical Oncology*, vol. 20, no. 10, pp. 2506–2513, 2002.

[3] L. B. Signorello, S. S. Cohen, and C. Bosetti, "Female survivors of childhood cancer: preterm birth and low birth weight among their children," *Journal of the National Cancer Institute*, vol. 98, no. 20, pp. 1453–1461, 2006.

[4] J. Y. Wo and A. N. Viswanathan, "Impact of radiotherapy on fertility, pregnancy, and neonatal outcomes in female cancer patients," *International Journal of Radiation Oncology, Biology, Physics*, vol. 73, no. 5, pp. 1304–1312, 2009.

[5] Publications Committee, Society for Maternal-Fetal Medicine, Belfort, MA, "Placenta accreta," *American Journal of Obstetrics and Gynecology*, vol. 203, no. 5, pp. 430–439, 2010.

[6] G. Pridjian, N. E. Rich, and A. G. Montag, "Pregnancy hemoperitoneum and placenta percreta in a patient with previous pelvic irradiation and ovarian failure," *American Journal of Obstetrics and Gynecology*, vol. 162, no. 5, pp. 1205–1206, 1990.

[7] E. R. Norwitz, H. M. Stern, H. Grier, and A. Lee-Parritz, "Placenta percreta and uterine rupture associated with prior whole body radiation therapy," *Obstetrics and Gynecology*, vol. 98, no. 5 Pt 2, pp. 929–931, 2001.

[8] E. de Menezes and S. M. Tuck, "Pelvic radiotherapy damage to the endometrium causing morbid adherence of placenta. A new risk factor?" *Journal of Obstetrics and Gynaecology*, vol. 27, no. 5, pp. 526–527, 2007.

[9] Z. S. Bowman, M. Simons, C. Sok, and M. L. Draper, "Cervical insufficiency and placenta accreta after prior pelvic radiation," *Journal of Obstetrics and Gynaecology*, vol. 34, no. 8, p. 735, 2014.

[10] H. Sudour, P. Chastagner, L. Claude et al., "Fertility and pregnancy outcome after abdominal irradiation that included or excluded the pelvis in childhood tumor survivors," *International Journal of Radiation Oncology, Biology, Physics*, vol. 76, no. 3, pp. 867–73, 2010.

[11] H. O. Critchley and W. H. Wallace, "Impact of cancer treatment on uterine function," *Journal of the National Cancer Institute Monographs*, vol. 34, pp. 64–68, 2005.

[12] C. Clausen, L. Lonn, and J. Langhoff-Roos, "Management of placenta percreta: a review of published cases," *Acta Obstetricia et Gynecologica Scandinavica*, vol. 93, no. 2, pp. 138–143, 2014.

[13] D. J. Brennan, B. Schulze, and N. Chetty, "Surgical management of abnormally invasive placenta: a retrospective cohort study demonstrating the benefits of a standardized operative approach," *Acta Obstetricia et Gynecologica Scandinavica*, vol. 94, no. 12, pp. 1380–1386, 2015.

[14] J. Wang, M. Boerma, and Q. Fu, "Radiation responses in skin and connective tissues: effect on wound healing and surgical outcome," *Hernia*, vol. 10, no. 6, pp. 502–506, 2006.

[15] J. Feddock, M. Randall, and M. Kudrimoti, "Impact of post-radiation biopsies on development of fistulae in patients with cervical cancer," *Gynecologic Oncology*, vol. 133, no. 2, pp. 263–267, 2014.

[16] J. M. O'Brien, J. R. Barton, and E. S. Donaldson, "The management of placenta percreta: conservative and operative strategies," *American Journal of Obstetrics and Gynecology*, vol. 175, no. 6, pp. 1632–1638, 1996.

[17] W. A. Goh and I. Zalud, "Placenta accreta: diagnosis, management and the molecular biology of the morbidly adherent placenta," *Journal of Maternal-Fetal and Neonatal Medicine*, vol. 29, no. 11, pp. 1795–1800, 2016.

[18] A. Lax, M. R. Prince, and K. W. Mennitt, "The value of specific MRI features in the evaluation of suspected placental invasion," *Magnetic Resonance Imaging*, vol. 25, no. 1, pp. 87–93, 2007.

[19] F. D'Antonio, C. Iacovella, and J. Palacios-Jaraquemada, "Prenatal identification of invasive placentation using magnetic resonance imaging: systematic review and meta-analysis," *Ultrasound in Obstetrics & Gynecology*, vol. 44, no. 1, pp. 8–16, 2014.

[20] E. C. Larsen, K. Schmiegelow, and C. Rechnitzer, "Radiotherapy at a young age reduces uterine volume of childhood cancer survivors," *Acta Obstetricia et Gynecologica Scandinavica*, vol. 83, no. 1, pp. 96–102, 2004.

[21] L. E. Bath, H. O. Critchley, S. E. Chambers, R. A. Anderson, C. J. H. Kelnar, and W. H. B. Wallace, "Ovarian and uterine characteristics after total body irradiation in childhood and adolescence: response to sex steroid replacement," *BJOG: An International Journal of Obstetrics and Gynaecology*, vol. 106, no. 12, pp. 1265–1272, 1999.

[22] N. Ledee-Bataille, F. Olivennes, and J. L. Lefaix, "Combined treatment by pentoxifylline and tocopherol for recipient women with a thin endometrium enrolled in an oocyte donation programme," *Human Reproduction*, vol. 17, no. 5, pp. 1249–1253, 2002.

51

Influenza A Viral Infection with Septic Shock in Pregnancy

Soe Lwin,[1] Myat San Yi,[1] May Shi Leong,[2] Haris Suharjono,[2] and Tin Moe Nwe[3]

[1]*Department of Obstetrics & Gynecology, Faculty of Medicine and Health Sciences, UNIMAS, Malaysia*
[2]*Department of Obstetrics & Gynecology, Sarawak General Hospital, Malaysia*
[3]*Department of Basic Health Sciences, Faculty of Medicine and Health Sciences, UNIMAS, Malaysia*

Correspondence should be addressed to Soe Lwin; lsoe@unimas.my

Academic Editor: Erich Cosmi

The influenza virus is RNA virus and is classified into four subtypes, influenza A, influenza B, influenza C, and influenza D. One of the subtypes of influenza A, the H1N1 strain, also known as swine flu, is especially of high risk for development of complications in pregnant women. The influenza A virus infection is difficult to diagnose clinically because its presenting symptoms are similar to those of the common cold but are more severe, last longer, and can be potentially life-threatening. This case also presented with common cold symptoms but her condition worsened later. Fortunately, obstetric health providers were vigilant enough to address the developing infection and its related complications. It was the cooperative effort of multidisciplinary team care which resulted in a favourable outcome in both mother and baby.

1. Introduction

Influenza virus is a single-stranded, enveloped RNA virus from *Orthomyxoviridae* family. Its incubation period is 2-5 days and the transmission is mainly air-borne, i.e., droplet inhalation or direct transmission or contact through hands and fomites. It is classified into four distinct generations such as influenza A, B, C, and D depending on antibody responses to glycoproteins, *hemagglutinin* (HA), and *neuraminidase* (NA) on the surface of the viruses [1].

One of the subtypes of influenza A, influenza A (H1N1) strain called swine flu was first identified in April 2009 and the outbreak has since reached pandemic status at that time [2, 3]. So far, there have been 4 pandemic attacks worldwide: Spain in 1918 (unknown strain but suggestive of avian-like H1N1), Asian flu in 1957 by H_2 N_2, in Hong Kong in 1968, and Mexico in 2009. After each pandemic attack, healthcare personnel have become more aware of its lethal complications. In Malaysia, the avian influenza virus (AIV) (H5N1) outbreaks occurred in 2004, 2006, 2007, and 2017 in the state of Kelantan, Perak, and Pulau Pinang [4].

The influenza virus infection presents with fever, cough, sore throat, rhinorrhea, headache, myalgia, vomiting, and diarrhea. Pregnant women are at especially high risk of the development of complications of H1N1 influenza A. This increased risk is related to several physiological changes during pregnancy including alterations in the cardiovascular, respiratory, and immune systems. The serious illness and hospitalization rates of women with influenza during pregnancy have a 4- to 5-fold increase compared to nonpregnant women [2, 5–8]. Qi et al. (2014) stated that pregnant women are particularly susceptible to severe complications from influenza and have a greater mortality risk.

Influenza A infection is diagnosed by obtaining an upper respiratory specimen (nasopharyngeal swab, nasal aspirate, or a combined nasopharyngeal swab with oropharyngeal swab or throat swab) to test for novel influenza A (H1N1) virus. The specimen should be placed into sterile viral transport media and immediately placed on ice or cold packs or at 4°C (refrigerator) for transport to the laboratory and the virus is identified by real-time polymerase chain reaction (RT-PCR) or viral culture method [9, 10].

2. Case Presentation

A 26-year-old female, period of gestation of 35 weeks and 6 days into her third pregnancy, presented with contraction pain which was increased in intensity and frequency. She denied any leaking liquor nor show. Fetal movements were well felt. She claimed that she had fever, headache, sore throat, and dry cough for one-day duration. She denied any travelling or any contact with live poultry. She also had no history of dysuria and frequency. Her booking visit was at 9th week of gestation and all routine antenatal tests were negative. Latest scan was done at 33-week follow-up and all parameters were corresponding to gestational age.

On physical examination, she appeared alert, conscious, with no tachypnea and no signs of dehydration. She was afebrile, with no cervical lymph nodes and tonsillar enlargement. The lungs were clear. She had tachycardia up to 110/min and blood pressure was 105/57 mmHg. The abdominal findings corresponded to gestational age, single fetus, longitudinal lie, and cephalic presentation with good fetal heart rate. The estimated fetal weight was 2 to 2.2 kg. The vaginal examination noted that os was closed. The ultrasound examination was repeated and it corresponded to respective gestation. The urine dip stick was suggestive of urinary tract infection. The urine specimen was sent for culture and sensitivity (C&S) before starting the antibiotics.

She was observed in the maternity ward. However, the patient was noted to be febrile with temperature of 39°C, tachycardia, and low blood pressure 80/50mmHg on next day leading to septic shock. Her blood pressure was maintained by intravenous noradrenaline infusion. A septic workup was done and initial resuscitative measures were performed. The blood test results came back with white cell count of 15.34 x 10^9/L and C-reactive protein level of 365mg/L. She went into active phase of labour at the same time.

Multidisciplinary input from anaesthetist for ICU backup, physician, and infectious disease teams was obtained, led by obstetric consultant shared care. The arterial blood gas showed metabolic acidosis. Her condition worsened as she became restless and breathless even with 2L/min oxygen under nasal prong. Four hours in labour, it was noted that the progress of labour was unsatisfactory with features of fetal distress. A decision was made to deliver by caesarean section in collaboration with anaesthetist and ICU team. An alive, female, 2.61 kg baby with Apgar score of 5 in 1 minute, 7 in 5 minutes and 8 in 10 minutes, was delivered and estimated blood loss was about 700 ml. A placental swab was taken for C & S. The anaesthetist noted on lungs auscultation that air entry at the left lower zone and a portable chest X- ray was ordered. The chest X-ray was reported as slight basal lobe collapse at left lobe with reactive pleural effusion (Figures 1 and 2). Tamiflu was started and she was diagnosed with Acute Respiratory Distress Syndrome (ARDS). The baby was admitted to the nursery for late prematurity with presumed sepsis. Antibiotic treatment was given. The placenta swab culture result came back as sterile; still the baby needed photo therapy as neonatal jaundice arose.

The patient was extubated after one day but continued support with Venturi mask 50% and 1.5L/min of oxygen. Once stable, she was transferred to High Dependency Unit and continued monitoring there. The throat swab was reported as influenza A positive and the message was relayed to both Infectious Diseases and Paediatric team. The recommendation was to continue tablet Tamiflu (oseltamivir

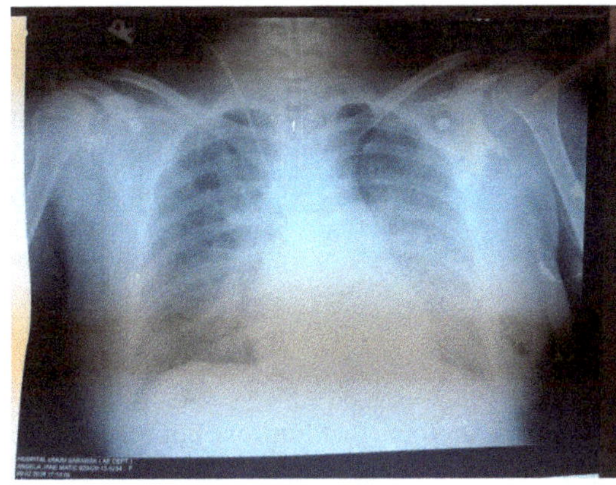

FIGURE 1

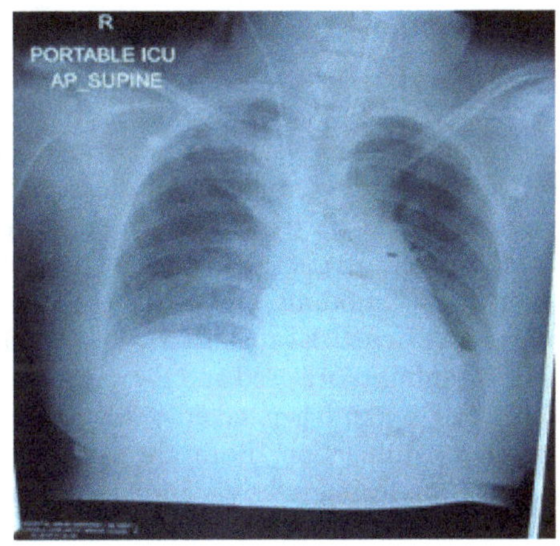

FIGURE 2

phosphate) for one week. Universal precaution and isolation of the patient were followed. The symptoms subsided with the treatment. The patient and baby were discharged on the fifth day postoperatively without complications.

3. Discussion

The patient presented with a seasonal flu; however, her conditions deteriorated quickly into septic shock with ARDS. Despite this, early awareness of the serious symptoms and a multidisciplinary team approach with appropriate and aggressive treatment resulted in favourable outcome for both mother and baby. Unfortunately, the subtyping of influenza A was not able to be carried out as our center lacked such facility. However, it did not change the management and its good outcome.

There are warning signs which should alert the clinicians to the diagnosis of an influenza A infection. Early recognition of warning signs will lead to timely treatment and a better prognosis.

Warning signs for the clinician are as follows:

(i) Difficulty breathing or shortness of breath

(ii) Pain or pressure in the chest or abdomen

(iii) Sudden dizziness

Table 1

Drug	Treatment	Chemoprophylaxis
Oseltamivir	75 mg twice a day for 5 days	75 mg once a day for 10 days
Zanamivir	5 mg inhalations twice per day for 5 days	5 mg inhalations daily for 10 days
Peramivir	One time intravenously over 15-30 mins	

From http://www.cdc.gov/hlnlflu/recommendation/html [12].

(iv) Confusion

(v) Severe or persistent vomiting

(vi) Flu-like symptoms that improve but then return with fever and worsening cough

(From flu symptoms: https://www.cdc.gov/flu/takingcare.html [11].)

4. Antiviral Medication

Pregnancy is a physiological state of relative immunosuppression and all pregnant women should be assumed to be at high risk and should be treated if the potential benefit outweighs the theoretical risk of the fetus. Antiviral drugs will help to relieve symptoms and reduce viral shedding, but therapy is more beneficial if started within 12-48 hours. Neuraminidase inhibitors are used and they are as an adjunct to immunization. Oseltamivir is taken orally and zanamivir is administered via inhalation. Both are category C drugs but oseltamivir is preferred over zanamivir due to its well-evidenced results from clinical experience with a guaranteed systemic absorption [9, 10]. See Table 1.

5. Isolation

The patients should continue to practice good hand hygiene and cough etiquette and wear a face mask for the next 7 days. The patients with suspected N1H1 should wear a face mask and be placed in an isolated room away from providers and other hospitalized patients [9]. Surveillance on the appearance of new symptoms as well as progress of current condition is necessary during isolation period.

6. Breastfeeding

Breastfeeding is encouraged in H1N1 influenza although H1N1 transmission through breast milk is unknown; breastfeeding strengthens the neonatal immune response and infants who are bottle fed may be prone to getting a viral infection [13]. If the infant needs to be isolated from the infected mother, the infant should receive bottle feedings of expressed breast milk until the mother and infant can be reunited. The patients should use a facemask and practice strict hand hygiene and cough etiquette [9, 10].

7. Immunization

Immunization is recommended to pregnant women especially during flu season (November–March). They are low-cost interventions that have been shown to have substantial benefits for both mother and baby [14, 15].

8. Life Style Changes

Personal hygiene is important in preventing transmission of viral influenza. Measures such as hand hygiene and wearing a face mask or N95 disposable respirator during close contact with a sick individual should be advised to patients and relatives. Household members should be monitored for influenza-like symptoms and should be advised to contact their healthcare provider if symptoms occur [16].

9. Conclusion

Pregnant women are at high risk of infection with the H1N1 influenza A virus at high risk of spontaneous miscarriage and associated neural tube defects, neonatal seizures, encephalopathy, cerebral palsy, and neonatal death [17–19]. The influenza A virus infection is difficult to be diagnosed clinically because the presenting symptoms of an influenza infection are similar to those of the common cold but they are more severe and protracted and can potentially be life-threatening. Therefore, early recognition and awareness of warning signs with appropriate, timely treatment, and multidisciplinary support matter to achieve the best outcome.

Abbreviations

AIV: Avian influenza virus
ARDS: Adult respiratory distress syndrome
CDC: Centers for Disease Control
C& S: Culture and sensitivity
CTG: Cardiotocogram
ICU: Intensive care unit
ID: Infectious disease
LSCS: Lower segment caesarean section
O&G: Obstetrics and gynecology
RT-PCR: Real-time polymerase chain reaction
US: United States
WHO: World Health Organization.

Consent

Written informed consent was obtained from the patient for publication of this case report and any accompanying images.

Acknowledgments

We would like to thank the Head of Department of Obstetrics

and Gynecology, Director of Sarawak General Hospital, and Director General of Ministry of Health for the approval to publish this case report in a medical journal.

References

[1] G. Neumann, T. Noda, and Y. Kawaoka, "Emergence and pandemic potential of swine-origin H1N1 influenza virus," *Nature*, vol. 459, no. 7249, pp. 931–939, 2009.

[2] F. S. Dawood, S. Jain, L. Finelli et al., "Emergence of a novel swine-origin influenza A (H1N1) virus in humans," *The New England Journal of Medicine*, vol. 360, no. 25, pp. 2605–2615, 2009.

[3] Centers for Disease Control and Prevention, *Pregnant Women and Novel Influenza A (H1N1) Considerations for Clinicians*, The Centers, Atlanta, GA, USA, 2009.

[4] Z. Hashim and S. S. Arshad, "Avian influenza outbreaks in Malaysia, 1980–2017," *Asia Pacific Environmental and Occupational Health Journal*, vol. 12, no. 3, p. 2, 2017.

[5] D. J. Jamieson, M. A. Honein, S. A. Rasmussen et al., "H1N1 2009 influenza virus infection during pregnancy in the USA," *The Lancet*, vol. 374, no. 9688, pp. 451–458, 2009.

[6] S. A. Rasmussen, D. J. Jamieson, and J. S. Bresee, "Pandemic influenza and pregnant women," *Emerging Infectious Diseases*, vol. 14, no. 1, pp. 95–100, 2008.

[7] T. Teke, Ü. Duran, E. Maden, K. Gezginç, M. D. Yavşan, and K. Uzun, "A pregnant case with severe influenza a (H1N1) virus infection-related ARDS," *European Journal of General Medicine*, vol. 8, no. 2, pp. 163–167, 2011.

[8] C. Hüzmeli, M. Saglam, A. Arıkan, B. Doner, G. Akıncı, and F. Candan, "Infrarenal aorta thrombosis associated with H1N1 influenza A virus infection," *Case Reports in Infectious Diseases*, vol. 2016, Article ID 9567495, 3 pages, 2016.

[9] K. Trevennec, V. Grosbois, F. Roger, T. H. Ho, C. Berthouly-Salazar, and V. Chevalier, "Evidence for freedom from swine influenza in a remote area of Northern Vietnam," *Acta Tropica*, vol. 122, no. 1, pp. 160–163, 2012.

[10] Centers for Disease Control and Prevention (CDC), "Interim guidance on antiviral recommendations for patients with novel influenza A (H1N1) virus infection and their close contacts," http://www.cdc.gov/h1n1flu/recommendations.htm, 2009.

[11] https://www.cdc.gov/flu/takingcare.html.

[12] http://www.cdc.gov/h1n1flu/recommendation/html.

[13] Centers for Disease Control and Prevention, "Pregnant women and novel influenza A (H1N1): considerations for clinicians," http://www.cdc.gov/h1n1flu/clinician_pregnant.htm, 2009.

[14] Centers for Disease Control and Prevention, "Considerations regarding novel H1N1 flu virus in obstetric settings," 2009.

[15] K. Q. Chen, E. H. Hayles, and J. Sinn, "Flu-like symptoms in pregnancy - A case study," *Australian Family Physician*, vol. 45, no. 5, pp. 307-308, 2016.

[16] Centers for Disease Control and Prevention, "Interim guidance on specimen collection, processing, and testing for patients with suspected swine-origin influenza A (H1N1) virus infection," http://www.cdc.gov/h1n1flu/specimencollection.htm, 2009.

[17] Centers for Disease Control and Prevention, "Interim recommendations for facemask and respirator use to reduce novel Influenza A (H1N1) virus transmission. Centers for Disease Control and Prevention, US Department of Health and Human Services, Public Health Service, Tuberculosis Control Division, Atlanta," http://www.cdc.gov/h1n1flu/masks.htm (accessed March 15, 2013), 2010.

[18] S. A. Rasmussen, D. J. Jamieson, K. MacFarlane, J. D. Cragan, J. Williams, and Z. Henderson, "Pandemic influenza and pregnant women: Summary of a meeting of experts," *American Journal of Public Health*, vol. 99, no. 2, pp. S248–S254, 2009.

[19] M. Rashid, R. Ara, and N. Akhter, "Novel influenza H1N1 in pregnancy: Report of a diagnosed case in Bangladesh," *Bangladesh Journal of Obstetrics and Gynecology*, vol. 24, no. 2, pp. 75–78, 2009.

52

Calcified Leiomyomata Presenting as Recurrent Pregnancy Loss

Mohammad Marwan Alhalabi[1] **Ameer Kakaje**[1] **and Marwan Alhalabi**[2]

[1]*Faculty of Medicine, Damascus University, Damascus, Syria*
[2]*Department of Reproductive Medicine, Genetics and Embryology, Damascus University, Damascus, Syria*

Correspondence should be addressed to Mohammad Marwan Alhalabi; mouhammadalhalabi@gmail.com

Academic Editor: Mehmet A. Osmana ao lu

Recurrent spontaneous abortion (RSA) is a problem that faces women for a variety of reasons. Although leiomyomata is relatively common, calcified leiomyomata which is called "womb stones" is a very rare cause of RSA. These womb stones are correlated with retained products from conception and osseous metaplasia. We report a very rare case of a large calcified leiomyomata which caused secondary infertility and pregnancy loss of 7 pregnancies due to spontaneous abortions.

1. Introduction

Recurrent spontaneous abortion (RSA) occurs in approximately 1% of females in the reproductive age and is of a wide variety in nomenclature (recurrent pregnancy loss, recurrent miscarriage) [1]. RSA is defined as two or more of pregnancy losses according to the American Society for Reproductive Medicine (ASRM) [2].

Calcification in the endometrium of the uterus is not very common in infertility cases, and it has a correlation with the products retained from conception and with osseous metaplasia. Ultrasonography is the most reliable method of diagnosis for endometrial calcifications [3]. Infertility and recurrent abortion are uncommonly caused by the calcific endometritis [4]. The existence of bone-like tissue within the uterine cavity is called endometrial osseous metaplasia and affects about 0.15% of the patients referred to obstetrics and gynecology clinics [5].

The term "womb stones" refers to calcified appearance of leiomyomata in radiological imaging [6–8]; such osseous endometrial metaplasia is also of a wide nomenclature (uterine bone, womb stones, and calcified fibroid) [4, 9, 10]. We present herein a case of a large calcified leiomyomata (womb stone) suspected to be the cause of secondary infertility and idiopathic pregnancy loss of 7 consecutive spontaneous abortions.

2. Case Report

A married couple presented to our fertility clinic complaining of recurrent pregnancy loss for ten years. The wife was 32 years old and had pregnancy loss for seven times occurring in the second trimester in each pregnancy with the last one being a year from the date of the clinic visit. In each pregnancy, her pregnancies were monitored by an obstetrician and the loss of pregnancy was verified by ultrasonography in each case. There was no history of primary infertility or any delay of conception. Menstrual cycles were regular with no dysmenorrhea or any other symptoms. Gynecological physical examination was unremarkable, and the uterus was normal in size, contour, and no tenderness was noted. It was also anteverted and anteflexed, all adnexae were normal, and hormonal and chemical parameters were also within normal range. The medical history was otherwise unremarkable. She had a surgical history of dilation and curettage (D&C) and an open ovarian cystectomy. An abdominal ultrasonography was conducted and showed a normal anatomy of the uterus with subendometrial calcifications in the frontal wall of the uterus, spanning 2 cm in diameter (Figure 1).

A later abdominal ultrasonography showed normal ovulation with both ovaries showing as normal in bulk, echotexture, and follicle maturation, and the calcified endometrium

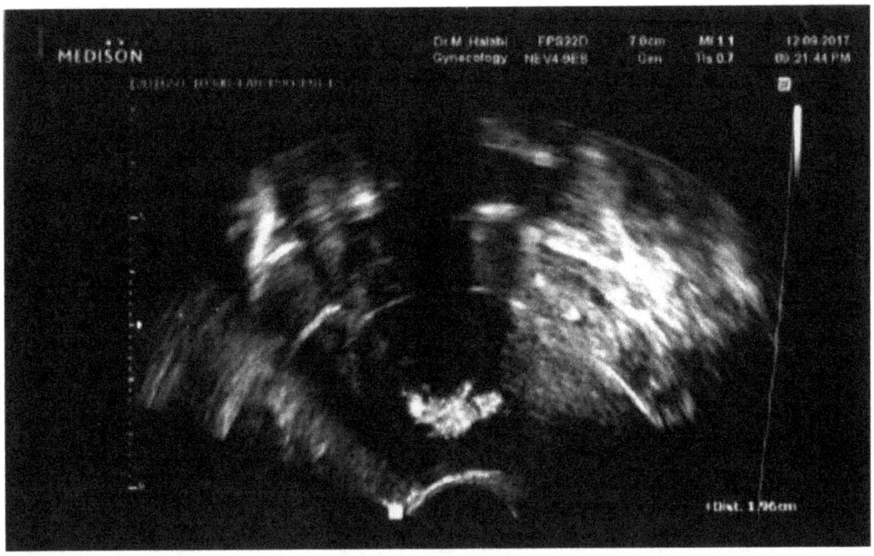

FIGURE 1: View of the uterus during abdominal ultrasonography.

was also seen. The patient underwent hysterosalpingogram which showed partial obstruction of the fallopian tubes. The patient was referred to conduct hysteroscopy for diagnosis and treatment. Hysteroscopy showed a large calcification with multiple calcific protrusions in the endometrium (Figure 2), and it was removed (Figure 3), and everything else was within normal limits. The calcification was sent to pathological analysis which concluded a leiomyoma with calcifications and no malignancy (Figures 4 and 5).

3. Discussion

Endometrial calcification is an uncommon finding, and the presence of uterine bone tissue has been reported in several reports in the past years [11–23], and the affected couples may have already suffered great emotional trauma and stress. One frequently mentioned theory about the formation of uterine bones is the fetal bone retention after miscarriage or pregnancy termination [11, 12, 16, 24–28], but this requires at least one previous 12-week-long pregnancy having the embryo reach endochondral ossification [11, 15, 24]. It was reported that osseous metaplasia usually presents itself as diffuse, sporadic ossification in the uterine endometrium without a reaction in the tissues around a retained fetus [13, 24]. Osseous metaplasia is also associated with uterine bone formation and is correlated with chronic inflammation and destruction of endometrial tissue which can cause endometrial stromal cell heteroplasia into bony tissue [13–15, 24]. Furthermore, chronic endometritis causes superoxides and tumor necrosis factor to be released, and the exposure in the long term negatively affects stromal cells especially in patients with superoxide dismutase deficiency [14]. Another theory suggests that there are retained embryonic cells without a previous pregnancy which underwent heteroplasia into bony tissue; this theory can also explain the presence of womb stone [29]. Although in our study the patient did not complain of secondary infertility, the patient complained of recurrent pregnancy loss of all previous pregnancies, and therefore, the uterine bone was not suspected to be caused by fetal bone retention and was more suspected to be caused by the theory of endometrial fibroid calcifying metaplasia, and the pathological report of the specimen obtained concluded the specimen to be a calcified endometrial leiomyoma.

Calcific endometritis has also been correlated with Asherman's syndrome [4, 9]. However, in our patient, despite having a history of D&C, the patient did not complain of any of the symptoms of endometritis or Asherman's syndrome.

Calcification of the endometrium has also been reported without a history of an intrauterine device (IUD) or malignancy [9, 10]. Osseous metaplasia of the endometrium is less commonly reported than uterine bone [4, 9, 10], and only few cases reported spontaneous abortion to be related to endometrial ossification [21]. ****Endometrial ossification was described to cause many gynecological disturbances such as symptoms of menorrhagia, metromenorrhagia, abnormal vaginal discharge, pain in the pelvis, and bone fragments passing through the vagina spontaneously [3, 12, 13, 16, 22–28]. Several cases reported that normal conception was achieved after repeat curettage or hysteroscopy of the uterine endometrium which led to removal of the ossification of the endometrium [3, 12, 13, 21–23, 25, 28], so we speculate that endometrial bone does permit the implantation of the embryo but prevents pregnancy from being sustained. It was also reported that uterine bone can act as an intrauterine contraceptive device causing failure of implantation [12]. It has been indicated by almost all previous publications that abnormal endometrial tissue has been handled by surgical removal [3, 11–14, 17, 19, 22–26, 30–33]. The removal of abnormal endometrial tissue either by D&C or hysteroscopy has also been reported in order to treat intrauterine adhesions through metroplasty and resection of submucous fibroids, therefore resolving problems relating to infertility and recurrent pregnancy loss [3, 12–14, 22, 23, 25, 28, 31, 32].

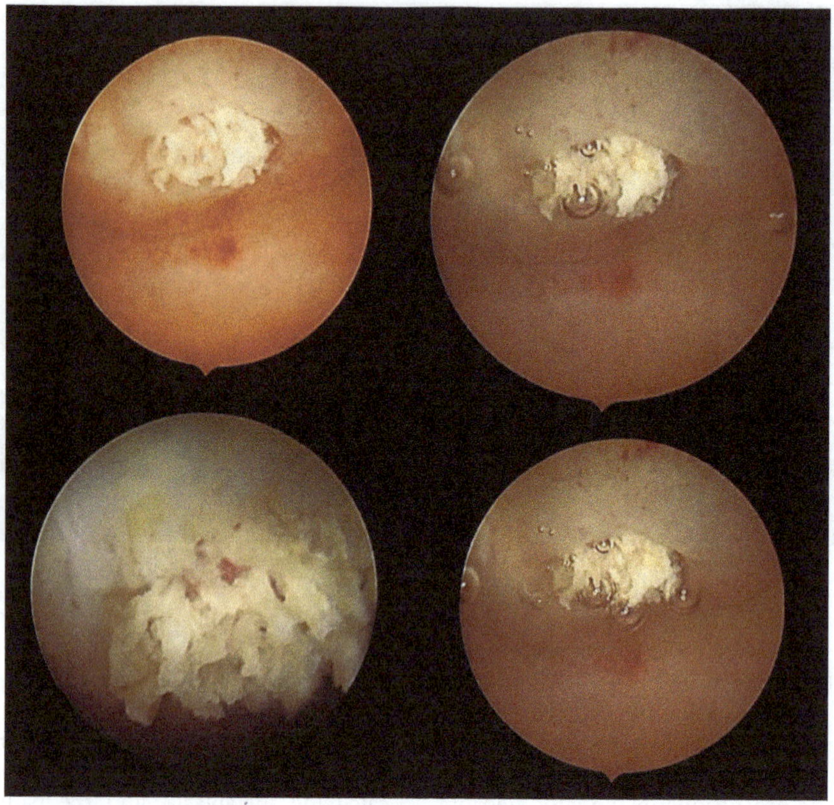

FIGURE 2: The large calcification shown during hysteroscopy.

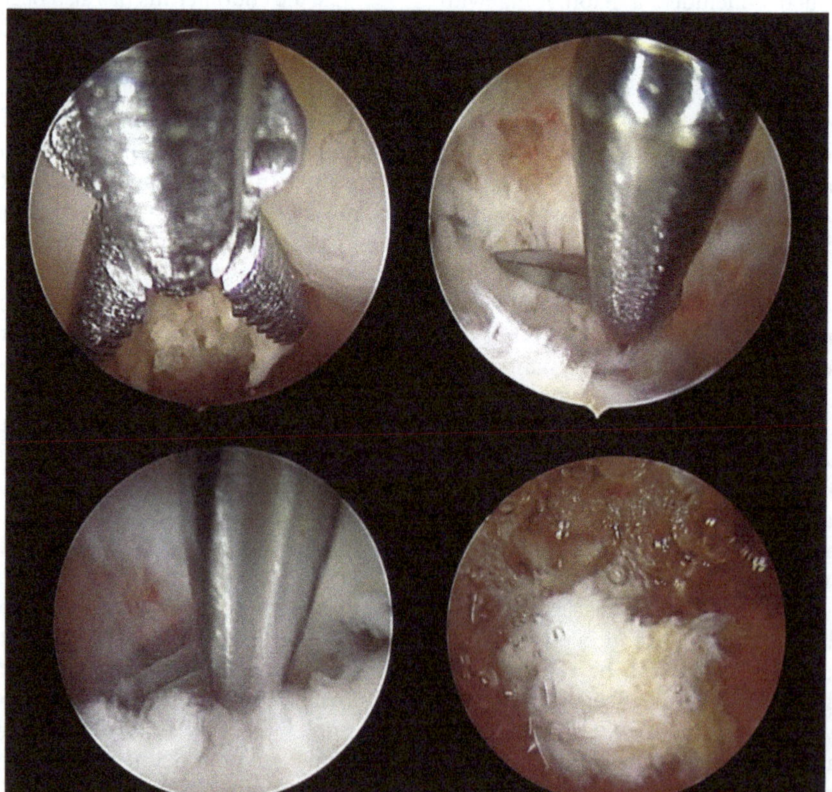

FIGURE 3: Showing the removal of the uterine bone through hysteroscopy.

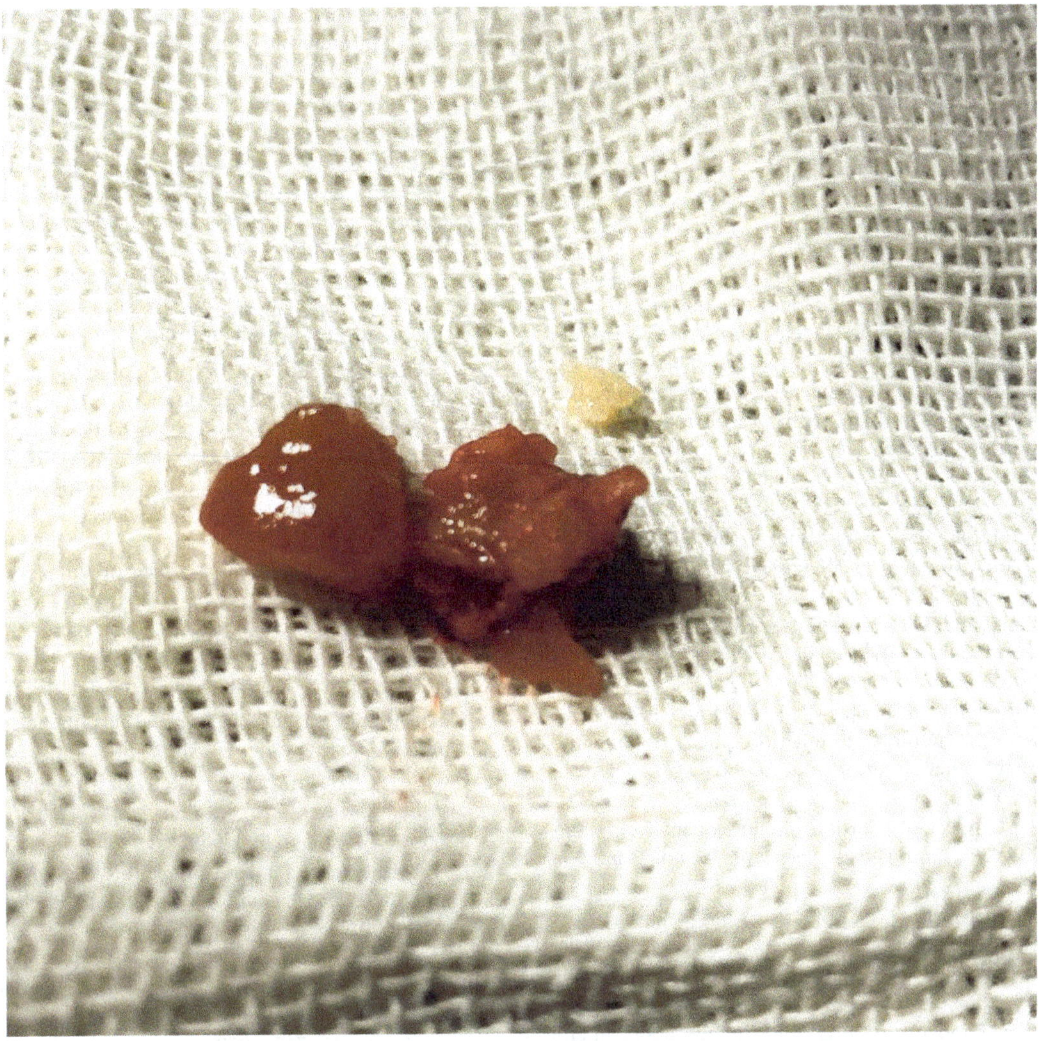

FIGURE 4: The gross view of the large calcification after removal.

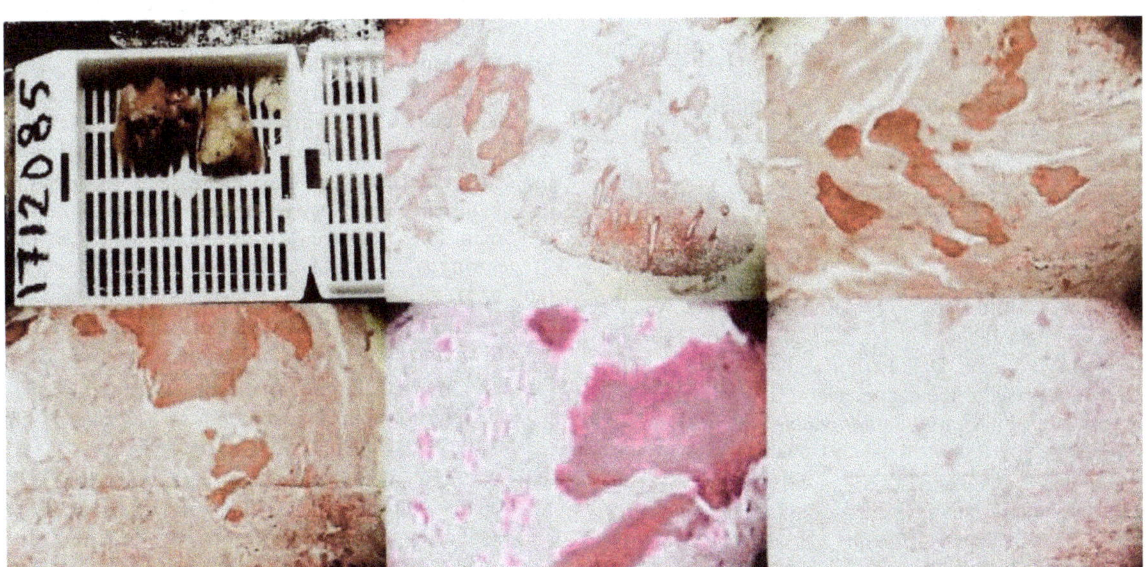

FIGURE 5: The microscopic pathological view of the calcification.

Consent

Informed consent was taken for this research. Consent for using and publishing the data was taken before participating in the research.

References

[1] E. Jauniaux, R. G. Farquharson, O. B. Christiansen, and N. Exalto, "Evidence-based guidelines for the investigation and medical treatment of recurrent miscarriage," *Human Reproduction*, vol. 21, no. 9, pp. 2216–2222, 2006.

[2] Practice Committee of the American Society for Reproductive Medicine, "Evaluation and treatment of recurrent pregnancy loss: a committee opinion," *Fertility and Sterility*, vol. 98, no. 5, pp. 1103–1111, 2012.

[3] S. F. Marcus, J. Bhattacharya, G. Williams, P. Brinsden, and J. Hamou, "Endometrial ossification: a cause of secondary infertility," *American Journal of Obstetrics and Gynecology*, vol. 170, no. 5, pp. 1381–1383, 1994.

[4] D. R. Herbold and D. M. Magrane, "Calcifications of the benign endometrium," *Archives of Pathology & Laboratory Medicine*, vol. 110, no. 7, pp. 666–669, 1986.

[5] R. C. M. Parente, V. d. Freitas, R. S. d. Moura Neto et al., "Metaplasia óssea endometrial: quadro clínico e seguimento após tratamento," *Revista Brasileira de Ginecologia e Obstetrícia*, vol. 32, no. 1, pp. 33–38, 2010.

[6] C. J. Hogue, "Impact of abortion on subsequent fecundity," *Clinics in Obstetrics and Gynaecology*, vol. 13, no. 1, pp. 95–103, 1986.

[7] S. Lurie, R. Levy, Z. Katz, Z. Appelman, and V. Insler, "The influence of midtrimester termination of pregnancy on subsequent fertility: four to five years follow-up," *Contraception*, vol. 50, no. 3, pp. 239–241, 1994.

[8] S. Lurie and Z. Shoham, "Induced midtrimester abortion and future fertility-where are we today?," *International journal of fertility and menopausal studies*, vol. 40, no. 6, pp. 311–315, 1995.

[9] V. G. Untawale, J. B. Gabriel Jr., and P. M. Chauhan, "Calcific endometritis," *American Journal of Obstetrics and Gynecology*, vol. 144, no. 4, pp. 482-483, 1982.

[10] J. F. Valicenti Jr. and S. K. Priester, "Psammoma bodies of benign endometrial origin in cervicovaginal cytology," *Acta Cytologica*, vol. 21, no. 4, pp. 550–552, 1977.

[11] M. Chanda and S. Power, "Womb stones a case report and literature review," *Journal SOGC*, vol. 21, no. 7, pp. 692–697, 1999.

[12] Y. F. Dajani and S. M. Khalaf, "Intrauterine bone contraceptive device: an accident of nature," *Fertility and Sterility*, vol. 43, no. 1, pp. 149-150, 1985.

[13] U. Acharya, S. B. Pinion, D. E. Parkin, and M. P. R. Hamilton, "Osseous metaplasia of the endometrium treated by hysteroscopic resection," *BJOG: An International Journal of Obstetrics & Gynaecology*, vol. 100, no. 4, pp. 391-392, 1993.

[14] M. Bahceci and L. C. Demirel, "Case report: Osseous metaplasia of the endometrium: a rare cause of infertility and its hysteroscopic management," *Human Reproduction*, vol. 11, no. 11, pp. 2537–2539, 1996.

[15] N. N. Bhatia and M. G. Hoshiko, "Uterine osseous metaplasia," *Obstetrics & Gynecology*, vol. 60, no. 2, pp. 256–259, 1982.

[16] F. A. Melius, T. M. Julian, and T. C. Nagel, "Prolonged retention of intrauterine bones," *Obstetrics & Gynecology*, vol. 78, 5 Part 2, pp. 919–921, 1991.

[17] C. Hsu, "Endometrial ossification," *British Journal of Obstetrics and Gynaecology*, vol. 82, no. 10, pp. 836–839, 1975.

[18] C. P. Shroff, N. G. Kudterkar, and V. R. Badhwar, "Endometrial ossification–report of three cases with literature review," *Indian Journal of Pathology & Microbiology*, vol. 28, no. 1, pp. 71–74, 1985.

[19] F. R. Bellingham, "Endometrial bone formation," *Australian and New Zealand Journal of Obstetrics and Gynaecology*, vol. 36, no. 1, pp. 109-110, 1996.

[20] L. Ceccacci and G. Clancy, "Endometrial ossification: Report of an additional case," *American Journal of Obstetrics and Gynecology*, vol. 141, no. 1, pp. 102-103, 1981.

[21] S. Degani, R. Gonen, K. d. Vries, and M. Sharf, "Endometrial Ossification Associated with Repeated Abortions," *Acta Obstetricia et Gynecologica Scandinavica*, vol. 62, no. 3, pp. 281-282, 1983.

[22] S. Dutt, "ENDOMETRIAL OSSIFICATION ASSOCIATED WITH SECONDARY INFERTILITY. CASE REPORT," *BJOG: An International Journal of Obstetrics and Gynaecology*, vol. 85, no. 10, pp. 787–789, 1978.

[23] P. J. Taylor, J. Hamou, and L. Mencaglia, "Hysteroscopic detection of heterotopic intrauterine bone formation," *Journal of Reproductive Medicine*, vol. 33, no. 4, pp. 337–339, 1988.

[24] N. S. T. Chan, "Intrauterine Retention of Fetal Bone," *The Australian and New Zealand Journal of Obstetrics and Gynaecology*, vol. 36, no. 3, pp. 368–371, 1996.

[25] F. A. Chervenak, H. K. Amin, and R. S. Neuwirth, "Symptomatic intrauterine retention of fetal bones," *Obstetrics & Gynecology*, vol. 59, 6 Suppl, pp. 58S–61S, 1982.

[26] M. Y. Dawood and J. C. Jarrett II, "Prolonged intrauterine retention of fetal bones after abortion causing infertility," *American Journal of Obstetrics and Gynecology*, vol. 143, no. 6, pp. 715–717, 1982.

[27] V. Lewis, F. Khan-Dawood, M. King, C. Beckmann, and M. Y. Dawood, "Retention of intrauterine fetal bone increases menstrual prostaglandins," *Obstetrics & Gynecology*, vol. 75, no. 3, pp. 561–563, 1990.

[28] H. S. Moon, Y. H. Park, H. Y. Kwon, S. H. Hong, and S. K. Kim, "Iatrogenic secondary infertility caused by residual intrauterine fetal bone after midtrimester abortion," *American Journal of Obstetrics and Gynecology*, vol. 176, no. 2, pp. 369-370, 1997.

[29] W. G. McCluggage, "Benign diseases of the endometrium," in *Blaustein's Pathology of the Female Genital Tract*, R. J. Kurman, L. H. Ellenson, and B. M. Ronnett, Eds., pp. 305–358, Springer, Boston, MA, 2011.

[30] B. D. Rodriguez and G. D. Adamson, "Hysteroscopic treatment of ectopic intrauterine bone. A case report," *Journal of Reproductive Medicine*, vol. 38, no. 7, pp. 515–520, 1993.

[31] W. Ombelet, "Endometrial ossification, an unusual finding in an infertility clinic. A case report," *Journal of Reproductive Medicine*, vol. 34, no. 4, pp. 303–306, 1989.

[32] V. Niccoli, C. Carillo, M. T. Caruso, A. Lippa, and L. Serrao, "Clinical-diagnostic considerations of a case of endometrial ossification as a cause of secondary infertility," *Minerva ginecologica*, vol. 49, no. 6, pp. 289–291, 1997.

[33] E. Roth and H. B. Taylor, "Heterotopic cartilage in the uterus," *Obstetrics & Gynecology*, vol. 27, no. 6, pp. 838–844, 1966.

A Rare Cause of Hypovolemic Shock in Prepubertal Girl: Vaginal Leech Infestation

W. Lahmini,[1] M. Bourrous,[1] and K. Harou[2]

[1]*Department of Paediatric Emergency, UHC Mohamed VI, Cadi Ayyad University, Marrakech, Morocco*
[2]*Department of Gynaecology and Obstetrics, UHC Mohamed VI, Cadi Ayyad University, Marrakech, Morocco*

Correspondence should be addressed to M. Bourrous; mounirbourrous@yahoo.fr

Academic Editor: Vorapong Phupong

Vaginal bleeding in girls is an alarming symptom for both parents and pediatricians. Serious underlying causes should be always evoked. *Case Report.* We describe here a 9-year-old girl who was admitted at our emergency department for vaginal bleeding and severe anemia. No history of trauma and no evidence of prior abuse were reported by the parents. Full Blood Count showed profound anemia (hemoglobin at 4 g/dl). The child was managed as a hypovolemic shock and resuscitated with intravenous fluids and urgent blood transfusion. Gynecologic examination found a live leech at the vulva and the extraction was facilitated by applying a saline solution. The child was clinically stable and discharged home the next day with ambulatory treatment. *Conclusion.* This case emphasizes that a through external genital exam with possible exam under anesthesia should be undertaken in all girls with unexplained vaginal bleeding and that in those living in rural areas without potable water, leech infection should be considered.

1. Introduction

Vaginal bleeding in girls is an alarming symptom for both parents and pediatricians. Serious underlying causes should be always evoked. The etiology of vaginal bleeding in young girls varies widely from sexual abuse, vulvovaginal infections, trauma, foreign bodies, urethral prolapse, precocious puberty, malignant tumors, and idiopathic bleeding [1]. Although there have been a few rare cases of vaginal bleeding due to leech infestation, this has never been reported in Morocco. We describe here the case of a girl admitted at the emergency department with a life-threatening hypovolemic shock secondary to vaginal bleeding. The physical examination revealed the presence of a leech in the vulva.

2. Case Report

A 9-year-old girl was admitted at our paediatric emergency department for vaginal bleeding spanning 10 days and severe anemia. She was initially treated by a general practitioner with oral antibiotics as a vulvovaginitis. Abdominal and pelvic ultrasound scan was normal. But, due to the persistence of vaginal bleeding and worsening of her condition, she was referred to the paediatric emergency department. No history of trauma and no evidence of abuse were reported by the parents. She had no bleeding from other areas of the body. She was acutely sick and had pale teguments. Her physical examination was as follows: temperature: 36,5°C, thready pulse and tachycardia (pulse rate:120/min), blood pressure: 70/40 in millimeters of mercury, respiratory rate: 28 breaths per minute, and oxygen saturation: 90% in room air. Full Blood Count showed profound anemia (hemoglobin at 4 g/dl). Biochemistry and coagulation parameters were normal. The child was managed as a hypovolemic shock and resuscitated with intravenous fluids and urgent blood transfusion. Gynecological examination found a live leech at the vulva on the fourchette; its extraction was facilitated by applying a saline solution (Figure 1). We interrogated the mother for a second time, and she revealed that the symptomatology appeared after a long day of swimming in a pond. The evolution saw a spectacular improvement and a stop to the bleeding. The child was clinically stable and discharged home the next day with ambulatory treatment.

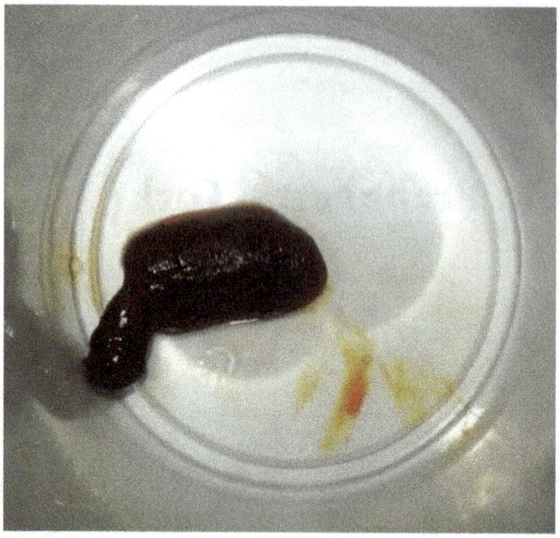

FIGURE 1: Live leech after its vulva extraction.

3. Discussion

Leeches are invertebrates of phylum Annelida and class Hirudinea. Their size varies from about 5 mm to nearly 45 cm. Leeches are found in rivers and ponds in tropical and subtropical regions. The leech has an oral sucker as a mouth and a caudal sucker for movement [2, 3]. Leeches can suck and store blood up to ten times its body size. The continuous bleeding after a leech bite is a result of the action of substances in the leech's saliva. Hirudin, a thrombin inhibitor, is an important enzyme, converting fibrinogen to fibrin in the coagulation cascade. It is secreted onto the wound and inhibits the coagulation of the sucked blood [4, 5]. Calin inhibits the platelet aggregation induced by collagen. In addition, calin has been shown to inhibit platelet adhesion [2, 5]. The coagulation profile in Kose et al. [6] case was disrupted (prothrombin time, international normalized ratio, and partial thromboplastin extremely increased). Cutaneous leech infestation is commonly encountered in children in tropical countries [2]. Human leech infestation is a disease of the rural areas where untreated water is used for drinking or swimming. Leech bites on various body sites including body orifices and internal body cavities with potentially life-threatening consequences. These include nasal cavity, pharynx, esophagus, larynx, trachea, bronchus, vagina, uterus, rectum, and urinary bladder [2, 7]. The mucosa of the lower genital tract can be infested by leeches when females use contaminated water for bathing.

The morbidity associated with a leech bite is mainly due to 2 factors: mechanical obstruction of a vital organ and/or persistent hemorrhage leading to severe anemia and shock [2, 7]. Complications of leech bites may range from minor bleeding to profound hypovolemic shock [7]. Similar cases have also been reported in adult women as demonstrated *in a case report of a postmenopausal woman* with hypovolemic shock and severe life-threatening anemia due to continuous vaginal bleeding that revealed vaginal leech infestation [8]. The authors recommend that the possibility of vaginal leech infestation must be considered in postmenopausal woman who use river water for bathing and present with vaginal bleeding. In this case reported in Morocco, the girl had profound life-threatening anemia with hypovolemic shock that needed emergency management and transfusion with compatible blood.

Although there have been a few rare cases of vaginal bleeding due to leech infestation especially in *tropical* areas [2, 7, 9, 10], this has never been reported in Morocco. Review of the literature reveals that most girls present with vaginal bleeding after swimming in local bodies of water and that the vaginal wall and the vulva were the most common sites of leech bite [7]. The girl described here in Morocco had also a long bath in a pond and the vulva was the site of leech bite. Saha reported a very rare case report of an intraperitoneal leech in a 2-year-old girl, which entered through vagina, perforated the uterus, and got into the peritoneal cavity [10].

Diagnosis of a leech bite can be made simply with the patient's history and clinical examination. This allays the anxiety of parents and reduces unnecessary investigations [2, 3, 11]. In contrast to recommendations, a large study of 86 girls found that genital examination was not performed in all cases of vaginal bleeding. The authors attributed this to the lack of knowledge among physicians to manage vaginal bleeding in prepubertal girls [1]. The same finding was noticed in our observation: the genital exam was insufficient and the patient was treated as a vulvovaginitis, without any improvement. This eventually led to the development of a severe life-threatening anemia. In most of the cases, the leech's removal can be facilitated by applying a saline solution. This is widely used in literature. Its removal by surgical forceps has also been reported [2, 7]. But, the leech should not be forcibly removed because its jaws may remain in the wound, causing continuous bleeding and infection [2, 7]. The leech, in our case, was simply dislodged by irrigation with a saline solution.

4. Conclusion

Vaginal leech infestation in girl can cause a life-threatening hypovolemic shock secondary to continuous vaginal bleeding. Thus, in patients presenting vaginal bleeding, it is of utmost importance to take a good history and perform a thorough physical examination.

References

[1] H. F. Söderström, A. Carlsson, A. Börjesson, and M. Elfving, "Vaginal bleeding in prepubertal girls: etiology and clinical management," *Journal of Pediatric & Adolescent Gynecology*, vol. 29, no. 3, pp. 280–285, 2016.

[2] P. K. Saha, S. Roy, D. Bhattacharya, P. Mukherjee, T. Naskar, and A. Bhuiya, "Leech bite: a rare gynecologic emergency," *MedGenMed*, vol. 7, no. 4, p. 73, 2005.

[3] A. Anek and P. Vorapong, "Vaginal bleeding in thai children due to the leech," *The Journal of Tropical Medicine and Parasitology*, vol. 22, pp. 77–79, 1999.

[4] E. Smoot, J. Ruiz-Inchaustegui, and A. Roth, "Mechanical Leech Therapy to Relieve Venous Congestion," *Journal of Reconstructive Microsurgery*, vol. 11, no. 1, pp. 51–55, 1995.

[5] M. D. Wells, R. T. Manktelow, J. Brian Boyd, and V. Bowen, "The medical leech: An old treatment revisited," *Microsurgery*, vol. 14, no. 3, pp. 183–186, 1993.

[6] A. Kose, S. Zengin, B. Kose et al., "Leech bites: massive bleeding, coagulation profile disorders, and severe anemia," *The American Journal of Emergency Medicine*, vol. 26, no. 9, pp. e3–e6, 2008.

[7] A. H. Karunaratne, B. T. Wijerathne, R. S. Wickramasinghe, A. K. Wijesinghe, and A. S. Liyanage, "A rare case of vaginal bleeding in a child due to a leech bite and review of the literature," *Wilderness & Environmental Medicine*, vol. 26, no. 4, pp. 579–584, 2015.

[8] T. Tilahun, "Vaginal leech infestation: a rare cause of hypovolumic shock in postmenopausal woman," *Ethiopian Journal of Health Sciences*, vol. 25, no. 4, pp. 377–380, 2015.

[9] A. Aribarg and V. Phupong, "Vaginal bleeding in young children," *Southeast Asian Journal of Tropical Medicine and Public Health*, vol. 34, no. 1, pp. 208–212, 2003.

[10] M. Saha and S. Nagi, "Intraperitoneal leech: A rare complication of leech bite," *Journal of Indian Association of Pediatric Surgeons*, vol. 16, no. 4, pp. 155–157, 2011.

[11] M. Dwiggins and V. Gomez-Lobo, "Current review of prepubertal vaginal bleeding," *Current Opinion in Obstetrics and Gynecology*, vol. 29, no. 5, pp. 322–327, 2017.

Permissions

All chapters in this book were first published by Hindawi Publishing Corporation; hereby published with permission under the Creative Commons Attribution License or equivalent. Every chapter published in this book has been scrutinized by our experts. Their significance has been extensively debated. The topics covered herein carry significant findings which will fuel the growth of the discipline. They may even be implemented as practical applications or may be referred to as a beginning point for another development.

The contributors of this book come from diverse backgrounds, making this book a truly international effort. This book will bring forth new frontiers with its revolutionizing research information and detailed analysis of the nascent developments around the world.

We would like to thank all the contributing authors for lending their expertise to make the book truly unique. They have played a crucial role in the development of this book. Without their invaluable contributions this book wouldn't have been possible. They have made vital efforts to compile up to date information on the varied aspects of this subject to make this book a valuable addition to the collection of many professionals and students.

This book was conceptualized with the vision of imparting up-to-date information and advanced data in this field. To ensure the same, a matchless editorial board was set up. Every individual on the board went through rigorous rounds of assessment to prove their worth. After which they invested a large part of their time researching and compiling the most relevant data for our readers.

The editorial board has been involved in producing this book since its inception. They have spent rigorous hours researching and exploring the diverse topics which have resulted in the successful publishing of this book. They have passed on their knowledge of decades through this book. To expedite this challenging task, the publisher supported the team at every step. A small team of assistant editors was also appointed to further simplify the editing procedure and attain best results for the readers.

Apart from the editorial board, the designing team has also invested a significant amount of their time in understanding the subject and creating the most relevant covers. They scrutinized every image to scout for the most suitable representation of the subject and create an appropriate cover for the book.

The publishing team has been an ardent support to the editorial, designing and production team. Their endless efforts to recruit the best for this project, has resulted in the accomplishment of this book. They are a veteran in the field of academics and their pool of knowledge is as vast as their experience in printing. Their expertise and guidance has proved useful at every step. Their uncompromising quality standards have made this book an exceptional effort. Their encouragement from time to time has been an inspiration for everyone.

The publisher and the editorial board hope that this book will prove to be a valuable piece of knowledge for researchers, students, practitioners and scholars across the globe.

List of Contributors

P. D. M. Pathiraja
Obstetrics and Gynaecology, Ministry of Health, Sri Lanka

S. K. Ranaraja
Teaching Hospital Peradeniya, Sri Lanka

Sae Yu, Koji Yamanoi, Masumi Sunada, Sachiko Kitamura, Naoki Horikawa, Yoshitsugu Chigusa, Ken Yamaguchi, Akihito Horie, Junzo Hamanishi, Eiji Kondoh and Masaki Mandai
Department of Gynecology and Obstetrics, Graduate School of Medicine, Kyoto University, 54 Shogoinkawahara-cho, Sakyo-ku, Kyoto City, Kyoto, Japan

Sofía Córdoba-Vives
Department of Maternal Fetal Medicine, Rafael Angel Calderón Guardia Hospital, San José, Costa Rica
University of Costa Rica, San José, Costa Rica

Patricia Pérez-Rodríguez
University of Costa Rica, San José, Costa Rica
Department of Obstetrics and Gynecology, Rafael Angel Calderón Guardia Hospital, San José, Costa Rica

Astrid Marín-Delgado and Adriana Arias-González
University of Costa Rica, San José, Costa Rica
Department of Pathology, Rafael Angel Calderón Guardia Hospital, San José, Costa Rica

Miguel Matus-Vargas
University of Costa Rica, San José, Costa Rica

Susana Patrícia Lima Oliveira, Ana Isabel Sousa and Nuno Nogueira Martins
Department of Obstetrics and Gynecology, Centro Hospitalar Tondela-Viseu, Viseu, Portugal

Rawad Halimeh, Marianne Bersaoui and Elie Anastasiadis
Obstetrics and Gynecology Department, Saint George Hospital University Medical Center, Beirut, Lebanon

Serge Tomassian, Maria El Hage and Nicole Metri
Faculty of Medicine and Medical Sciences, University of Balamand, El-Koura, Lebanon

Rafi Daou
Faculty of Medicine, University of London, St. Georges, Nicosia, Cyprus

Mojgan Javedani Masroor and Anna Zarei
Shahid Akbar Abadi Clinical Research Development Unit, School of Medicine, Iran University of Medical Sciences, Tehran, Iran

Hossein Sheibani
Clinical Research Development Unit, Imam Hossein Hospital, Shahroud University of Medical Sciences, Shahroud, Iran

Shadi Rezai, Elise Bardawil and Xiaoming Guan
Division of Minimally Invasive Gynecologic Surgery, Department of Obstetrics and Gynecology, Baylor College of Medicine, 6651 Main Street, 10th Floor, Houston, TX 77030, USA

Richard A. Giovane and Tiffanie Mann
University of Alabama, Department of Family Medicine, 801 Campus Drive, Tuscaloosa, AL 35487, USA

Ninad M. Patil
Department of Pathology & Immunology, Baylor College of Medicine, 6651 Main Street, Suite F0455.10, Houston, TX 77030, USA

Cassandra E. Henderson
Maternal and Fetal Medicine, Department of Obstetrics and Gynecology, Lincoln Medical and Mental Health Center, 234 East 149th Street, Bronx, NY 10451, USA

Natalja Haninger-Vacariu, Sarah El-Hadi, Marina Foretnik, Alice Schmidt and Gere Sunder-Plassmann
Division of Nephrology and Dialysis, Department of Medicine III, Medical University of Vienna, Vienna, Austria

Udo Pauler
Department of Medicine I, University Hospital St. Pölten, Lower Austria, Austria

Renate Kain
Department of Pathology, Medical University of Vienna, Vienna, Austria

Zoltán Prohászka
Semmelweis University, Research Laboratory, Third Department of Internal Medicine, Budapest, Hungary

Nina Skuban and Jay A. Barth
Amicus Therapeutics, Inc., Cranbury, NJ, USA

Priya V. Patel, Recia Frenn and Thaddeus P. Waters
Department of Obstetrics and Gynecology, Loyola University Medical Center, Maywood, IL, USA

Raanan Alter
Department of Gynecology Oncology, University of Chicago, Chicago, IL, USA

Funda Gungor Ugurlucan, Cenk Yasa, Omer Demir, Ozlem Dural and Suleyman Engin Akhan
Istanbul University Istanbul Faculty of Medicine, Department of Obstetrics and Gynecology, Turkey

Ekrem Yavuz
Istanbul University Istanbul Faculty of Medicine, Department of Pathology, Turkey

Guiwen Wang, Hiroshi Ishikawa, Asuka Sato and Makio Shozu
Department of Reproductive Medicine, Graduate School of Medicine, Chiba University, Chiba 260-8670, Japan

Geoffrey D. Towers, Candace Benoit, Rose Maxwell and Jerome Yaklic
Department of Obstetrics and Gynecology, Wright State University Boonshoft School of Medicine, 128 E. Apple Street, Suite 3800 CHE, Dayton, OH 45409, USA

Krystal Koh
Department of Obstetrics and Gynecology, KK Women's and Children's Hospital, Singapore

Devendra Kanagalingam
Department of Obstetrics and Gynecology, Singapore General Hospital, Singapore

Rajeswari Kathirvel
Department of Obstetrics and Gynecology, KK Women's and Children's Hospital, Lee Kong Chian School of Medicine, Duke NUS Medical School and Yong Loo Lin School of Medicine, Singapore

Courtney T. Connolly, Olivia Grubman and Zainab Al-Ibraheemi
Department of Obstetrics, Gynecology and Reproductive Science, Icahn School of Medicine at Mount Sinai, New York City, USA

Tatyana Kushner
Department of Medicine and Liver Disease, Icahn School of Medicine at Mount Sinai, New York City, USA

Melese Gezahegn Tesemma
Arsi University, College of Health Science, Department of Obstetrics & Gynecology, Asella, Ethiopia

A. Jayawardane
Obstetrics and Gynaecology, Faculty of Medicine, University of Colombo, Colombo, Sri Lanka

M. Patabendige
Obstetrician and Gynaecologist, Base Hospital, Mahaoya, Sri Lanka

C. Gunathilaka
National Hospital of Sri Lanka, Colombo, Sri Lanka

Haruka Suzuki, Koji Yamanoi, Jumpei Ogura, Takahiro Hirayama, Koji Yasumoto, Shimpei Shitanaka, Yoshihide Inayama, Mie Sakai, Tsutomu Ohara and Koh Suginami
Department of Obstetrics and Gynecology, Toyooka Public Hospital, 1094, Tobera, Toyooka City, Hyogo 6680065, Japan

Yuki Ito, Taizan Kamide, Akiko Konishi, Hiroshi Kishi, Osamu Samura and Aikou Okamoto
Department of Obstetrics and Gynaecology, The Jikei University School of Medicine, 3-25-8, Nishi-Shinbashi, Minato-ku, Tokyo, Japan 105-8461

Kosuke Taniguchi and Kenichiro Hata
Department of Maternal-Fetal Biology, National Research Institute for Child Health and Development, 2-10-1, Okura, Setagayaku, Tokyo 157-8535, Japan

Taisuke Sato, Michihiro Yamamura and Ken Takahashi
Department of Obstetrics and Gynaecology, The Jikei University School of Medicine, 3-25-8, Nishi-Shinbashi, Minato-ku, Tokyo, Japan 105-8461
Department of Maternal-Fetal Biology, National Research Institute for Child Health and Development, 2-10-1, Okura, Setagayaku, Tokyo 157-8535, Japan

Momoko Owada, Yoshie Shibata and Shunji Suzuki
Department of Obstetrics and Gynecology, Japanese Red Cross Katsushika Maternity Hospital, Tokyo, Japan

Manuel Sánchez-Prieto, María Jesús Puy, Núria Barbany, Betlem Graupera, Maria Angela Pascual and Pere Barri-Soldevila
Department of Obstetrics and Gynecology, Instituto Universitario Dexeus, Barcelona, Spain

Silvia F. Navarro-Perez
Unidad de Investigación en Ginecología y Alto Riesgo Obstétrico, División de Ginecología y Obstetricia del Hospital General de Occidente, Av. Zoquipan #1050, Col. Seattle, 45170, Mexico

Karen Corona-Fernandez and María G. Zavala-Cerna
Immunology Research Laboratory, International Program of Medicine, Universidad Autonoma de Guadalajara, 44100, Mexico

José L. Rodriguez-Chavez and A. Bañuelos-Franco
Unidad de Investigación en Ginecología y Alto Riesgo Obstétrico, División de Ginecología y Obstetricia del Hospital General de Occidente, Mexico

William M. Curtin
Division of Maternal-Fetal Medicine, Penn State University Milton S. Hershey Medical Center, Penn State College of Medicine, Hershey, Pennsylvania, USA
Department of Pathology & Laboratory Medicine, Penn State University Milton S. Hershey Medical Center, Penn State College of Medicine, Hershey, Pennsylvania, USA

Jaimie L. Maines and Niamh A. Condon
Division of Maternal-Fetal Medicine, Penn State University Milton S. Hershey Medical Center, Penn State College of Medicine, Hershey, Pennsylvania, USA

Christina T. DeAngelis
Department of Obstetrics & Gynecology, Penn State University Milton S. Hershey Medical Center, Penn State College of Medicine, Hershey, Pennsylvania, USA

Serdar H. Ural
Division of Maternal-Fetal Medicine, Penn State University Milton S. Hershey Medical Center, Penn State College of Medicine, Hershey, Pennsylvania, USA
Department of Radiology, Penn State University Milton S. Hershey Medical Center, Penn State College of Medicine, Hershey, Pennsylvania, USA

Karmaine A. Millington
Department of Pathology & Laboratory Medicine, Penn State University Milton S. Hershey Medical Center, Penn State College of Medicine, Hershey, Pennsylvania, USA
Department of Pathology, Perinatal Pathology, North well Health/Cohen Children's Medical Center/Long Island Jewish Medical Center, New Hyde Park, New York, USA

Laurence Carmant, Sandrine Wavrant and Elisabeth Codsi
Department of Obstetrics and Gynecology, Division of Maternal Fetal Medicine, Sainte-Justine Mother and Child University Hospital, 3175 Chemin de la Côte Sainte Catherine, Montreal, QC, Canada

Gloria Calagna, Salvatore Polito, Francesco Labate and Giuseppe Calì
Obstetrics and Gynecology, "Villa Sofia-Cervello" Hospital, Palermo, Italy

Rosa Anna Guiglia, Francesca De Maria and Chiara Bisso
University of Palermo, Palermo, Italy

Gaspare Cucinella
Obstetrics and Gynecology, "Villa Sofia-Cervello" Hospital, University of Palermo, Palermo, Italy

Phoy Cheng Chun, Ka-Hee Chua, Mohamed Siraj Shahul Hameed, Manisha Mathur and Wai Kheong Ryan Lee
Department of Obstetrics and Gynecology, Kandang Kerbau Women's and Children's Hospital, 229899, Singapore

Meredith S. Campbell and Jeff Reese
Division of Neonatology, Department of Pediatrics, Monroe Carell Jr. Children's Hospital at Vanderbilt, Nashville, TN, USA

Amanda M. Craig
Department of Obstetrics and Gynecology, Vanderbilt University Medical Center, Nashville, TN, USA

Alicia K. Crum and Soha S. Patel
Department of Obstetrics and Gynecology, Vanderbilt University Medical Center, Nashville, TN, USA
Division of Maternal-Fetal Medicine, Department of Obstetrics and Gynecology, Vanderbilt University Medical Center, Nashville, TN, USA

Marjorie H. Thompson
University of Washington School of Medicine, USA

Nathaniel R. Miller
Providence Sacred Heart Maternal and Fetal Medicine, USA

Shelby L. Haugan
Billings Clinic Bozeman, USA

Michael C. Gordon
Billings Clinic Maternal Fetal Medicine, USA

Beatriz Féria, Maria João Palma and Filipa Passos
Obstetrics and Gynecology, Hospital Garcia de Orta, Almada, Portugal

Madalena Trindade and Joana Figueiredo
General Surgery, Hospital Garcia de Orta, Almada, Portugal

Sarah McGriff, Paige Percer, Iberia Sosa, Hector Mendez-Figueroa, Joseph L. Mills and Manisha Gandhi
Baylor College of Medicine, Texas Children's Hospital, Houston, Texas, USA

Jamal Ouachaou, Hamza Mimouni, Mohammed Maarad, Yassine Mellagui, Houssam Bkiyar and Brahim Housni
Intensive Care Unit, Mohammed VI University Hospital Center, Faculty of Medicine and Pharmacy of Oujda, Mohammed I University, Oujda, Morocco

Asmae Oulad Amar and Imane Kamaoui
Radiology Department, Mohammed VI University Hospital Center, Faculty of Medicine and Pharmacy of Oujda, Mohammed I University, Oujda, Morocco

Haruka Suzuki, Yoshitsugu Chigusa, Junzo Hamanishi, Masaki Mandai and Eiji Kondoh
Department of Gynecology and Obstetrics, Kyoto University, 54 Shogoin Kawahara-cho, Sakyo, Kyoto 606-8507, Japan

Evangelos Petrakis, Ioannis Chatzipapas, Ioannis K. Papapanagiotou, Panagiotis Fotinopoulos, Panagiota Siemou, Konstantinos Ntzeros and Dimitrios Loutradis
1st Department of Obstetrics and Gynaecology, School of Medicine, National and Kapodistrian University of Athens, Alexandra General Hospital, Lourou and Vasilisis Soas Avenue, 11528 Athens, Greece

Nozomi Ouchi, Yoshimitsu Kuwabara, Mirei Yonezawa, Ryuhei Kurashina, Tomoko Ichikawa, Rintaro Sawa and Toshiyuki Takeshita
Department of Obstetrics and Gynecology, Nippon Medical School Hospital, 1-1-5 Sendagi, Bunkyo-ku, Tokyo, Japan

P. D. M. Pathiraja
Ministry of Health, Sri Lanka

Junaid Rafi, Emily Woolnough and Anna Clare
St John of God Midland Public and Private Hospitals, Australia

Kaori Morimoto and Luke O'Rourke
Western University of Health Sciences College of Osteopathic Medicine Pacific Northwest, 200 Mullins Dr., Lebanon OR 97355, USA

Charles Gallaher
Emergency Department, St Helier Hospital, Wrythe Ln, Sutton, Carshalton SM5 1AA, UK

Farshad Tahmasebi, Ahmad Sayasneh and Gautam Mehra
Obstetrics and Gynaecology, Guy's & St Thomas' NHS Foundation Trust, Westminster Bridge Rd, London SE1 7EH, UK

Gregory W. Kirschen
Medical Scientist Training Program, Stony Brook Medicine, USA

Natalie Semenyuk
Albert Einstein College of Medicine, Montefiore Medical Center, USA

Antoine Naem
Faculty of Medicine of Damascus University, Damascus, Syria

Baraa Ahmad and Bashar Al-Kurdy
Faculty of Medicine of Damascus University, Damascus, Syria
University Hospital of Obstetrics and Gynecology of Damascus, Damascus, Syria

Kathryn L. Ponder, Rosa Won and Laurel Clymer
John Muir Medical Center, Walnut Creek, CA 94598, USA

Olivia Grubman, Farrah Naz Hussain, Zoe Nelson and Lois Brustman
Department of Obstetrics and Gynecology, Mount Sinai West, Icahn School of Medicine at Mount Sinai, New York, NY 10019, USA

Midori Yoshikawa, Takahiro Seyama, Takayuki Iriyama, Seisuke Sayama, Tatsuya Fujii, Masatake Toshimitsu, Keiichi Kumasawa, Takeshi Nagamatsu, Kaori Koga and Yutaka Osuga
Department of Obstetrics and Gynecology, Faculty of Medicine, The University of Tokyo, 7-3-1 Hongo, Bunkyo-ku, Tokyo 113-8655, Japan

Moto Nakaya, Ryo Kurokawa, Eisuke Shibata and Takeyuki Watadani
Department of Radiology, Faculty of Medicine, The University of Tokyo, 7-3-1 Hongo, Bunkyo-ku, Tokyo 113-8655, Japan

K. C. Janga, Pavani Chitamanni, Shraddha Raghavan, Kamlesh Kumar, Sheldon Greenberg and Kundan Jana
Maimonides Medical Center, Brooklyn, NY 11219, USA

Déborah Wernly
Department of Obstetrics and Gynecology, Sion's Hospital, Valais, Switzerland

Valérie Besse
Department of Radiology, Sion's Hospital, Valais, Switzerland

Daniela Huber
Department of Obstetrics and Gynecology, Sion's Hospital, Valais, Switzerland
Department of Pediatrics, Obstetrics and Gynecology, Geneva University Hospitals, Switzerland

Ryan Farias and Janice Hartnett
University of Connecticut Obstetrics and Gynecology, USA

Craig V. Towers and Heather Deisher
Obstetrics and Gynecology, Maternal-Fetal Medicine, High Risk Obstetrical Consultants, Knoxville, Tennessee 37920, USA

Alicia Martínez-Varea, Clara Martínez-Sáez and Vicente Diago-Almela
Department of Obstetrics and Gynaecology, La Fe University and Polytechnic Hospital, Avenida Fernando Abril Martorell 106, 46026 Valencia, Spain

María Patrocinio Tarrazó-Millet
Department of Obstetrics and Gynaecology, Dr. Peset University Hospital, Avenida de Gaspar Aguilar 90, 46017 Valencia, Spain

Katie P. Nguyen
Department of Family Medicine, Riverside Community Hospital, HCA Healthcare, Riverside, CA, USA

Marlekah Hudspeth
University of California Riverside, School of Medicine, Riverside, CA, USA

Honey Milestone
Department of Obstetrics & Gynecology, University of California Riverside, School of Medicine, Riverside Community Hospital, Riverside, CA, USA

Mie Sakai, Jumpei Ogura, Koji Yamanoi, Takahiro Hirayama, Tsutomu Ohara, Haruka Suzuki, Yoshihide Inayama, Koji Yasumoto and Koh Suginami
Department of Obstetrics and Gynecology, Toyooka Public Hospital, Japan

Jayesh Tigdi
Department of Obstetrics & Gynecology, McMaster University, Hamilton, Ontario, Canada

Cynthia Chan
Department of Obstetrics&Gynecology, Western University, London, Ontario, Canada

Nanayo Sasagasako, Hirohiko Tani, Yoshitsugu Chigusa, Shingo Io, Haruta Mogami, Junzo Hamanishi, Akihito Horie, Eiji Kondoh, Yukiyasu Sato and Masaki Mandai
Department of Obstetrics and Gynecology, Kyoto University Hospital, Kyoto, Japan

Soe Lwin and Myat San Yi
Department of Obstetrics & Gynecology, Faculty of Medicine and Health Sciences, UNIMAS, Malaysia

May Shi Leong and Haris Suharjono
Department of Obstetrics & Gynecology, Sarawak General Hospital, Malaysia

Tin Moe Nwe
Department of Basic Health Sciences, Faculty of Medicine and Health Sciences, UNIMAS, Malaysia

Mohammad Marwan Alhalabi and Ameer Kakaje
Faculty of Medicine, Damascus University, Damascus, Syria

Marwan Alhalabi
Department of Reproductive Medicine, Genetics and Embryology, Damascus University, Damascus, Syria

W. Lahmini and M. Bourrous
Department of Paediatric Emergency, UHC Mohamed VI, Cadi Ayyad University, Marrakech, Morocco

K. Harou
Department of Gynaecology and Obstetrics, UHC Mohamed VI, Cadi Ayyad University, Marrakech, Morocco

Index